Pediatric Trauma Life Support

For Prehospital Care Providers

Ann Marie Dietrich, MD, FACEP, FAAP
Steven Shaner, EMT-P
Ohio Chapter
American College of Emergency Physicians

John Campbell, MD, FACEP,
Editor

3rd Edition

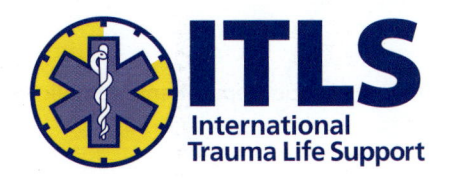

ITLS
International
Trauma Life Support

Copyright © 2009 by International Trauma Life Support

All rights reserved under International and Pan-American Copyright Conventions. No part of the material protected by this copyright notice may be reproduced or utilized in any form, electronic or mechanical, including photocopying, recording or by any information storage and retrieval system, without permission from the copyright owner ITLS. All inquiries should be addressed to:

International Trauma Life Support
3000 Woodcreek Drive, Suite 200
Downers Grove, IL 60515 USA
Phone: 888.495.4857
630.495.6442 (international)
Fax: 630.495.6404
Web: www.itrauma.org
Email: info@itrauma.org

Published in the United States
by International Trauma Life Support
Downers Grove, Illinois

ISBN-13 978-0-9647418-5-0
ISBN-10 0-9647418-5-7

Notice on Care Procedures

It is the intent of the authors, editors and publisher that this textbook be used as part of an education program taught by qualified instructors and supervised by a licensed physician. The procedures described in this textbook are based upon consultation with paramedics, nurses, and physicians. The authors, editors, and publisher have take care to make certain that these procedures reflect currently accepted clinical practice; however, they cannot be considered absolute recommendations.

The material in this textbook contains the most current information available at the time of publication. However, federal, state, and local guidelines concerning clinical practices, including, without limitation, those governing infection control and universal precautions, change rapidly. The reader should note, therefore, that new regulations may require changes in some procedures.

It is the responsibility of the reader to familiarize himself or herself with the policies and procedures set by federal, state, and local agencies as well as the institution or agency where the reader is employed. The authors, editors, and publisher of this textbook and the supplements written to accompany it disclaim any liability, loss, or risk resulting directly or indirectly from the suggested procedures and theory, from any undetected errors, or from the reader's misunderstanding of the text. It is the reader's responsibility to stay informed of any new changes or recommendations made by any federal, state, and local agency as well as by his or her employing institution or agency.

Notice on Gender Usage

The English language has historically given preference to the male gender. Among many words, the pronouns he and his are commonly used to describe both genders. Society evolves faster than language, and the male pronouns still predominate our speech. The authors have made great effort to treat the two genders equally, recognizing that a significant percentage of prehospital providers are female. However, in some instances, male pronouns may be used to describe both males and females solely for the purpose of brevity. This is not intended to offend any readers of the female gender.

Cover and Publication Design by Norcom Inc.

Supported in part by a grant from the Illinois Department of Public Health (Contract #87820408)

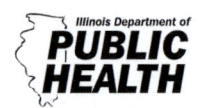

Illinois Department of
PUBLIC HEALTH

ISBN-13   978-0-9647418-5-0
ISBN-10   0-9647418-5-7

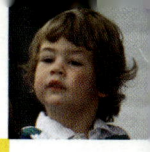

CONTENTS

FOREWORD ix
CONTRIBUTORS x
ABOUT ITLS xv

Chapter 1 The Injured Child

Objectives • Case Study 1
Introduction 2
Communicating with Children 3
    Infancy 4
    Toddlers 4
    Preschool Age 5
    School Age 6
    Adolescents 7
Trauma in Children 7
    Type of Trauma 8
    Mechanism of Injury 9
Injury Prevention by Age Group 13
    Infancy 14
    Toddlers 14
    Preschool Age 15
    School Age 15
    Adolescents 16
Transport Considerations 17
Confident Approach 17
Equipment 18
Recommended Reading 22

Chapter 2 Assessment of the Pediatric Patient

Objectives • Case Study 23
Introduction 24
Preparations for Assessment of the Pediatric Patient 24
Patient Assessment 24
    ITLS Primary Survey 25
    ITLS Secondary Survey 33
    ITLS Ongoing Exam 34
Recommended Reading 37

Chapter 3 Patient Assessment Skills

Objectives 39
ITLS Primary Survey 40
    Scene Size-Up 40
    Initial Assessment 40
    Rapid Trauma Survey or Focused Exam 43
    Critical Interventions and Transport Decisions 45
    Contacting Medical Direction 46

ITLS Secondary Survey 46
ITLS Ongoing Exam 48

Chapter 4 The Pediatric Airway

Objectives • Case Study 51
Introduction 52
Anatomy and Physiology 52
Patient Assessment 54
    ITLS Primary Survey 54
    ITLS Secondary Survey 62
Recommended Reading 64

Chapter 5 Pediatric Thoracic Trauma

Objectives • Case Study 65
Introduction 66
Anatomy and Pathophysiology 66
Patient Assessment 68
    ITLS Primary Survey 69
    ITLS Secondary Survey 77
Recommended Reading 81

Chapter 6 Airway Management and Thoracic Trauma Skills

Objectives 83
Basic Airway Management 84
    Airway Assessment 84
    Supplemental Oxygen 84
    Oropharyngeal Airway 85
    Bag-Valve-Mask Ventilation 86
Advanced Airway Management 88
    Airway Assessment 88
    Oral Intubation 88
    Blind Nasotracheal Intubation 90
    Needle Cricothyroidotomy 90
    Needle Decompression of the Chest 92

Chapter 7 Pediatric Shock and Fluid Resuscitation

Objectives • Case Study 95
Introduction 96
Anatomy and Pathophysiology 96
Patient Assessment 97
    ITLS Primary Survey 98
    ITLS Secondary Survey 102
Recommended Reading 104

Pediatric Trauma Life Support

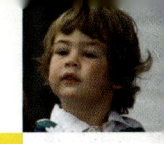

Chapter 8 Fluid Resuscitation Skills

Objectives 105
Intravenous Access Via Peripheral Cannulation 106
    Indications 106
    Contraindications 106
    Equipment 106
    Procedure 107
Intraosseous Infusion 107
    Indications 107
    Contraindications 107
    Equipment 108
    Procedure 108
Fluid Bolus Administration 109
    Indications 109
    Contraindications 109
    Equipment 109
    Procedure 110

Chapter 9 Pediatric Abdominal Trauma

Objectives • Case Study 111
Introduction 112
Anatomy and Pathophysiology 113
Patient Assessment 114
    ITLS Primary Survey 114
    ITLS Secondary Survey 116
Recommended Reading 120

Chapter 10 Pediatric Head Trauma

Objectives • Case Study 121
Introduction 122
Anatomy and Pathophysiology 122
    Brain Injuries 123
    Head Injuries 125
Patient Assessment 128
    ITLS Primary Survey 128
    ITLS Secondary Survey 132
Recommended Reading 135

Chapter 11 Pediatric Spinal Trauma

Objectives • Case Study 137
Introduction 138
Anatomy and Pathohysiology 138
Patient Assessment 139
    ITLS Primary Survey 140
    ITLS Secondary Survey 144
Recommended Reading 147

Chapter 12 Spinal Motion Restriction and Extrication Skills

Objectives 149
Introduction 150
Spinal Motion Restriction 150
    Cervical Collar Application.. 150
    Selecting Appropriate Equipment 152
    Head Motion Restriction Device... 153
Child Passenger Restraint Devices... 153
    Extrication for a Normal Assessment—No Abnormalities Found 155
    Extrication for an Abnormal Assessment—Injury Suspected.................... 155

Chapter 13 Pediatric Extremity Trauma

Objectives • Case Study 157
Introduction 158
Anatomy and Pathophysiology 158
Patient Assessment 159
    ITLS Primary Survey 159
    ITLS Secondary Survey 161
Fractures and Dislocations 161
    Signs and Symptoms 162
    Treatment 162
Sprains and Strains 165
    Signs and Symptoms 165
    Treatment 165
Compartment Syndrome 165
    Signs and Symptoms 165
    Treatment 165
Amputations 166
    Signs and Symptoms 166
    Treatment 166
Recommended Reading 169

Chapter 14 Pediatric Burns

Objectives • Case Study 171
Introduction 172
Anatomy and Pathophysiology 174
    Burn Depth 174
    Extent of Injury 176
Patient Assessment 177
    ITLS Primary Survey 178
    ITLS Secondary Survey 181
Burn Wound Management 181
    Fluid Resuscitation 182
    Pharmacologic Therapy 182
    Special Problems in Burn Management 182
Burn Prevention 184
    Smoke Detectors 184

Pediatric Trauma Life Support

Education 184
Recommended Reading 187

Chapter 15 Pediatric Submersion Injuries

Objectives • Case Study 189
Introduction 190
Anatomy and Pathophysiology 191
    Submersion Injury 191
    Immersion Syndrome 192
Patient Assessment 192
    ITLS Primary Survey 192
    ITLS Secondary Survey 196
Special Considerations 196
Prognosis 197
    Warm-Water Drowning 197
    Cold-Water Drowning 197
Prevention 197
    Pool Enclosures, Covers, and Alarms 198
    Public Information Campaigns 198
Recommended Reading 202

Chapter 16 Pediatric Traumatic Cardiopulmonary Arrest

Objectives • Case Study 203
Introduction 204
Patient Assessment 205
    ITLS Primary Survey 206
    ITLS Secondary Survey and Ongoing Exam 209
Recommended Reading 210

Chapter 17 Child Abuse

Objectives • Case Study 211
Introduction 212
Suspecting Child Abuse 213
Care and Safety Issues 215
Prehospital Provider Considerations 216
Family Members' Emotions 216
Arrival to the Emergency Department 217
Recommended Reading 220

Chapter 18 Death of a Child

Objectives • Case Study 221
Introduction 222
Grief Reactions 224
Critical Incident Stress Debriefing (CISD) 226
Recommendations for How to Help 226
Recommended Reading 229

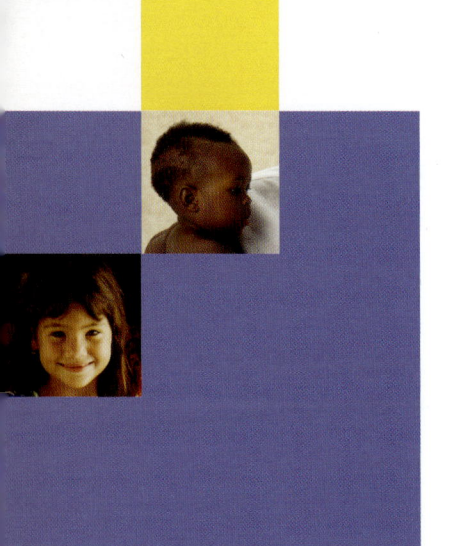

Chapter 19 Trauma in the Newborn

Objectives • Case Study 231
Introduction 232
Advances in Trauma Care of the Newly Born Infant...232
Neonatal Resuscitation 234
Patient Assessment 236
Initial Stabilization and Assessment..236
Approach to the Newly Born Infant with an Abnormal Initial Assessment 238
    Airway 238
    Breathing 239
    Circulation 240
    Drug Therapy 242
Ongoing Assessment of the Resuscitated Newly Born Infant 244
Recommended Reading 246

Chapter 20 Children with Special Health Care Needs

Objectives • Case Study 247
Introduction 248
Evaluation 249
    CSHCN Medical Equipment..250
Recommended Reading 258

Appendix A Use of Specialized Pediatric Care Centers

Objectives 259
Introduction 260
Decision Process..260
    Suggested Criteria for Transfer 260
Recommended Reading 264

Appendix B Pediatric Trauma Triage and Multiple Casualty Incident Management

Objectives 265
Introduction 266
Planning for Pediatric Major Incidents 266
Managing Pediatric Multiple Casualty Incidents..267
    Triage Considerations 269
    Treatment Considerations 270
    Communications Considerations...272
    Pediatric Consent and Major Incident Management...273
    Equipment Considerations 273
    Transportation and Destination Decision Making 274
Psychological Effects 274
Recommended Reading 276

PHOTO & ILLUSTRATION CREDITS 277
INDEX 282

FOREWORD

There is nothing as tragic as the death of a child. For a child who dies of injuries, this tragedy often has a devastating effect, not only on family and friends, but also on those prehospital providers who tried to save the child. For most emergency medical services providers, there is nothing more dreaded than having to care for a critically injured child. Since trauma is the leading cause of death in children, all responders face this situation at some time. Unfortunately, most responders don't treat injured children often enough to develop the kind of expertise that is desired.

Though the care of the pediatric patient is taught in the ITLS provider course, there is much more to know about the injured child than can be covered in one chapter of an already intensive course. Pediatric trauma care is unique is several ways. Prehospital providers must learn not only how to communicate with various ages of pediatric patients, but also with the parents and family that accompany them. Because children's anatomy and activities are different than adults, they suffer different injuries. Assessment of the small child is often difficult because the patient is frightened and struggling, can't communicate verbally, and has vital signs that are not only difficult to obtain, but whose normal ranges are unfamiliar. Add to this an emotional family standing by, and the job becomes almost overwhelming.

In 1995, under the leadership of Ann Marie Dietrich, MD, FACEP, FAAP, Steven J. Shaner, EMT-P, and the Ohio Chapter of the American College of Emergency Physicians, the first short course to cover the special needs of the injured child was introduced. Pediatric ITLS is intended for EMS providers who have already had ITLS or PHTLS training and are familiar with adult trauma care. This course focuses on the practical training needed to make responders feel confident and competent when faced with caring for the critically injured child.

This 3rd edition of the Pediatric ITLS textbook is a companion to the 6th edition *ITLS for Prehospital Care Providers* manual and reflects the same ITLS method of assessment and management but with an emphasis on the special needs of the pediatric patient. The text has been updated and refined to reflect the latest and most effective approaches to the care of the pediatric trauma patient. The text also has been revised to conform to the newest American Heart Association guidelines for artificial ventilation and CPR. As introduced in the 6th edition ITLS provider manual, the text's "Pearls" feature has been repositioned so that it consistently appears in the margins beside relevant text, and many of the illustrations have been redrawn for a more up-to-date look.

On behalf of ITLS, I hope you'll find this latest edition of *Pediatric Trauma Life Support for Prehospital Care Providers* a useful and complete resource for prehospital pediatric trauma care and training.

John E. Campbell, MD, FACEP
August 2009

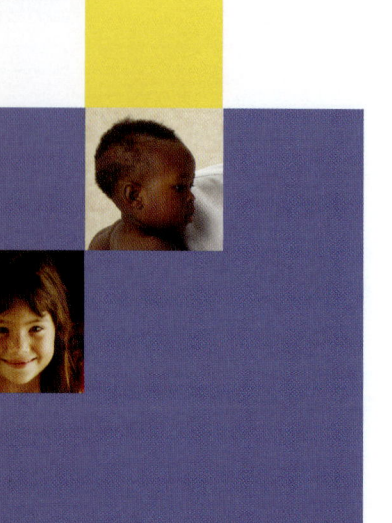

Contributors

EDITORS

Ann Marie Dietrich, MD, FACEP, FAAP
Professor of Pediatrics, The Ohio State University College of Medicine and Public Health
Pediatric Associate Medical Director, MedFlight of Ohio
Risk Manager, Section of Pediatric Emergency Medicine, Nationwide Children's Hospital
Columbus, Ohio

Steven J. Shaner, EMT-P
Staff Captain, Division of Fire, City of Grandview Heights
Grandview Heights, Ohio

John E. Campbell, MD, FACEP
President, International Trauma Life Support
Medical Director, EMS and Trauma, State of Alabama
Auburn, Alabama

AUTHORS

Nancy Asp, RN, EMT
Columbus, Ohio

Mary Jo Bowman, MD, FAAP
Associate Professor of Clinical Pediatrics, The Ohio State University College of Medicine
Pediatric Emergency Medicine Fellowship Director, Associate Director, Emergency
Department, Nationwide Children's Hospital
Columbus, Ohio

John E. Campbell, MD, FACEP
President, International Trauma Life Support
Medical Director, EMS and Trauma, State of Alabama
Auburn, Alabama

William Cotton, MD
Clinical Professor Pediatrics, Nationwide Children's Hospital
Columbus, Ohio

John P. Crow, MD, FACS
Trauma Medical Director, Attending Pediatric Surgeon, Akron Children's Hospital
Associate Prof of Clinical Surgery, NEOUCOM
Akron, Ohio

Lori Dandrea, MD
Savannah, Georgia

Sharon Deppe, BSN, RN
Emergency Department, Dublin Methodist Hospital
Columbus, Ohio

Ann Marie Dietrich, MD, FACEP, FAAP
Professor of Pediatrics, The Ohio State University College of Medicine and Public Health
Pediatric Associate Medical Director, MedFlight of Ohio
Risk Manager, Section of Pediatric Emergency Medicine, Nationwide Children's Hospital
Columbus, Ohio

Robert E. Falcone, MD, FACS
Clinical Professor of Surgery, The Ohio State University
Columbus, Ohio

Jeanette Foster, MSW, LISW-S
Columbus, Ohio

Kathy J. Haley, RN, BSN
Trauma Program Manager, Nationwide Children's Hospital
Columbus, Ohio

Sharon Hammond, RN, BSN, MA, EMT-P
Flight Nurse, MedFlight of Ohio
Regional STEMI Program Coordinator, The Ohio State University Medical Center
Columbus, Ohio

Debi Hastilow, EMT-P, RN
Flight Nurse, MedFlight of Ohio
Columbus, Ohio

Holly Herron MS, RN, CNS, EMT-P
Grant Medical Center, Ohio Health
Manager, LifeLink and EMS Education
Columbus, Ohio

Patricia M. Hicks, MS, NREMT-P
Washington, DC

Ann Hoffman, RN, CPN
Staff Nurse and EMS Coordinator, Nationwide Children's Hospital
Columbus, Ohio

Jeffrey Kempf, DO
Director, Pediatric Residency Program, Emergency Medicine Department,
Akron Children's Hospital
Akron, Ohio

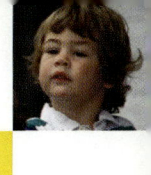

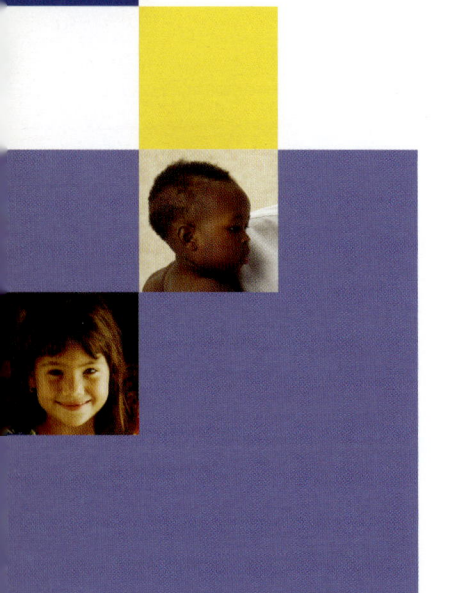

Sherri Kovach, RN, EMT-B
Nationwide Children's Hospital
Columbus, Ohio

Joanne E. Lapetina, MD, MS, FAAP, FACEP
Pediatric Emergency Physician, CJW Medical Center- Chippenham Campus
Richmond, Virginia
Emergency Department Medical Director, TeamHealth MidSouth, DePaul Medical Center
Norfolk, Virginia

Linda Manley, RN, BSN
Columbus, Ohio

Ronald R. McWilliams, NREMT–P
Columbus, Ohio

Francis R. Mencl, MD, FACEP
Akron, Ohio

Nancy B. Nelson, MSW, LISW
Clinical Social Worker, Pediatric Intensive Care Unit, Child Assessment Team,
Nationwide Children's Hospital
Columbus, Ohio

Richard N. Nelson, MD, FACEP
Professor and Vice Chair, Department of Emergency Medicine,
The Ohio State University College of Medicine
Columbus, Ohio

Kathryn E. Nuss, MD
Associate Professor of Pediatrics, The Ohio State University College of Medicine
Associate Trauma Medical Director, Associate Director of Emergency Medicine,
Operations Medical Director, Nationwide Children's Hospital
Columbus, Ohio

Randy L. Orsborn, MPAS, PA-C, NREMT-P
Fellow, APAC
Diplomate, ACCL
Knox Cardiology Associates
Mount Vernon, Ohio

Wendy J. Pomerantz, MD, MS
Associate Professor of Clinical Pediatrics, Cincinnati Children's Hospital
University of Cincinnati
Cincinnati, Ohio

Katherine Shaner, RN, BSN, EMT-B
Columbus, Ohio

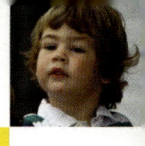

Steven J. Shaner, EMT-P
Staff Captain, Division of Fire, City of Grandview Heights
Grandview Heights, Ohio

Michael J. Stoner, MD
Assistant Professor of Clinical Pediatrics, The Ohio State University
Attending Physician of Pediatric Emergency Medicine, Nationwide Children's Hospital
Columbus, Ohio

George Waterman, MD
Clinical Assistant Professor of Pediatrics, The Ohio State University College of Medicine
Attending Physician, Emergency Department, Nationwide Children's Hospital
Columbus, Ohio

Laurie Weaver, RN, BSN, EMT-P
EMS Coordinator, Wooster Community Hospital
Wooster, Ohio

Howard A. Werman, MD, FACEP
Professor of Clinical Emergency Medicine, The Ohio State University
Medical Director, MedFlight of Ohio
Columbus, Ohio

REVIEWERS

Kyee Han, MBBS, FRCS, FFAEM
Editorial Board, International Trauma Life Support
Chair, Pediatric Task Force, Editorial Board, International Trauma Life Support
Consultant in Accident and Emergency Medicine, The James Cook University Hospital
Honorary Senior Clinical Lecturer, University of Newcastle Upon Tyne
Middlesbrough. England

Donna Hastings, MA, EMT-P
Chair, Editorial Board, International Trauma Life Support
Vice President, Health and Research, Heart and Stroke Foundation of Alberta, NWT & Nunavut
Calgary, Alberta, Canada

Eduardo Romero Hicks, MD
Editorial Board, International Trauma Life Support
Guanajuato, Mexico

David Maatman, NREMT-P/IC, CCEMT-P
Editorial Board, International Trauma Life Support
Educator, American Medical Response—West Michigan
Grand Rapids, Michigan

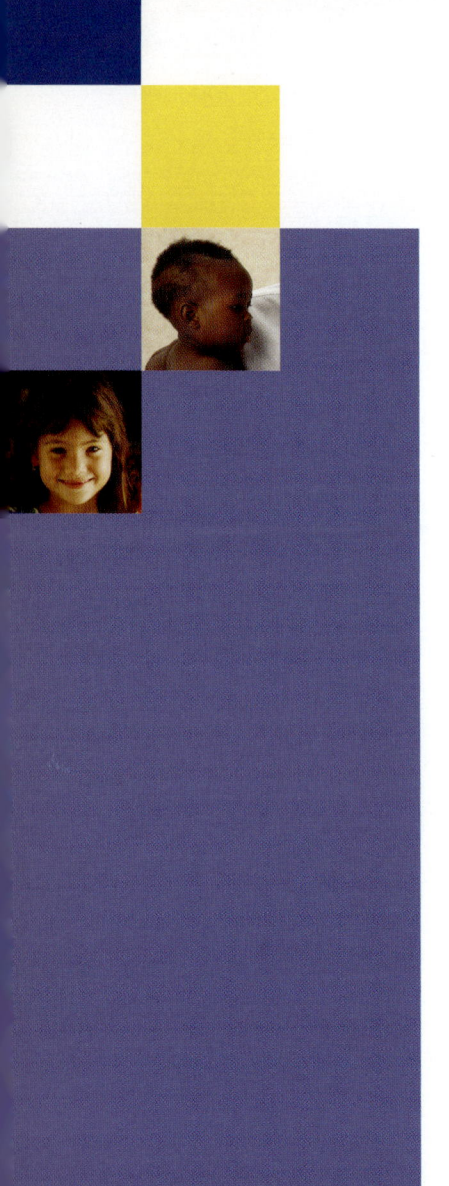

John Mohler, RN
Board of Directors, International Trauma Life Support
Flight Nurse, REMSA Care Flight
Reno, Nevada
Owner, John Mohler & Company
Sparks, Nevada

William Pfeifer III, MD, FACS
Board of Directors and Editorial Board, International Trauma Life Support
Col. MC USAR (Trauma Surgery)
Littleton, Colorado

Roberto Rivera, RN, BSN, EMT-B
Editorial Board, International Trauma Life Support
Trauma Nurse/Flight Nurse
Coordinator, ITLS Puerto Rico Training Centre
Manati, Puerto Rico

S. Robert Seitz, MEd, RN, NREMT-P
Editorial Board, International Trauma Life Support
Assistant Professor/ Study Coordinator, University of Pittsburgh, School of Health and Rehabilitation Sciences, Emergency Medicine Program
Pittsburgh, Pennsylvania

John T. Stevens, NREMT-P (ret.)
Editorial Board, International Trauma Life Support
Douglasville, Georgia

Art Editor

John Mohler, RN
Board of Directors, International Trauma Life Support
Flight Nurse, REMSA Care Flight
Reno, Nevada
Owner, John Mohler & Company
Sparks, Nevada

Pearls Editor

Susan M. Hohenhaus, MA, RN, FAEN
President, Hohenhaus & Associates, Inc.
Wellsboro, Pennsylvania

Managing Editor

Kate Blackwelder
Communications Manager, International Trauma Life Support
Downers Grove, Illinois

About ITLS

International Trauma Life Support is a global not-for-profit organization dedicated to preventing death and disability from trauma through education and emergency trauma care. Founded in 1985 as Basic Trauma Life Support, ITLS adopted its new name in 2005 to better reflect its global role and impact.

The ITLS framework is a global standard that enables providers to master the latest techniques in rapid assessment, appropriate intervention, and identification of immediate life-threatening injuries. ITLS is accepted internationally as the standard training course for prehospital trauma care. It is used as a state-of-the-art continuing education course and as an essential curriculum in many paramedic, EMT, and First Responder training programs.

Today, ITLS has more than 70 chapters and training centres worldwide. Through ITLS, hundreds of thousands of trauma care professionals have learned proven techniques endorsed by the American College of Emergency Physicians.

ITLS LEADERSHIP

Board of Directors

John E. Campbell, MD, FACEP
President
Auburn, Alabama

Peter Gianas, MD
Chair
Starke, Florida

Sabina Braithwaite, MD, FACEP
Vice Chair
Charlottesville, Virginia

Anthony Connelly, EMT-P, BHSc, PGCEd.
Secretary Treasurer
Edmonton, Alberta, Canada

William Pfeifer III, MD, FACS
Member-at-Large
Littleton, Colorado

Russell Bieniek, MD, FACEP
Erie, Pennsylvania

Amy Boise, NREMT-P
Phoenix, Arizona

Neil Christen, MD, FACEP
Anniston, Alabama

Martin Friedberg, MD, CCFP(EM)
Toronto, Ontario, Canada

John Mohler, RN
Sparks, Nevada

Wilhelmina Elsabe Nel, MD
Bloemfontein, Free State, South Africa

Bob Page, AAS, NREMT-P, CCEMT-P, NCEE
Springfield, Missouri

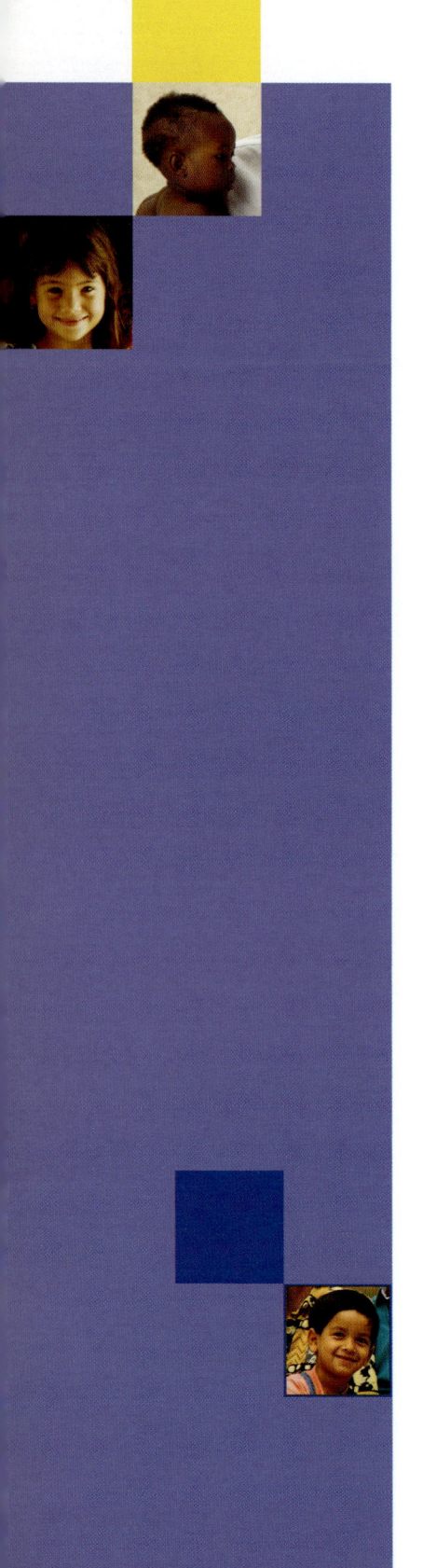

Editorial Board

Donna Hastings, MA, EMT-P
Chair
Calgary, Alberta, Canada

John E. Campbell, MD, FACEP
Chair Emeritus
Auburn, Alabama

Roy L. Alson, PhD, MD, FACEP
Winston-Salem, North Carolina

Sabina Braithwaite, MD, FACEP
Charlottesville, Virginia

Kyee Han, MBBS, FRCS, FFAEM
Middlesbrough, England

Eduardo Romero Hicks, MD
Guanajuato, Mexico

David Maatman, NREMT-P/IC, CCEMT-P
Grand Rapids, Michigan

William Pfeifer III, MD, FACS
Littleton, Colorado

Art Proust, MD, FACEP
Saint Charles, Illinois

Roberto Rivera, RN, BSN, EMT-B
Manati, Puerto Rico

S. Robert Seitz, MEd, RN, NREMT-P
Pittsburgh, Pennsylvania

J.T. Stevens, NREMT-P
Douglasville, Georgia

Executive Director

Virginia Kennedy Palys, JD
Downers Grove, Illinois

WHAT MAKES ITLS BETTER?

Since its beginnings more than 25 years ago as Basic Trauma Life Support, ITLS has become a global force for excellence in trauma education and response, with more than 70 chapters and training centres worldwide. What makes ITLS a better choice for trauma training? Here are just a few of the reasons.

- **Evidence-based.** ITLS is based on current science and research.
- **Practical.** ITLS training is a realistic, hands-on approach proven to work in the field "from scene to surgery."
- **Dynamic.** ITLS content is current, relevant, and responsive to the latest thinking in trauma management.
- **Flexible.** ITLS courses are taught through a strong network of chapters and training centres that customize content to reflect local needs and priorities.
- **Recognized.** ITLS is an internationally recognized certification that is the standard for prehospital trauma education.
- **Team centered.** ITLS emphasizes a cohesive teach approach that works in the real world and recognizes the importance of the emergency care provider's role.
- **Grounded in emergency medicine.** Practicing emergency physicians—medicine's front-line responders—lead ITLS's efforts to deliver stimulating content that has its base in solid emergency medicine.
- **Challenging.** ITLS course content raises the bar on performance in the field by integrating classroom knowledge with practical application of skills through interactive stations.
- **Confidence building.** The unique ITLS course format builds confidence in new providers and knowledge in experienced providers.

FOCUSED CONTENT THAT DELIVERS

ITLS is accepted internationally as the standard training course for prehospital trauma care. It is taught not only as a continuing education course, but also used as essential curriculum in many paramedic, EMT, and First Responder training programs.

ITLS courses combine classroom learning and hands-on skill stations. The courses also challenge the student with scenario assessment stations where learning is put to work in simulated trauma situations. ITLS courses are designed, managed, and delivered by course directors, coordinators, and instructors experienced in EMS, prehospital care, and the ITLS approach.

ITLS is synonymous with training EMS personnel to provide optimal care for the injured in the prehospital setting. The program provides a variety of training options to suit the requirements of all levels and backgrounds of prehospital emergency personnel around the world.

CHAPTER 1
The Injured Child

Sharon Hammond, RN, BSN, CEN, EMT-P
Randy Orsborn, PA-C, MPAS, NREMT-P
Katherine Shaner, RN, BSN, CEN, EMT-B

Objectives

Upon completion of this chapter, you should be able to:

1. Identify factors that are important when dealing with children and their families.
2. Identify the stages of development in children.
3. Discuss the importance of understanding mechanisms of injury for traumatic events.
4. Discuss injury prevention measures.

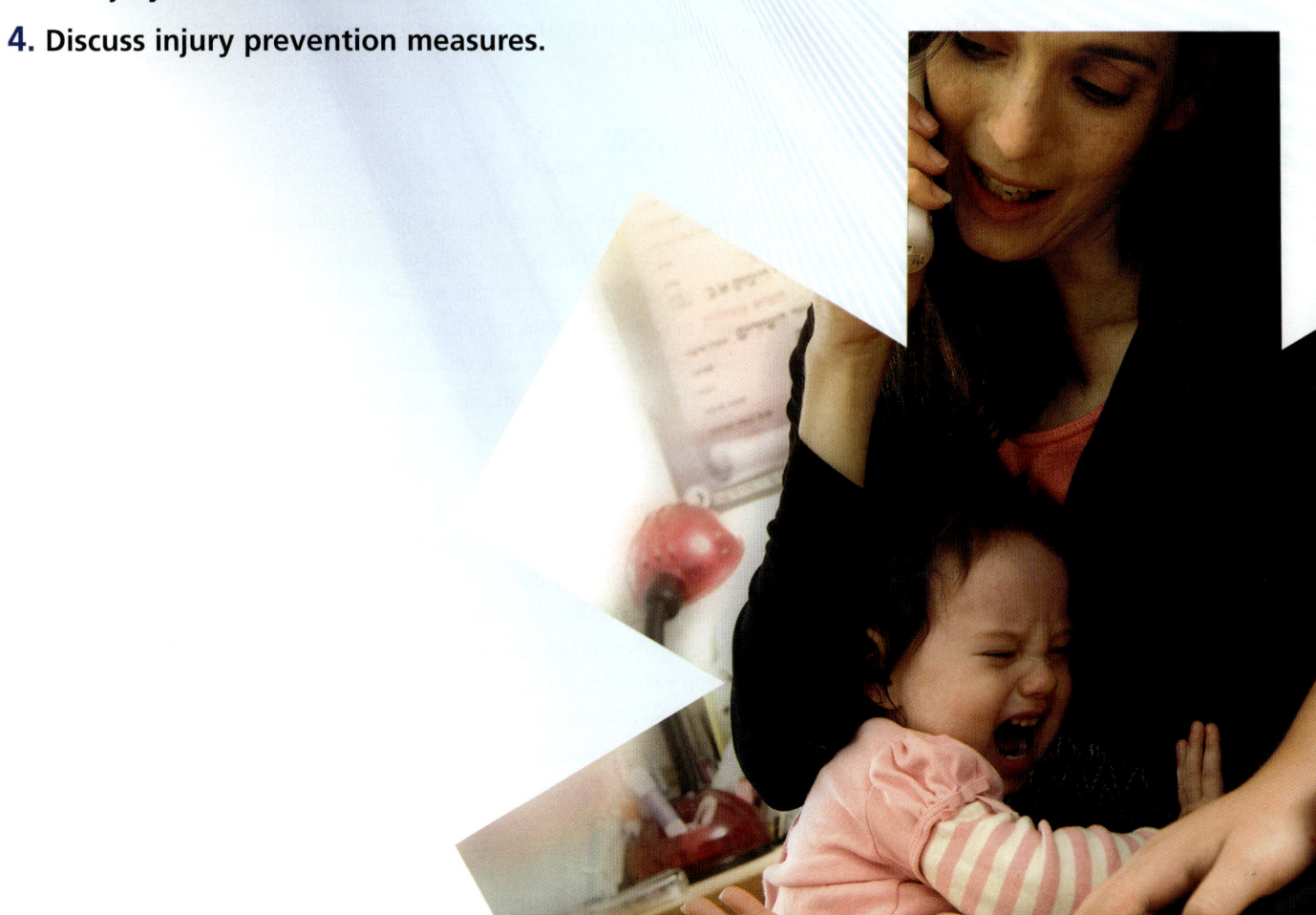

Case Study

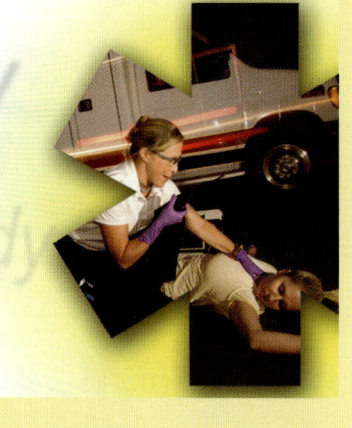

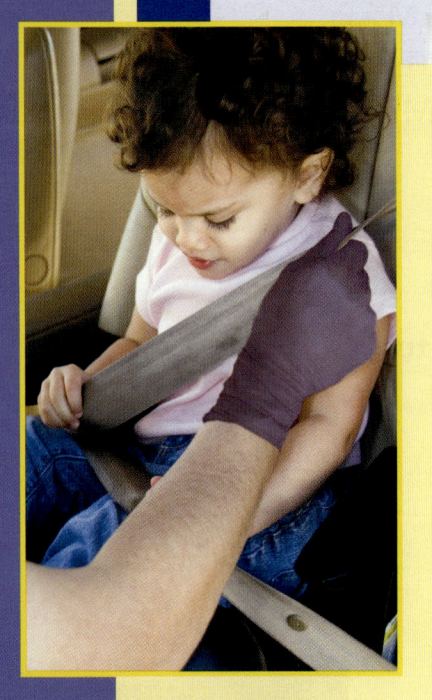

John, Susan, and Bob of the Emergency Transport System (ETS) are called to the scene of a motor vehicle collision reportedly involving more than one child. On the team's arrival, they see a minivan with significant damage to the front driver's side of the vehicle with entrapment of passengers. After assuring that the scene is safe, the team approaches the vehicle and finds two small children secured in child safety seats next to each other in the middle seat. Both children are crying; one is telling the team to "go away" and the second child is screaming, "I want my mommy!" Firefighters are extricating an adult female from the driver's seat. How should the team approach these children? How do they estimate their age? What do they need to understand about the mechanism of injury related to the pediatric patient? Keep these questions in mind as you read the chapter. Then, at the end of the chapter, find out how the rescuers completed this call.

PEARLS

When a child is injured, parents feel powerless and lose their sense of control. Include the family as part of your team.

INTRODUCTION

Contemporary health care providers are faced with caring for children from not only all age groups, but also varied backgrounds (e.g., culture, religion, or race). In order to provide care in such a diverse world, you must learn to interact with children of all ages in all settings. Communication is the key to providing excellent care to children and their families. As compared to adults, children have a very different style of communication, in order to make the "big" world understand them. They also have significantly different fears and stressors than do adults. Remember an important concept when caring for a sick or injured child: You must treat not only the child, but also the family. The child comes with an extra "package"— the child's parents and other family members are an important part of the child's care.

Family-centered care is an ideal based on the concept that a child's family is the one constant in his life. Facilitating parent–professional collaboration and honoring cultural/ethnic diversity will greatly enhance the child's and his family's medical experience. In other words, families need to be involved in the care of their children. According to Dr. Donald Brunquell of Minnesota Children's Hospital, "A family that feels explicitly involved is less likely to react in anger to fear and can be of great support to the child." Families who are included in the child's care will be much less frightened and therefore more willing and able to provide pertinent information about the child and to comfort the child than those families who are pushed to the side.

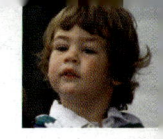

Basic communication skills are invaluable in health care situations and make parents feel that they are part of the "team," and are making a positive difference for their child. Remember that parents feel responsible for their child, and it is their job to help and protect the child. When a child is injured and the health care system takes over, parents feel powerless and lose their sense of control. Including parents in the care (i.e., "Would you like to ride in the ambulance with Billy to the hospital? He needs you to be with him right now") give them a sense of control.

COMMUNICATING WITH CHILDREN

In order to communicate with children, you must first understand how a child's communication changes with the child's developmental stage. In the following section, the child's communication techniques and fears are addressed by age group. Table 1.1 provides a summary of developmental milestones, issues, and coping strategies that may assist you in caring for the injured child.

> **PEARLS**
>
> **Communicating with children requires knowledge of typical developmental milestones.**

Table 1.1: Pediatric Treatment Issues by Age Group

Age	Development Issues	Important Fears	Useful Techniques
Infancy (0–12 months)	Minimal language Feel an extension of parents Sensitive to physical environment	Stranger anxiety	Keep parents in sight Avoid hunger Use warm hands Keep room warm
Toddlers (12–30 months)	Receptive language more advanced than expressive See themselves as individuals Assertive will	Brief separation Pain	Maintain verbal communication Examine with parent when possible Allow some choices when possible
Preschool (30 months–5 years)	Excellent expressive skill for thoughts and feelings Rich fantasy life Magical thinking Strong concept of self	Long separation Pain Disfigurement	Allow expression Encourage fantasy and play Encourage participation in care
School age (5–12 years)	Fully developed language Understanding of body structure and function Able to reason and compromise Incomplete understanding of death	Disfigurement Loss of function Death	Explain procedures Explain pathophysiology and treatment Project positive outcome Stress child's ability to master situation Respect physical modesty
Adolescence (12–18 years)	Self-determination Decision making Peer group important Realistic view of death	Loss of autonomy Loss of peer acceptance Death	Allow choices and control Stress acceptance by peers Respect autonomy

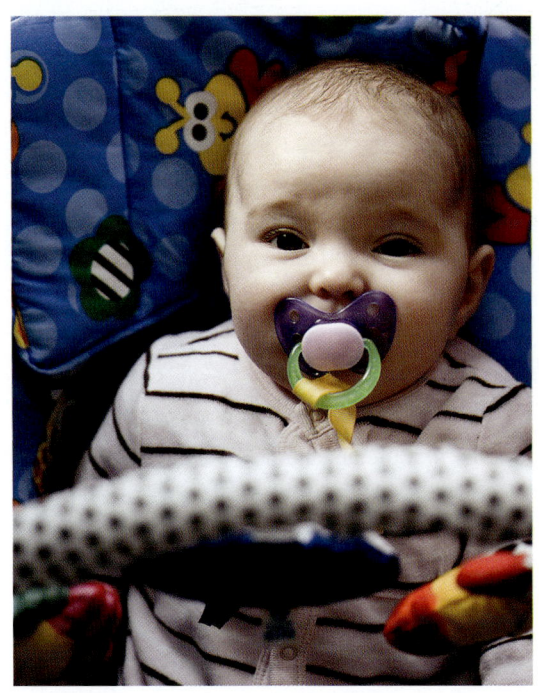

Figure 1.1 *The largest stressor to an infant is separation from the parent or caregiver.*

Infancy

Infancy is the period between birth and 12 months (Fig. 1.1). It is a time of rapid change and growth. By the age of three months, the infant will smile, make eye contact, and coo. An infant also will react to voices and follow visual stimuli. The infant will suck strongly and may hold a rattle briefly. As the child gets older, he learns to ambulate, first sitting (six months of age), then crawling (nine months of age), and then walking (one year of age).

In infancy, the largest stressor to an infant is separation from the parent or caregiver. Whenever possible, the child should remain in contact with the parent while receiving medical care. In addition to providing comfort for the child, the parent can assist in the child's assessment. Parents may assist with the care of their child, but they should not be expected to provide health care. Much like with adults, careful reassessment is needed for infants to ensure early recognition and proper management of injuries.

Toddlers

Toddlers range in age from 12 months to 30 months (Fig. 1.2). Normally, toddlers will walk and run. They are very inquisitive and like to investigate everything. They say words and phrases and may ask for things. They may even follow simple directions when asked to do so. Communication with these children should be in quiet, calming tones of voice. Avoid overly dramatic facial expressions, such as huge grins. Imagine the world from toddlers' point of view; for example, it is very frightening to a toddler to see unfamiliar faces yelling instructions at them.

As with infants, the greatest stress to a toddler is also parental separation. Allowing parents to provide comfort is of utmost importance. This age group needs to see their parents, hear their voices, and/or touch them. If the child must be transported, allow the parent to accompany the child to help keep him calm. Ensure that the child can clearly see

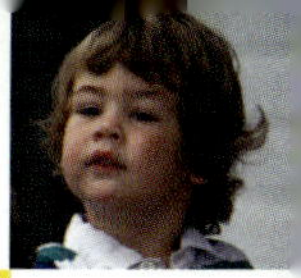

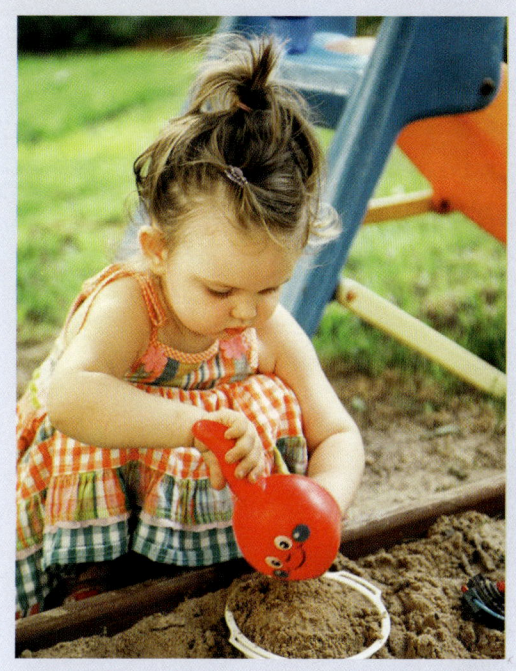

Figure 1.2 *Parental separation is the greatest source of stress for toddlers (12 months to 30 months) as well.*

the parent; if that is not possible, ensure that the child, at the very least, can easily hear the parent. Familiar items such as a blanket or favorite toy may also be helpful in comforting the child. Many traumatic injuries can be worsened by increasing the child's stress levels. Allowing the parents to accompany their children is actually considered a part of their treatment.

Always be honest when performing interventions on children. Tell them, "This is an ouchie" and "It's okay if you want to cry." Be careful not to say "all done" unless you know for a fact that all painful procedures are completed. As a kind gesture to a toddler, you can ask the parent if the child sucks a thumb or fingers and on which hand. Thumb sucking is a very popular self-calming measure in this age group; if possible, avoid placing an IV in that hand. Also be aware that because toddlers have a great fear of restriction of movement, spinal motion restriction can also be an ordeal. Again, whenever the situation allows, allow a parent to be present to comfort, reassure, and ease the child's stress during this procedure.

Preschool Age

Preschool-age children range in age from 30 months to five years (Fig. 1.3). Children in this age group can tell you what they want, when they want it, and ask "why?" for what seems like a thousand times. These children may fear body mutilation. Give them more preparatory information about what is happening to them, any procedures that are necessary, and how it will involve their bodies.

Preschoolers may still have a favorite blanket or toy that would make them more comfortable. Allow these children to keep these items with them at all times, when possible.

Parental involvement is still imperative with this age group. As always, honesty is crucial with children and their families, and acceptance of their feelings is also very important. Never say to a child, "Why are you crying? It's not that bad." Remember to speak calmly and constantly reassure both the injured child and his family.

The Injured Child

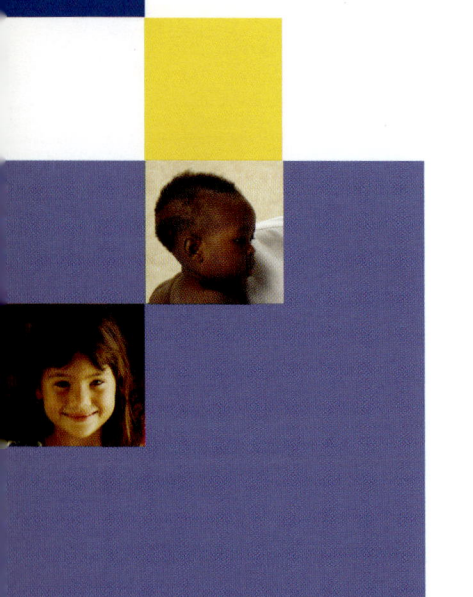

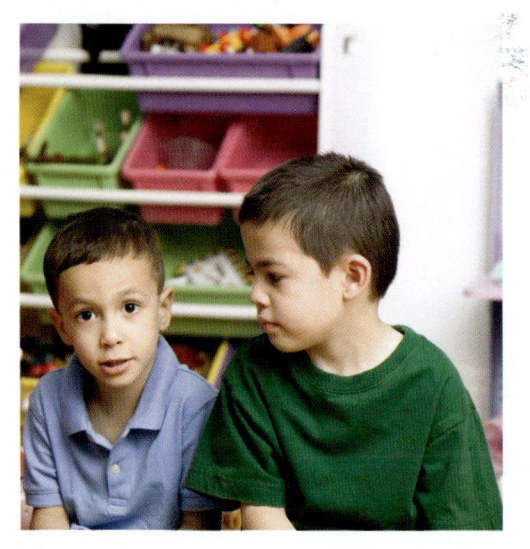

Figure 1.3 *Preschool-age children (30 months to five years old) need preparatory information about what prehospital procedures may take place.*

School Age

School-age children range in age from five years to 12 years (Fig. 1.4). These children are very good storytellers and historians. They can tell you what is wrong with them and how they were injured. Communication should not be a large problem with school-age children because they are beginning to think more concretely and actively like to talk.

The greatest stress for these children is loss of bodily control. Allow them to make some decisions, when possible, about their care. If possible, ask them in which hand they would like to have their IV. Are they right-handed or left-handed? What seems like a small choice to an adult may mean the world to the school-age child.

As with the younger children, parents also play a large part in a school-age child's life. Involve parents in decision-making along with the child. Again, always be honest about procedures. The easiest way to lose their trust is to not tell the truth. When in doubt, "I don't know" is the best answer.

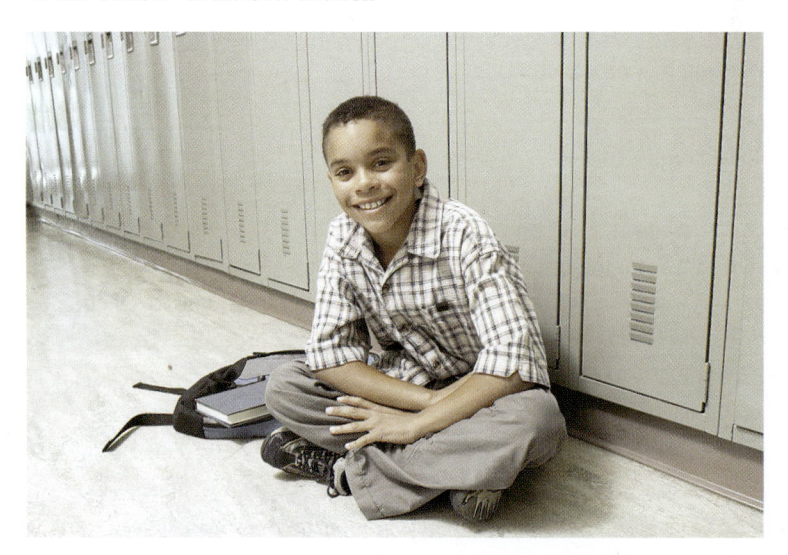

Figure 1.4 *Allow school-age children (five years to 12 years old) to make some decisions about their care whenever possible.*

Pediatric Trauma Life Support

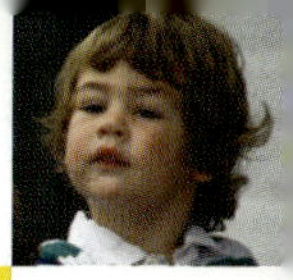

Adolescents

Adolescents range in age from 12 years to 18 years (Fig. 1.5). They are notoriously labeled as "difficult," as they are fighting to establish their independence and show that they are a valuable part of society. They often have many inner conflicts about whether they want to be treated as children or adults. Remember that they are indeed children, but it is imperative to involve them in their own care whenever possible.

The largest stressors to this age group are a lack of trust and enforced dependence. They do not like to think that they are dependent on anyone. Health care will be easier on everyone involved if, when possible, adolescents can make decisions about their care. This age group is very particular about parents. Some want their parents with them; others do not. This is an individual choice; do not force this issue with an adolescent.

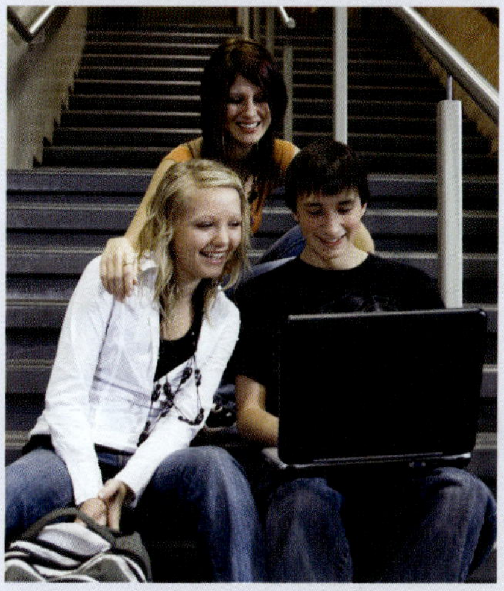

Figure 1.5 *Adolescents (ages 12 to 18 years) do not like to admit to dependence on anyone.*

TRAUMA IN CHILDREN

Emergency Medical Services (EMS) systems are designed primarily for the adult population. Training modalities, equipment design, and overall patient orientation have been developed to meet the needs of the ill and injured adult.

Nationally, five percent to ten percent of all EMS runs involve pediatric patients. Although children suffer critical injury far less frequently than adults do (a 1:10 ratio), nearly 50 percent of all pediatric EMS runs are trauma related.

Trauma remains the leading cause of death and disability for children over the age of one year. Each year, trauma kills 22,000 children, a large percentage of whom die before reaching the hospital. A sizeable number of the survivors suffer significant neurological damage. In addition, pediatric injuries account for more than 600,000 hospital admissions and 16 million emergency department visits, with a combined cost of over $7.5 billion. Therefore, providers must take part in community efforts to help prevent injury in the pediatric population.

The problem is evident: Pediatric trauma is a disease process that has reached epidemic proportions. As a prehospital provider, it is essential that, in addition to identifying obvious injuries, you learn to anticipate and identify "hidden" injuries based on how the accident occurred (mechanism of injury). This is accomplished through a quick scene survey upon arrival.

> **PEARLS**
>
> **Trauma remains the leading cause of death and disability for children over the age of one year. Carefully survey the scene and assess the child for "hidden" injuries.**

The Injured Child

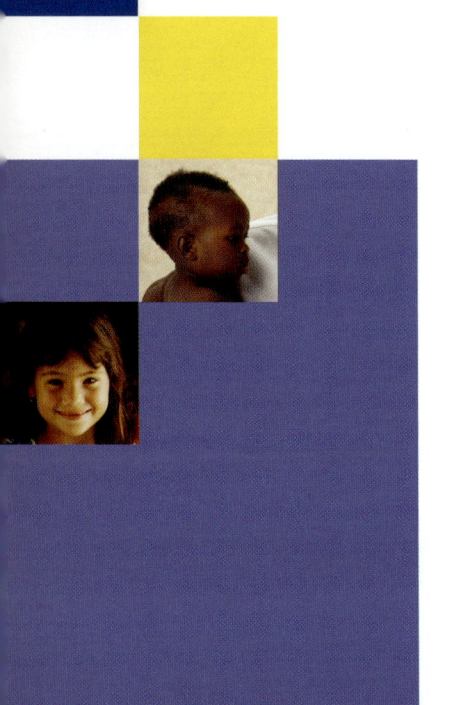

Over the past several decades, the "science" of injury mechanism (also known as the kinetics of trauma) has been refined, increasing our awareness of how accidents occur and the injuries that they produce. Numerous texts have addressed the subject, but few are dedicated to the pediatric patient. This next section focuses on the common pediatric injuries and the associated mechanisms of injury.

Types of Trauma

Trauma is generally divided into two categories: blunt and penetrating.

Blunt

Blunt trauma refers to the type of injury resulting from deceleration and/or compression forces (motor vehicle collisions, falls, and sports injuries), which produce internal injury to the underlying tissues. These forces compress and/or stretch the tissue beneath the skin, causing hollow organs (e.g., intestines and stomach) to rupture and spill their contents into the intra-abdominal cavity and causing solid organs (e.g., liver and spleen) to bleed profusely.

In children, common sites of blunt injury are "points of fixation." These are areas where organs or body structures are suspended by ligaments or held in place by bone (Table 1.2).

Table 1.2: Organs and Fixation Points

Organ	Fixation Point
Brain	Cranial nerves and blood vessels
Cervical spine	Thoracic spine
Lumbar spine	Sacral spine
Lower trachea	Upper trachea
Descending aorta	Ligamentum arteriosum
Kidneys	Renal vasculature
Liver	Ligamentum teres and hepatic vessels
Urethra	Urogenital diaphragm

Penetrating

Penetrating trauma (e.g., stabbings and gunshot wounds) occurs when the skin is broken and the injury extends beneath the open wound (Fig. 1.6). This is usually caused by direct contact with the injury source. Gunshot wounds typically cause associated tissue injury (i.e., injury to the area around the wound itself) from transmitted energy. This transmission is dependent on the size and type of weapon and speed of the projectile. Penetrating injury is seen more commonly in the urban setting but may occur anywhere and at any time.

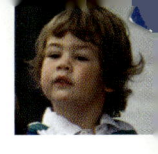

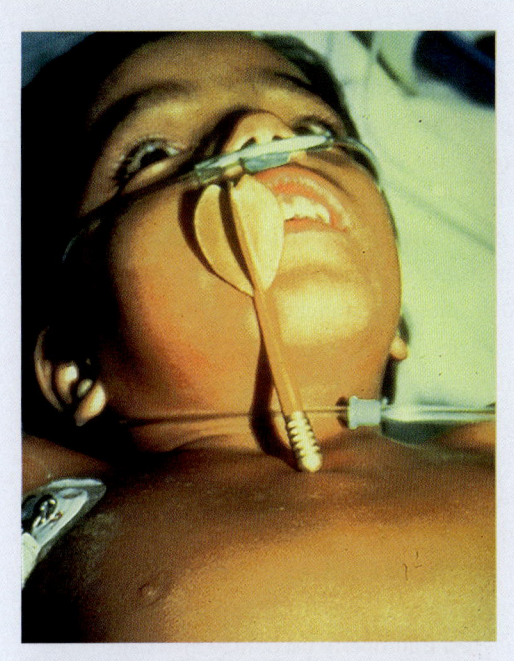

Figure 1.6 *A dart in the chest is an example of penetrating trauma.*

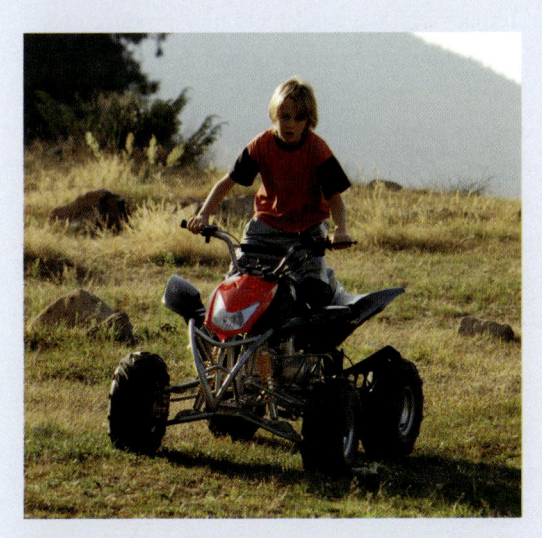

Figure 1.7 *ATV accidents are one type of motor vehicle collision.*

Mechanisms of Injury

Motor Vehicle Collision

Motor vehicle collision (MVC)–related traumatic events account for approximately 47 percent of all pediatric injuries and deaths. Contributing factors include failure to use (or improper use of) passenger restraint devices, alcohol use, and adolescent drivers. Half of all adolescent MVC deaths are attributed to alcohol. In younger children, a large number of MVC deaths are attributed to drunk drivers.

MVCs may involve automobiles, motorcycles, all-terrain vehicles (ATVs), or tractors (Fig. 1.7). As the prehospital provider, you must first identify the mode of transport in order to properly identify the pathway of injury. Predictable injury patterns are best recognized by maintaining a high degree of suspicion.

The Injured Child

For example, if the child was involved in a MVC, attempt to obtain as much information about the accident as possible. Conduct a visual inspection of the vehicle to help reveal both expected and unexpected injuries. Damage to the vehicle serves as an indicator of the forces involved. Deformity of the interior of the vehicle helps to indicate the impact to the patient, based on the child's positioning, and offers clues to possible injuries. In other words, the extent of damage to the vehicle corresponds to the extent of injury to the child.

Observe inside the vehicle for the type and position of restraint devices. Most automobile manufacturers have preinstalled restraint devices designed for the adult passenger. One study has demonstrated that approximately 60 percent of the U.S. population uses auto safety restraint devices improperly. Unused or improperly positioned restraints may subject the child to additional injury during the accident. If the infant is correctly restrained in a car seat, but the car seat is not properly restrained, the child may be ejected from the car or strike various structures in the car. Note whether the car seat is found still restrained. Even if a child has been restrained properly, do not assume the child is uninjured; maintain a high index of suspicion for serious injuries, because using a restraint device does not guarantee the child will not be injured. Seat belts, when improperly used, may also cause injuries to the abdomen and the lumbar spine of a child (see Chapter 9).

Pediatric MVC patients often appear unharmed. However, it is important to watch for hidden injury, especially abdominal trauma. Impact with the windshield may produce obvious head and facial injuries, so prepare for airway intervention as well as spinal motion restriction.

Suspect chest injuries such as flail chest, myocardial contusion, pulmonary contusion, simple and tension pneumothoraces, and great-vessel trauma if the child forcefully struck the dash, rear of the front seat, or other object inside the vehicle.

Ejection from the motor vehicle accounts for approximately 27 percent of all vehicular deaths. Impact with the ground, a tree, or other fixed object increases the child's risk for significant cervical spine injury. Partial ejection carries an increased risk of extremity trauma.

Pedestrian Injuries

Many children each year are struck by moving vehicles. Assess the child for injuries based on the speed of the vehicle, point of contact, and damage to the vehicle. Waddell's triad of injuries has been taught to prehospital providers for years (Fig. 1.8). It describes a "triad" of injuries (head, chest/abdomen, and extremity fracture) that may result from a collision between a pedestrian and a motor vehicle. It has been shown that only 2.4 percent of the children involved in this type of accident suffered the "triad" of injuries. Although the concept of Waddell's triad may not be universally applicable, a high index of suspicion for serious injury should be maintained any time a child is struck by a motor vehicle. Obviously, the smaller the child and the faster the vehicle, the greater the likelihood a serious injury will occur.

Cycling Injuries

There are more than 100 million bicyclists in the United States, and bicycle collisions account for an estimated 200,000 injuries and over 600 deaths of children each year (Fig. 1.9). Approximately 80 percent of all childhood bicycling accidents occur on residential streets within five blocks of the patient's home. Most bicycle riders involved in accidents have less than one year of riding experience.

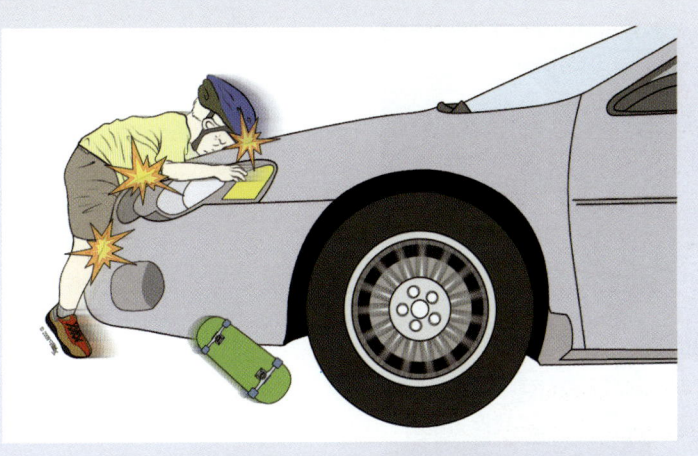

Figure 1.8a *Waddell's triad of injuries is often seen in injuries that result from a collision between a pedestrian and a motor vehicle.*

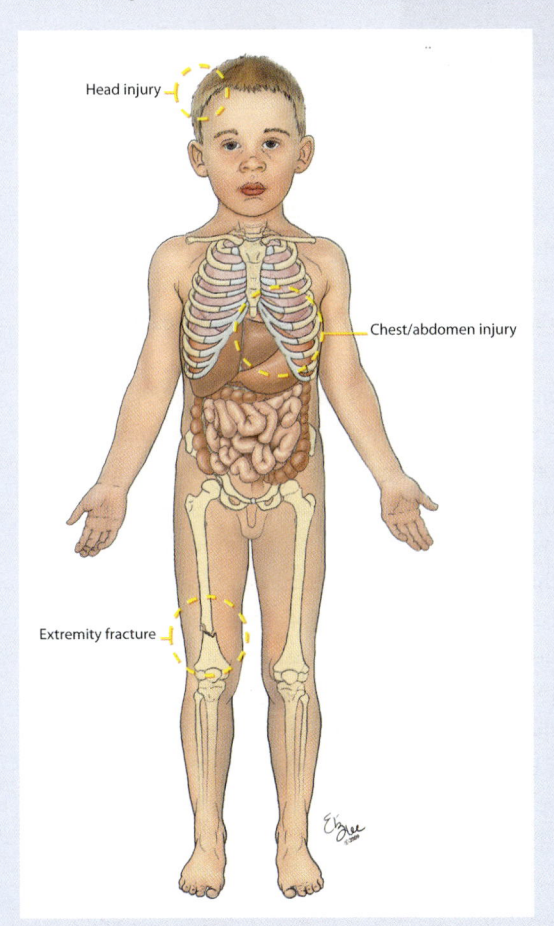

Figure 1.8b *Waddell's triad is defined by head injury, chest or abdomen injury, and extremity fracture.*

Collisions between motor vehicles and bicycles are commonly associated with children who are violating a traffic law (e.g., riding on the wrong side of the road and riding into traffic from alleys, side streets, driveways, and so on). In children younger than 12 years of age, death may occur more commonly when the victim is struck from the left, after riding in front of an oncoming vehicle. Older children tend to be struck from behind.

Head trauma is the leading cause of injury and death in most bicycle-related accidents. One study revealed that 69 percent of bicycle collision patients suffered head injuries, 23 percent suffered orthopedic injuries, and 25 percent were admitted for soft-tissue injuries and lacerations (the overlap was attributed to victims with multiple-system injury).

The Injured Child

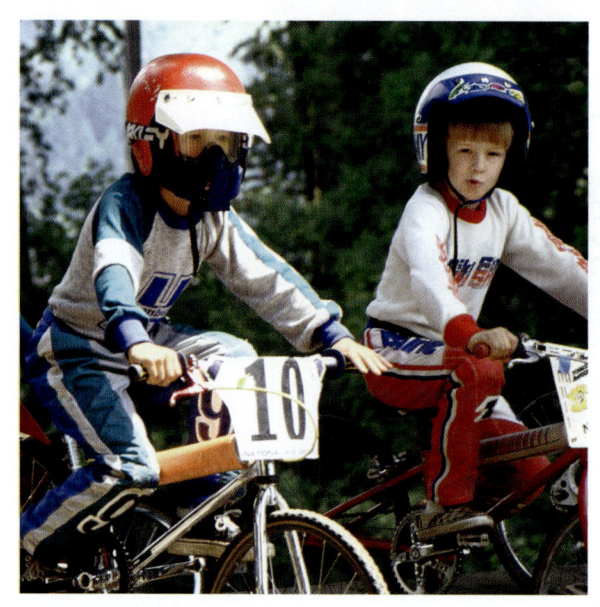

Figure 1.9 *Head trauma is the leading cause of injury and death in most bicycle-related accidents.*

Because the child's head is relatively large in relation to the rest of the body (25 percent of body weight), he is more likely to suffer significant head trauma. For this reason, you should anticipate that there is serious injury to the head and should direct resuscitation efforts accordingly. (Remember that any injury above the level of the clavicles may have an associated cervical spine injury.)

Bicycle helmets can prevent an estimated 85 percent of head trauma and 88 percent of brain injuries. Because many parents are unaware of the need for helmets, attempts to increase bicycle helmet usage should be made through public education. Children, family members, and health care providers need to be educated continually on helmet availability and the advantages of helmet use. Even with aggressive education regarding the advantages of bicycle helmet usage, it is estimated that only 25 percent of children wear helmets.

ATV accidents are more likely to occur during the months of April through September. Almost 70 percent of ATV riders have multiple injuries and 40 percent of those injured require an operation. The majority of ATV injuries, greater than 90 percent, occur in children under the age of 16 years, and the average age of a child involved in a crash is 11 years old. The American Academy of Pediatrics (AAP) and ATV manufacturers recommend that children who are not licensed drivers or at least 16 years of age should not be allowed to operate ATVs.

Falls

Falls are the single most common cause of injury in the pediatric population and account for approximately one-third of all trauma admissions. These children tend to be less than three years of age and are usually playing at the time of injury (Fig. 1.10). Fortunately, the mortality rate is low (0.7 percent) but morbidity is high, with over 60 percent of the children sustaining a fracture and some of those children left neurologically impaired from a head injury. Important factors to consider in a fall are the height from which the child fell, the mass (weight) of the child, and the surface the child contacted (e.g., if the child fell onto a wet grass surface, the probability of serious injury is much lower than if he contacted cement). Note the way the child landed and on what part of the body.

In urban areas, falls account for a significant number of serious injuries, particularly head trauma. In New York City, falls resulted in 20 percent of all unintentional traumatic deaths. Following a simple epidemiological study that demonstrated a clear relationship

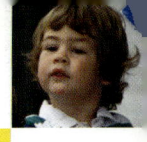

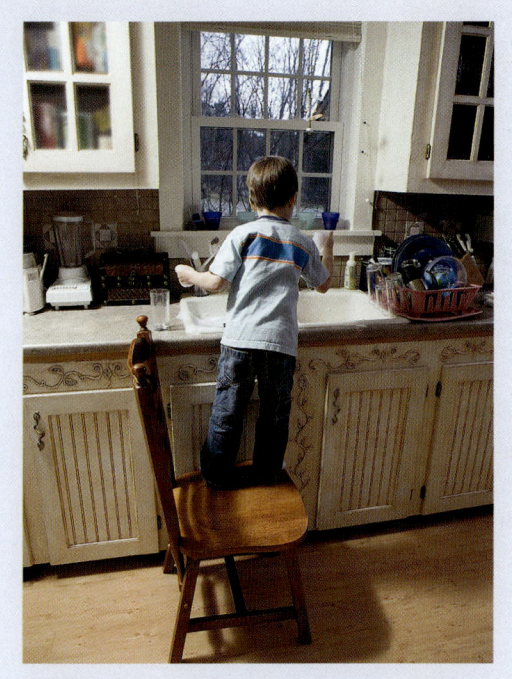

Figure 1.10 *Falls are a common cause of injury for children under age three.*

between warm weather and falls from windows, the city undertook a program to install window guards in apartments housing young children. Deaths caused by falls decreased markedly following the institution of this program. Other areas of the country have identified the serious morbidity that may result from falls, particularly in younger children, and are in the process of developing injury-prevention strategies.

Firearms

Firearms, handguns in particular, produce the most common form of penetrating injury in most of the world. Gunshot wounds are the sixth leading cause of accidental death in the United States. In fact, the United States has the highest firearm-related homicide rate of any nation, more than four times that of any other country.

Fifty percent of all U.S. homes have firearms, with one in four having a handgun. In a recent study, 34 percent of all high school students indicated that they could easily obtain a gun. When evaluating the mechanism of firearm-related injury, note, if possible, whether the injury was from an accidental (unintentional) or an intentional cause. This determination usually has a direct relationship to the scene itself. For example, the majority of unintentional shootings occur at home. The shooting may have been the result of a curious child at the wrong end of the weapon. The availability of a gun at home has also been linked to an increase in adolescent suicide.

When evaluating the mechanism of injury of penetrating trauma, take into consideration wound ballistics. Trajectory of the object, energy dissipation, and the type of projectile will influence injury severity.

INJURY PREVENTION BY AGE GROUP

Mechanisms of injury overlap age groups. When treating these injuries, do not treat only the injuries, but also treat the child based upon the child's age and developmental level. An EMS call for a preventable injury is an opportunity to teach or reinforce safety and prevention strategies.

> **PEARLS**
>
> A pediatric EMS call may represent a "teachable moment" to reinforce safety and prevention strategies.

The Injured Child

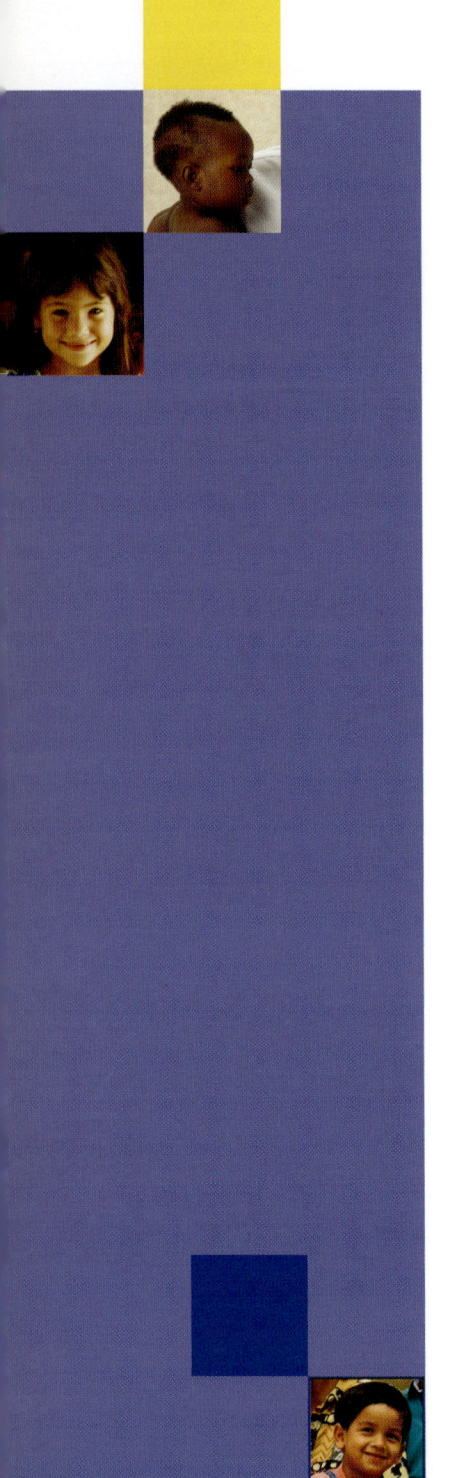

Infancy

Mechanisms of Injury

Because infants are dependent on adults for all of their needs, it is rare that infants cause injury to themselves. Instead, child abuse is a leading cause of injury for this age group. As these children become progressively mobile during the ages of six months to one year, other common mechanisms of injury are MVCs, falls, drowning, and burns.

Prevention

Focus prevention activities on caregivers. Some parents may need parenting classes and help to avoid the tendency to become violent. Educate parents on how to properly use restraint devices in automobiles. Many parents are not aware of developmental milestones for infants, and health care providers must educate them to become more aware of dangers to their children with respect to falls, drowning, and burns.

Toddlers

Mechanisms of Injury

Falls are the leading cause of injury in toddlers. MVCs, drowning, and burns are also major causes of injury in toddlers. As toddlers become progressively independent, especially as they begin to ride bicycles, they are often injured in pedestrian and bicycle accidents (Fig. 1.11).

Prevention

Again, concentrate prevention activities on the child's caregivers. Toddlers must be appropriately restrained in motor vehicles. Also, parents need to understand that, although these children are becoming more independent, they need constant supervision and guidance. This is the perfect age to begin teaching the children the importance of seat belts, bicycle safety, proper use of helmets, and so on.

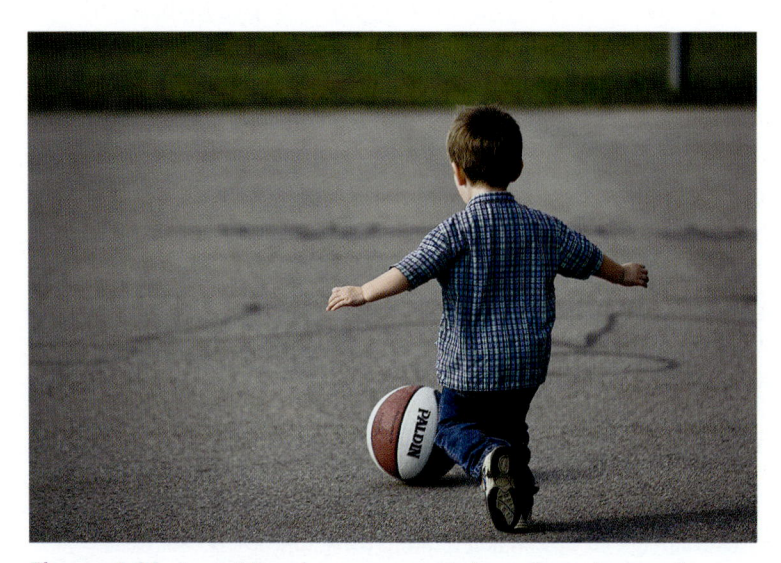

Figure 1.11 *As toddlers become more independent, they need constant supervision and guidance to prevent accidents.*

Pediatric Trauma Life Support

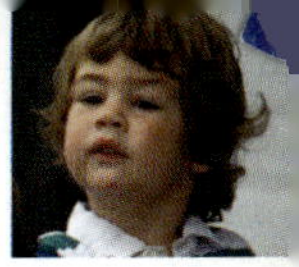

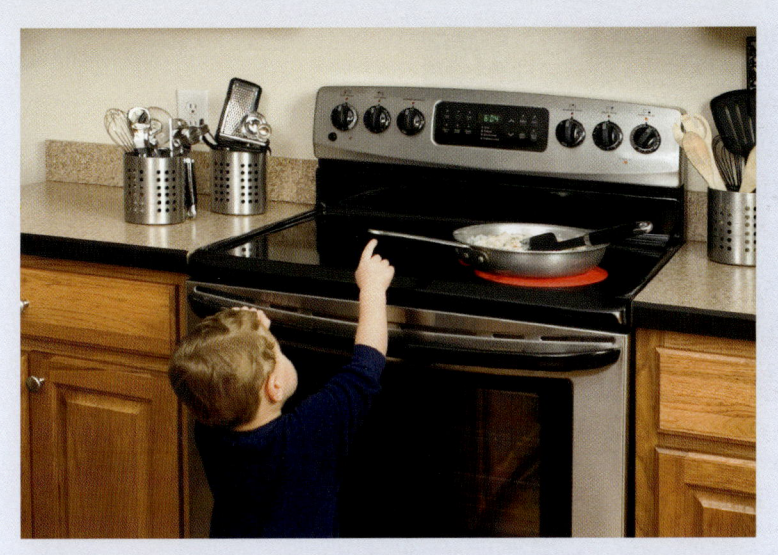

Figure 1.12 *Preschool-age children are very curious and tend to have no fear of potentially dangerous situations.*

Preschool-Age Children

Mechanisms of Injury

Preschool-age children tend to be very independent. They are commonly injured in MVCs, pedestrian accidents, and bicycle accidents. It is estimated that 50 percent of all pediatric MVC injuries and deaths can be prevented by proper use of child seat and lap-shoulder restraint devices. For children under the age of four years, it is estimated that 70 percent of serious injuries and deaths could have been prevented with the use of child restraint devices. Preschool-age children are also very curious and tend to have no fear (Fig. 1.12). Although MVCs are a common cause of injury, fire, drowning, and firearms hurt many preschool-age children. If the child finds a firearm in a home, the consequences could be deadly.

Prevention

Involve the parents of preschool-age children in prevention activities, but also educate the children themselves. This age is a perfect time to involve the children in prevention education, especially in the areas of bicycle and car safety. Many of these children can begin to understand that fire and water can be very dangerous. Although the concept of death is not truly understood, educate these children about firearms since these weapons are a leading cause of death in the United States.

School-Age Children

Mechanisms of Injury

Common mechanisms of injury for school-age children continue to be MVCs, bicycle accidents, falls, burns, and drowning (Fig. 1.13). School-age children are at the greatest risk of being struck and killed by a motor vehicle. Injuries commonly occur when a child runs out into the street. Because children are easily distracted and lack quick reflexive action, they often are injured while chasing a toy, friend, or pet into the path of an oncoming vehicle.

The Injured Child

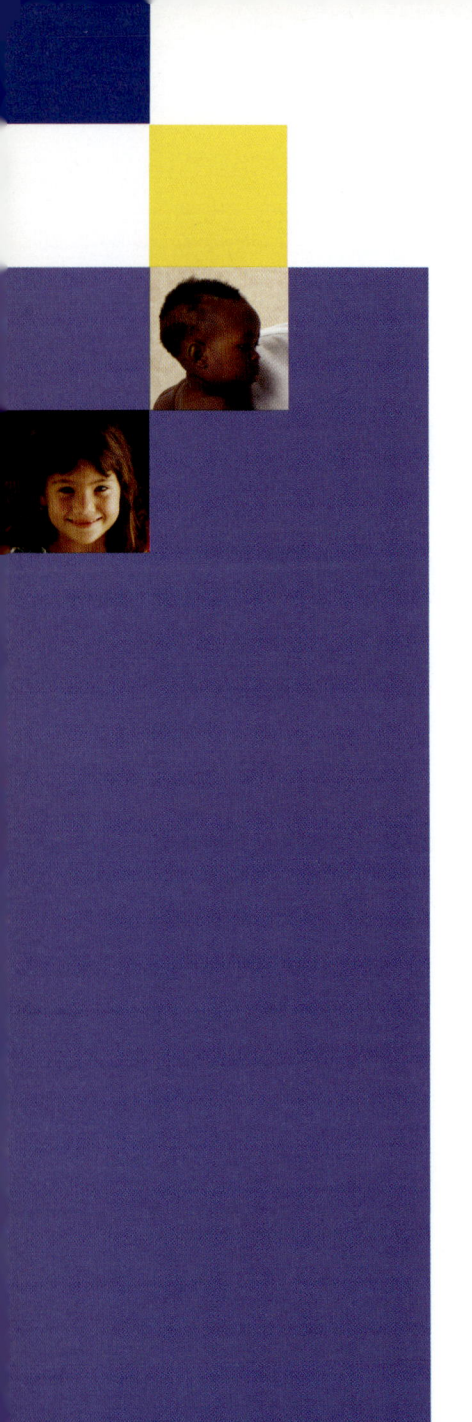

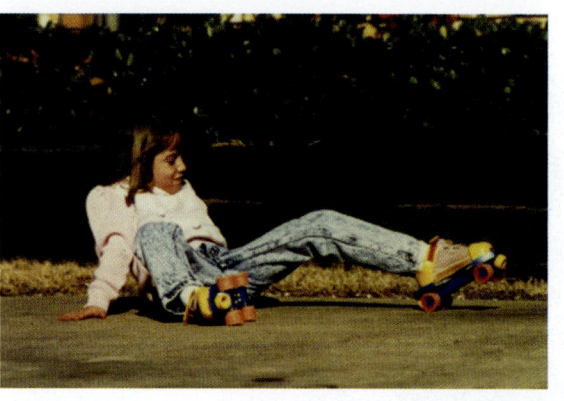

Figure 1.13 *Falls are a common mechanism of injury for school-age children.*

Prevention

Although parents still need to take an active role in prevention education, school-age children must begin to learn to take responsibility for their own actions. Prevention activities still need to stress the areas of motor vehicle, bicycle, and firearm safety. Many of these prevention activities are taught in the school system, but need to be continually reinforced at home.

Adolescents

Mechanisms of Injury

Adolescents are frequently involved in risky behaviors. The use of drugs and alcohol and "extreme sporting" activities are common precipitants for behavior that results in injury (Fig.1.14). Common mechanisms of injury include MVCs and firearm injuries. Though firearm injuries and MVCs are the leading causes of injury, these children are still at risk for other types of injuries including drowning and falls.

Prevention

Prevention activities must be concentrated toward areas of motor vehicle safety and abstinence from drugs and alcohol. Again, many of these prevention activities are reinforced at school, but parents and the lay community also need to be active in prevention activities. Prehospital personnel must assume the prevention role, as well.

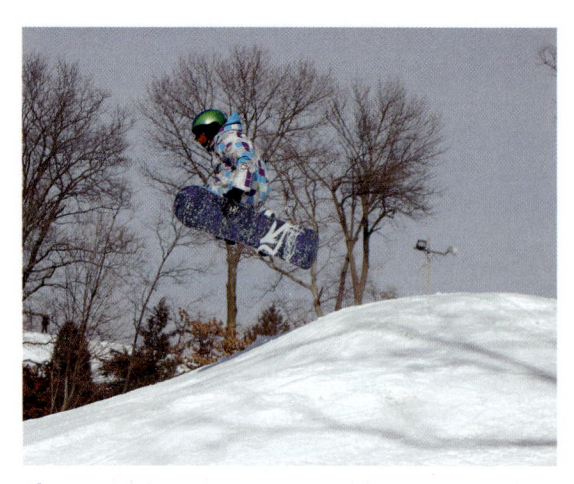

Figure 1.14 *"Extreme sporting" activities are a cause of injury commonly seen in adolescents.*

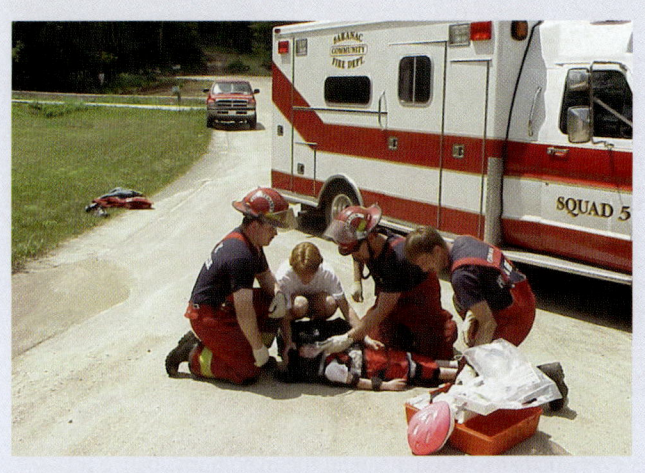

Figure 1.15 *Parents provide comfort to their child on the scene and should accompany the child to the hospital if possible.*

TRANSPORT CONSIDERATIONS

A common stressor that parents often identify following an injury is transporting their child to the hospital. Nothing terrifies parents more than the thought of their child being critically ill or injured and being transported to the hospital alone and frightened. This is compounded by the parents' fears that the child may not survive the transport to the hospital and that they may not see their child alive again.

If possible, parents or guardians should accompany the child to the hospital (Fig. 1.15). Not only are they the best historians regarding the child, they are also the most welcome source of comfort to the child. Make accommodations for parents to accompany children to the hospital, whether it is by ambulance, helicopter, or fixed-wing aircraft. Open and continued communication is imperative in this situation. Tell parents what interventions are needed and why. They are not interested in doing a critique on medical care; they are interested in seeing caring people work hard to make their child well again. Some parents may prefer to follow the emergency vehicle. This may be an acceptable alternative for parents who do not wish to accompany their child; however, stress caution to a family who chooses to follow the ambulance. The parents must remain a safe distance from the ambulance and not follow the ambulance if lights and sirens are utilized.

CONFIDENT APPROACH

Although managing pediatric trauma may be challenging for some caregivers, a confident, well-organized, systematic approach will allow you to provide the best care when evaluating the pediatric patient for life-threatening injuries. You must be objective, yet understanding. The ITLS patient assessment will provide you with a safe, efficient, organized and effective method. As with care of adults, the key to optimal pediatric patient care is maintaining a high index of suspicion for potential injury, using a careful assessment technique, having knowledge of the disease process, recognizing life-threatening injuries, and initiating early interventions. This standardized process has demonstrated a significant increase in the patient's chances for a successful outcome.

Even the most difficult case can be managed when an objective, systematic approach is used. A chaotic situation can be calmed if you are confident and well-organized. The team approach to pediatric trauma is essential. The following is an example of an effective prehospital team, and applies to pediatric as well as adult care.

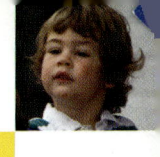

> **PEARLS**
>
> Prehospital providers should practice and encourage safe transport of children and families. Proper restraint in the ambulance or instruction regarding safe following is essential to prevent additional injury.

The Injured Child

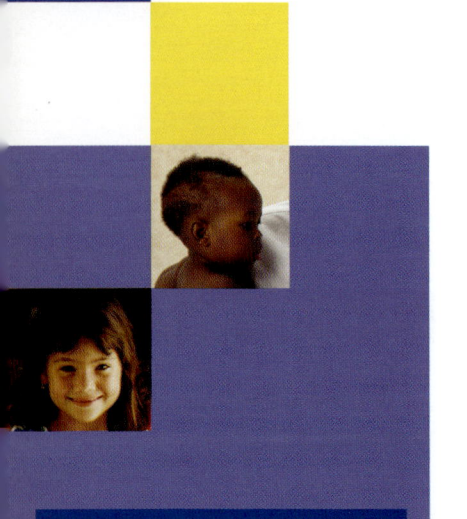

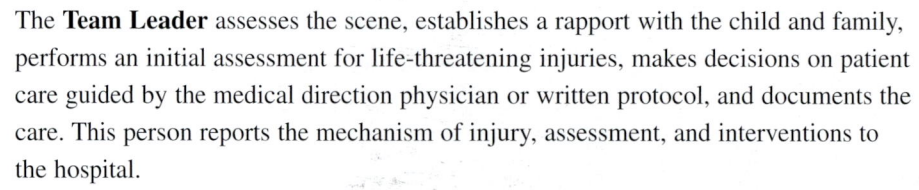

The **Team Leader** assesses the scene, establishes a rapport with the child and family, performs an initial assessment for life-threatening injuries, makes decisions on patient care guided by the medical direction physician or written protocol, and documents the care. This person reports the mechanism of injury, assessment, and interventions to the hospital.

Rescuer 2 stabilizes the cervical spine and performs airway maneuvers and management as directed by the Team Leader.

Rescuer 3 selects appropriate equipment and initiates interventions as directed by the Team Leader.

A well-organized team gives every pediatric trauma patient the maximum chance for survival. Assess every trauma patient, whether an injured bicyclist or an ejected MVC patient, in the same manner after any traumatic event. If assessment is performed in the same way every time, it is less likely that a life-threatening injury will be undetected. Remember that "practice makes perfect." Training and retraining serves to reinforce this concept of the confident approach.

EQUIPMENT

Trauma is no accident, nor is good patient care. Interventions performed in children, although similar to those performed in adults, are of a different nature and require different techniques.

Children cannot be expanded to fit onto, or into, adult-sized equipment, and adult-sized equipment cannot be condensed in the field (Fig.1.16). Use appropriate pediatric-sized equipment for every child as much as possible (Table 1.3). A variety of manufacturers offer equipment designed especially for children. Child-size airway equipment and pediatric spinal motion restriction devices are available (Fig.1.17). When the equipment is not quite suitable, you may use improvisational techniques, ensuring that you meet the objectives of the interventions. The skill stations of this book can assist in the selection of appropriate equipment.

PEARLS

A standardized team approach to pediatric trauma care is essential and requires routine practice to maintain skills.

PEARLS

Advocate for your pediatric patients and assure that proper child-sized equipment is available and in working order.

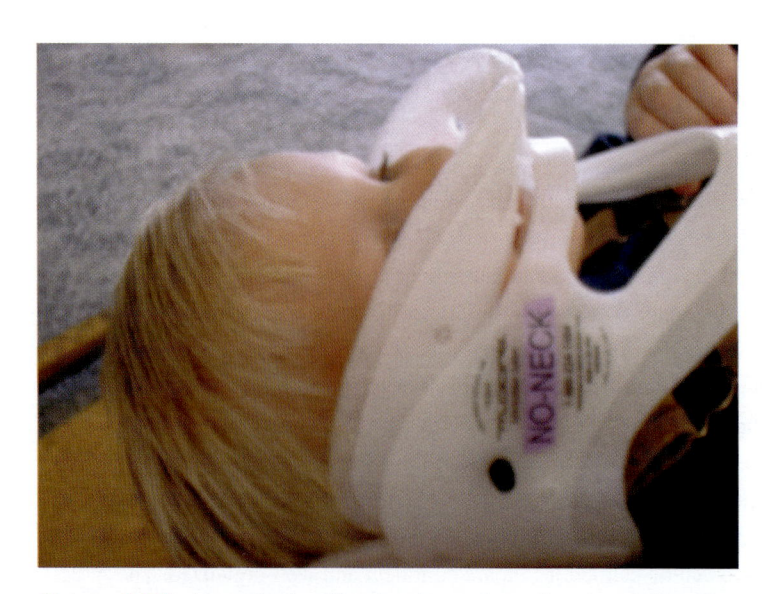

Figure 1.16 *A cervical collar that is too large for the child will not help to restrict the patient's movements.*

Table 1.3: Equipment

Airway

- Bag-valve device and mask sizes # 0, 1, 2, 3
- Laryngoscope handle with extra batteries and bulbs
- Laryngoscope blades — straight and/or curved, # 0, 1, 2, 3
- Stylettes — pediatric
- Endotracheal tubes
   – Uncuffed 2.5 – 6.0
   – Cuffed 6.0 – 8.0
- Magill forceps
- Water-soluble lubricating jelly
- Nasogastric tubes, sizes 5F to 18F
- Suction machine and catheters

Vascular Access

- Intravenous catheters, sizes 24g to 14g
- Intraosseous needles, sizes 16 and 18
- Tourniquets, rubber bands
- Three-way stop cocks
- Syringes
- Blood sample tubes
- Intravenous tubing, large-bore and regular

Intravenous Solutions and Medications

- Normal saline
- 25% dextrose solution
- Atropine
- Sodium bicarbonate
- Diazepam
- Epinephrine
- Lidocaine
- Naloxone
- Pain control medication

Monitoring Equipment

- Cardiac monitor/defibrillator
- Pulse oximeter
- Glucose analyzer

Spinal Motion Restriction Equipment

- Pediatric spine immobilizer
- Cervical collars, pediatric sizes
- Cervical immobilization device
- Straps to secure patient on board
- Pediatric backboard

The Injured Child

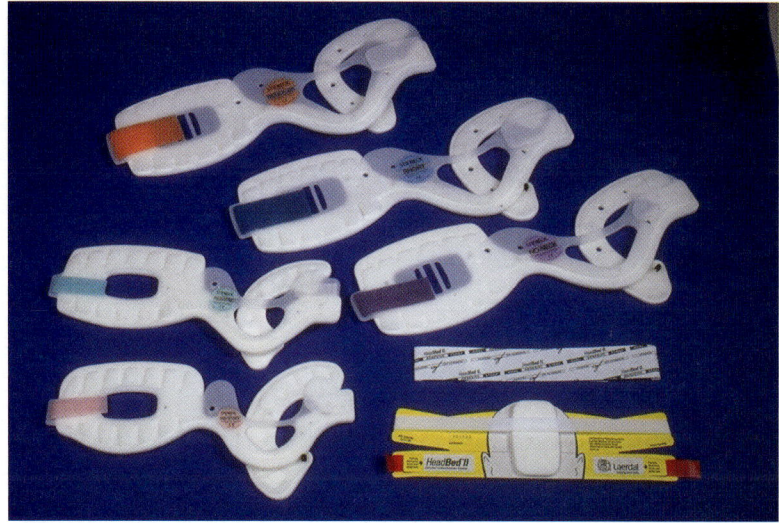

Figure 1.17 *Cervical collars come in multiple sizes to accommodate the needs of pediatric patients, including infants.*

Case Study *continued*

John, Susan, and Bob of the Emergency Transport Service (ETS) were called to the scene of a motor vehicle collision and found a mother with two young children in a minivan with significant damage to the front driver's side of the vehicle with entrapment of passengers. After assuring that the scene was safe, the team approached the vehicle and found two toddlers secured in child safety seats next to each other in the middle seat. Firefighters have extricated the mother from the driver's seat. Both children are crying; the smaller child is screaming over and over, "I want my mommy!" Based upon size and language, John estimates her to be a toddler about 2 years old who is kicking vigorously and struggling to get out of the car seat as she strains to see her mother. The second child's head is at the top of the car seat with his legs hanging down and he tells the team to "go away," then asks "why" after every instruction given. Based upon his size, language and interactions, John estimates him to be 4 years old. Upon inspection you find no damage to the interior compartment of the vehicle where the children are located. Both car seats are properly installed and both children are securely restrained in their car seats. Initial assessment reveals no injuries; however, there is only one ambulance at the scene so John makes the decision to transport the children in their car seats in the ambulance along with their mother who is unconscious. Both children settled noticeably as Susan talked with them in a calm reassuring voice and once they could see their mother. The four-year-old tells John, "Mommy is sleeping, so be quiet."

Pediatric Trauma Life Support

Case Study *wrap-up*

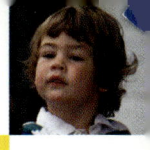

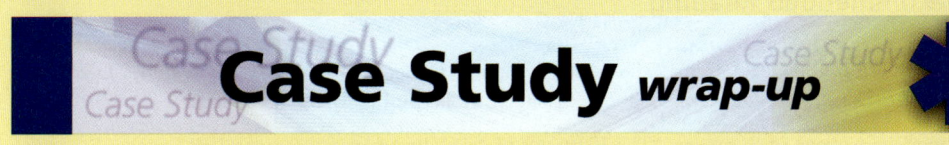

Although necessity required transporting all three patients together in this case because there was only one ambulance at the scene, it is always preferable to transport a family together if logistically possible. Children are comforted by their parents' presence and parents are reassured by seeing and knowing that their child is receiving the best of care. Using age-appropriate language and a calm voice and minimizing exaggerated facial expressions and gestures will help establish rapport with a child. Remember to commend parents who have properly installed child car seats and securely restrained their child. Let them know that their conscientious actions have prevented injury. When you come upon children who are not properly restrained, create a teachable moment for the adult who is with them and let them know they can make a real difference insuring the safety of the children entrusted to them.

SUMMARY

1. It is essential to communicate with children in a manner that is appropriate for the child's developmental stage, which will make assessment easier and more accurate.
2. A well-organized trauma team that uses a systemic approach and treats every situation in the same way will optimize patient care.
3. In an intense pediatric trauma situation, some caregivers panic instead of remembering the basics of trauma care. If you apply the techniques described in this textbook, the injured child will have the best chance for a successful resuscitation and full recovery from the injuries sustained.
4. Millions of children are victims of trauma. The four most common forms of childhood unintentional injury are MVCs, pedestrian injuries, bicycle accidents, and gunshot wounds.
5. When assessing children, remember that many of their injuries will be obvious, but some will not be obvious. Understanding the mechanism of injury will help you to recognize the hidden, less-obvious injuries.
6. Trauma is the leading cause of death and disability in children over the age of one year; in addition, the care required is very expensive. Fortunately, in most cases, trauma is preventable. Take an active part in not only the treatment of pediatric trauma, but also in its prevention.

The Injured Child

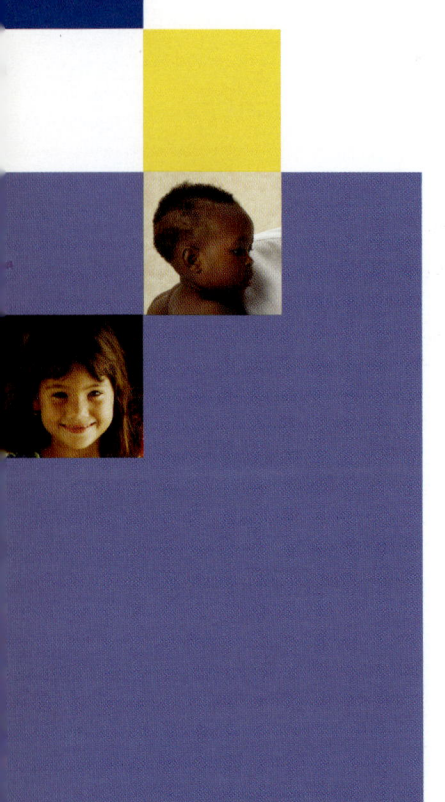

Recommended Reading

Advanced Life Support Group. "The Seriously Injured Child." In *Pre-Hospital Paediatric Life Support: The Practical Approach*, 2nd ed. London: Blackwell BMJ Books, 2005.

American College of Surgeons. "The Extremes of Age." In *Advanced Trauma Life Support Program for Doctors*, 8th ed. Chicago: Author, 2008.

Brown, Wesley, S. Kenneth Thurman, and Lynda Pearl. "Family Centered Early Interventions with Infants and Toddlers." In *Innovative Cross Disciplinary Approaches*. Baltimore: Paul H. Brooks Publishing, 1993.

Brunquell, Donald and Daniel P. Kohen. "Emotions in Pediatric Emergencies: What We Know, What We Can Do." *Children's Health Care* 20 (4, 1991): 240–47.

Campbell, John Emory, ed. "Trauma in Children." In *International Trauma Life Support for Prehospital Care Providers*, 6th ed., 258–77. Upper Saddle River, N.J.: Pearson/Prentice Hall, 2008.

Division of Injury Control Center for Environmental Health and Injury Control, Centers for Disease Control. "Childhood Injuries in the United States." *American Journal of Diseases in Children* 144 (1990): 627–46.

European Resuscitation Council (UK). "The Injured Child." In *European Paediatric Life Support*, 2nd ed. Antwerp, Belguin: Author, 2006.

Johnson, Kendall. "Trauma in the Lives of Children." In *Crisis and Stress Management for Counselors-Other Professionals*. Alameda, C.A.: Hunter House Inc., 1989.

Thornton, Susan M., et al. Child Health Care Communications: *Enhancing Interactions among Professionals, Parents and Children*. Langhorne, P.A.: Johnson and Johnson, 1983.

CHAPTER 2
Assessment of the Pediatric Patient

John E. Campbell, MD, FACEP
Ann Marie Dietrich, MD, FACEP, FAAP
Steven J. Shaner, EMT-P

Objectives

Upon completion of this chapter, you should be able to:

1. Describe the steps in trauma assessment and management.

2. Describe the ITLS Primary Survey and explain how it relates to the Rapid Trauma Survey and the Focused Exam.

3. Describe when the ITLS Primary Survey can be interrupted.

4. Describe when critical interventions should be made and where to make them.

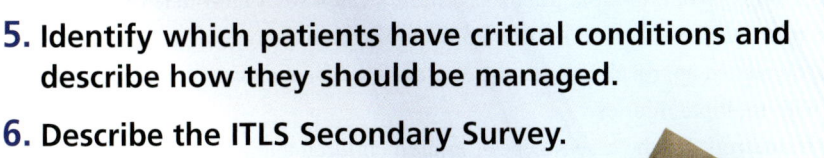

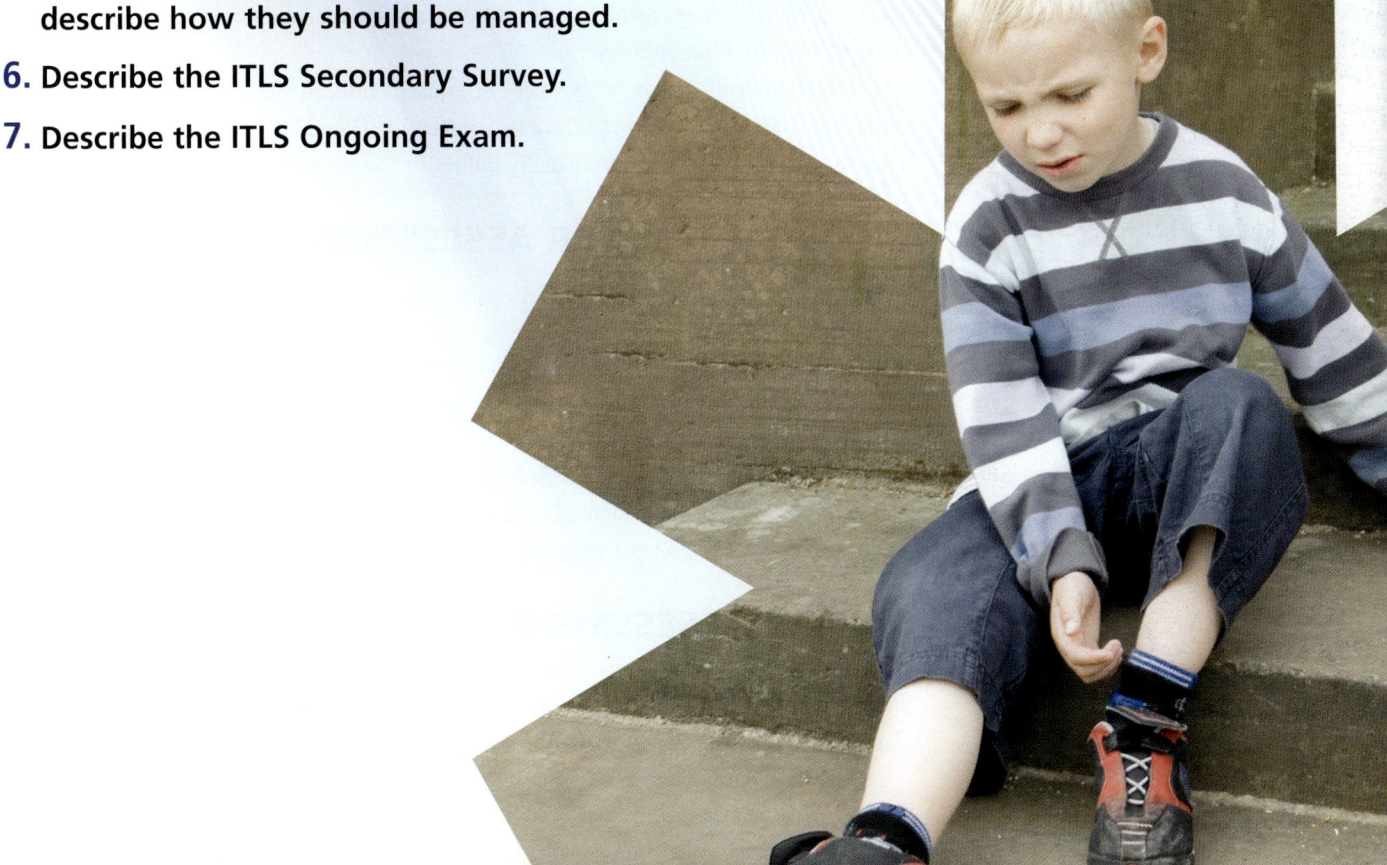

5. Identify which patients have critical conditions and describe how they should be managed.

6. Describe the ITLS Secondary Survey.

7. Describe the ITLS Ongoing Exam.

Case Study

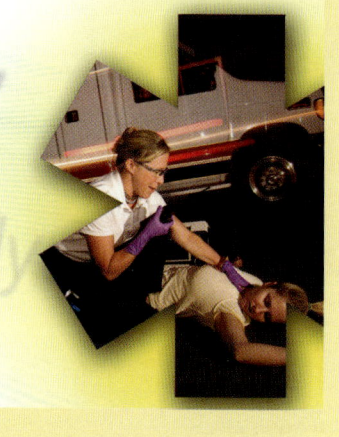

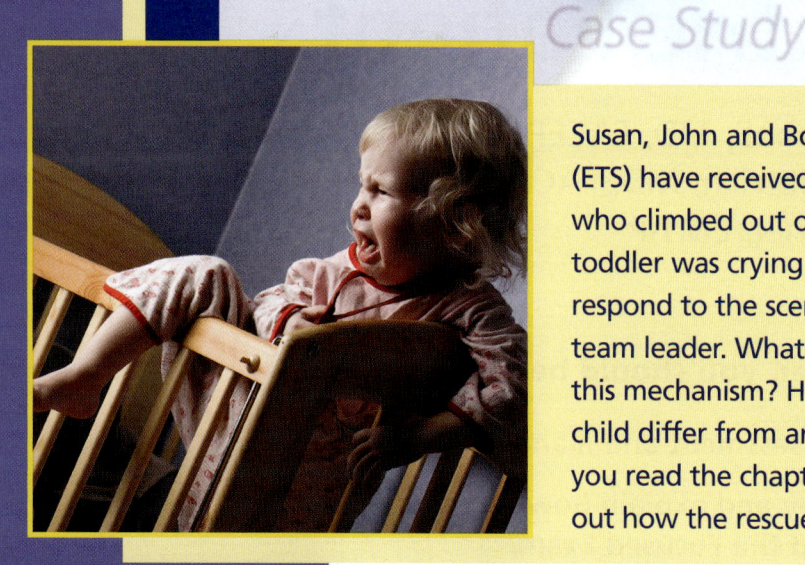

Susan, John and Bob of the Emergency Transport Service (ETS) have received a call to a home of an 18-month-old child who climbed out of her crib and fell. They are told that the toddler was crying and appears to be in pain. As they respond to the scene, they decide that Susan will be the team leader. What sort of injuries should they expect from this mechanism? How does evaluation and treatment of a child differ from an adult? Keep these questions in mind as you read the chapter. Then, at the end of the chapter, find out how the rescuers completed this call.

INTRODUCTION

Trauma is the leading cause of death among children over the age of one year, with most fatalities resulting from multiple traumas. Children can have a multitude of serious injuries, and most medical personnel are inexperienced in the management of young patients. A standard, organized approach ensures the appropriate management of unstable pediatric patients with multiple injuries.

The framework for the assessment of injured children and adults is similar, but the child's physiologic response to trauma is different. The child's normal vital signs vary with age, so even normal values are usually unfamiliar to rescuers.

PREPARATIONS FOR ASSESSMENT OF THE PEDIATRIC PATIENT

One of the most important things to do prior to arrival at the scene is to correctly prepare the necessary equipment (Review "Equipment" in Chapter 1). Ensure that appropriately sized equipment is easily accessible.

Because children vary in size, a length-based tape may be used to estimate weight and to appropriately size equipment (Fig. 2.1). Normal vital signs for different age groups are shown in Table 2.1. Do not trust your memory; carry a card with the normal values for age.

PATIENT ASSESSMENT

Pediatric ITLS emphasizes using the standard approach to assessment of the trauma patient. Patient assessment is divided into three exams (the ITLS Primary Survey, ITLS

> **PEARLS**
>
> **Follow the same standard, organized ITLS approach in children as in adults to ensure the appropriate management of pediatric patients.**

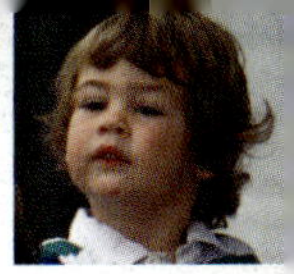

Secondary Survey, and ITLS Ongoing Exam), and each exam is comprised of certain steps (Figure 2.2). Survival of critical trauma pediatric patients depends on how quickly the patient is delivered to definitive care. To make the most efficient use of time, these exams are performed in a certain sequence. The usual order is as follows: the ITLS Primary Survey is performed first, then the ITLS Secondary Survey, and then the ITLS Ongoing Exam. However, depending on circumstances and transport time, the ITLS Secondary Survey may not be performed in every case.

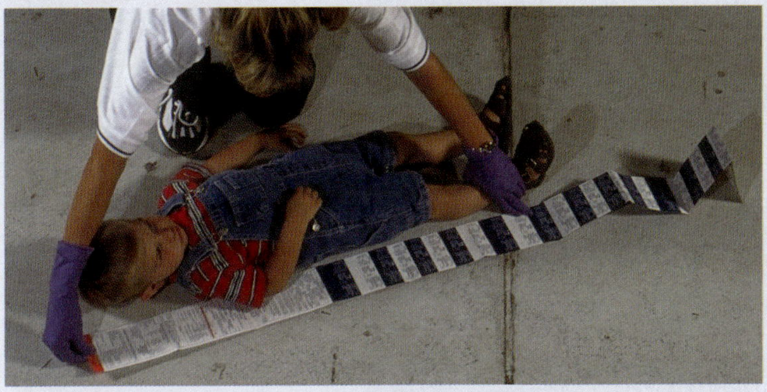

> **PEARLS**
>
> Do not trust your memory; carry a card with the normal values for age and use a length-based tape to determine equipment sizes and medication doses.

Figure 2.1 *A length-based tape helps determine equipment sizes and medication dosages.*

Table 2.1: Weight and Vital Signs by Age Group

Age	Weight in kg (lb)	Respirations (breaths per minute)	Pulse (beats per minute)	Systolic Blood (mmHg) Pressure
Newborn	3-4 kg (6-9 lb)	30-50	120-160	60-80
6 mo-1 yr	8-10 kg (16-22 lb)	30-40	120-140	70-80
2-4 yr	12-16 kg (24-34 lb)	20-30	100-110	80-95
5-8 yr	18-26 kg (36-55 lb)	14-20	90-100	90-100
8-12 yr	26-50 kg (55-110 lb)	12-20	80-100	100-110
>12 yr	>50 kg (110 lb)	12-16	60-90	100-120

ITLS Primary Survey

During the ITLS Primary Survey, identify all life-threatening injuries and determine the need for immediate transport. Complete the ITLS Primary Survey in two minutes or less. Do not interrupt the ITLS Primary Survey except for an obstructed airway, cardiopulmonary arrest, or if the scene becomes too unsafe to continue.

The ITLS Primary Survey consists of Scene Size-Up; Initial Assessment of the child's level of consciousness, airway, breathing, and circulation (ABCs); either a Rapid Trauma Survey (head-to-toe exam when the mechanism is generalized or the patient is unconscious) or Focused Exam (when the mechanism is very focused, such as a single gunshot wound to the leg, or if the mechanism is insignificant); and a decision about the need for early transport. If an ITLS Secondary Survey (thorough head-to-toe exam) is necessary, it may be performed en route to the hospital. Perform an ITLS Ongoing Exam during transport to monitor changes in the patient's condition.

Assessment of the Pediatric Patient

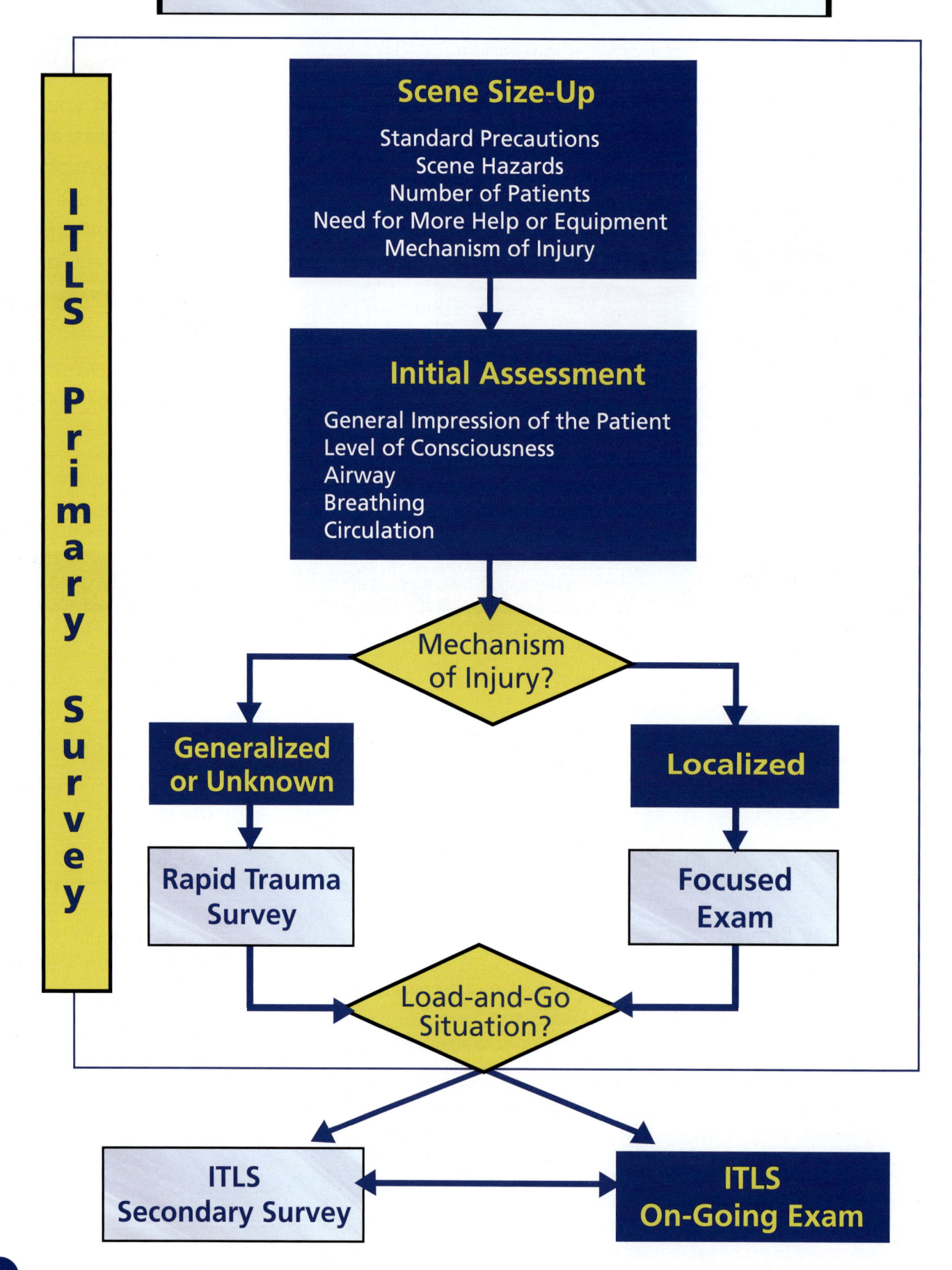

ITLS Patient Assessment

ITLS Primary Survey

Scene Size-Up
Standard Precautions
Scene Hazards
Number of Patients
Need for More Help or Equipment
Mechanism of Injury

↓

Initial Assessment
General Impression of the Patient
Level of Consciousness
Airway
Breathing
Circulation

↓

Mechanism of Injury?

- Generalized or Unknown → Rapid Trauma Survey
- Localized → Focused Exam

Load-and-Go Situation?

→ ITLS Secondary Survey ↔ ITLS On-Going Exam

Figure 2.2 *ITLS Patient Assessment diagram*

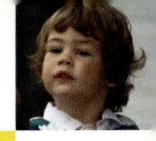

Scene Size-Up

Scene Size-Up requires rescuers to prepare prior to approaching the incident. All rescuers must have proper personal protective equipment (PPE) available. Rescuers should follow standard precautions for body fluid/infectious exposures.

It is important to scan the area for dangers and other patients. This gives the rescuers a chance to note possible mechanisms of injury. This is also the time to call for more help or special equipment if necessary to complete the rescue. The most common ways in which children are injured are motor vehicle crashes, as pedestrians or bicycle riders struck by a vehicle, falls, abuse, burns, and drowning. As indicated in Chapter 1, always consider the mechanism of injury in relation to the size of the child.

If a parent or guardian is at the scene, introduce and present yourself in an organized, efficient manner. Parents may be helpful during your assessment of a child (Fig. 2.3). They know what is normal for the child and they know the child's medical history. They also know how to keep their child calm so rescuers can complete an assessment. It is difficult for parents or guardians to see their child injured. However, it is their child and, under most circumstances, they need to be kept informed of any necessary medical intervention. Various age groups respond differently to strangers and medical personnel. If the child is critically injured, obtain a very brief history and explain to the parents the importance of rapid package and transport for an injured child. Move quickly to the child and begin a rapid assessment.

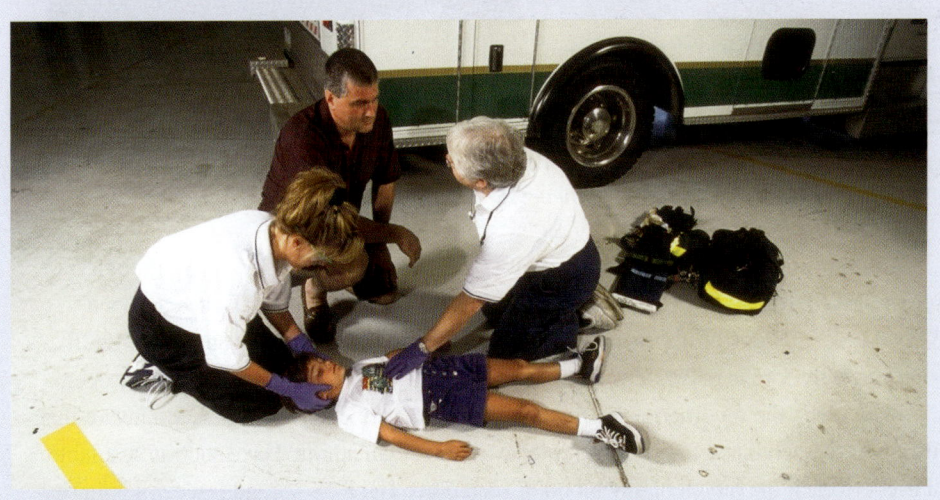

Figure 2.3 *Parents can be helpful during the assessment. They know the child's history and can help keep their child calm.*

Initial Assessment

General Impression

The rescuer forms a general impression on every scene. The impression becomes more precise with experience. This holds true for pediatric patients. As you provide care for pediatric patients, you become more comfortable and better prepared to deal with injuries to infants and children. As you begin your approach to the patient, you can see the child's position, estimate the child's age, and note the child's general appearance. You can often form an impression about whether the child is critical or stable by this information alone. This is called "street smarts." Experienced rescuers recognize that these "gut feelings" are usually correct.

> **PEARLS**
>
> Do not interrupt the ITLS Primary Survey except for an obstructed airway, cardiopulmonary arrest, or if the scene becomes too unsafe to continue. If a problem is found in the ITLS Primary Survey, provide rapid transport to the most appropriate setting. Continue to reassess the child.

> **PEARLS**
>
> Listen to parents and caregivers. They know what is normal for the child.

Assessment of the Pediatric Patient

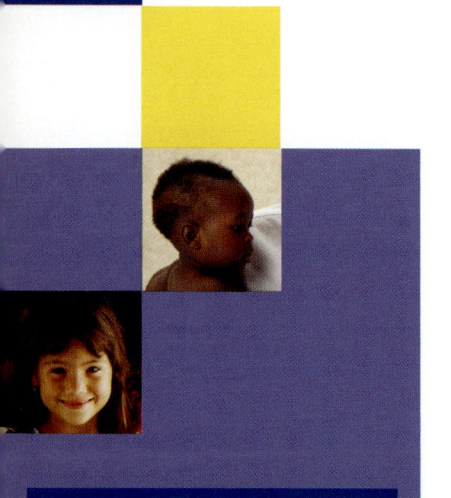

Level of Consciousness

Observe the child. The first few seconds of evaluation reveal valuable information. Is the child looking at you? Does he recognize his parents? Note whether the child is alert (A), responds to verbal command (V), responds only to pain (P), or is unresponsive (U). Continue to observe the child for the entire ITLS Primary Survey.

Airway and Cervical Spine

While assessing the airway, it is imperative to manually restrict movement of the cervical spine. In children, the head is relatively large compared to the rest of the body, so you may have to add padding under the shoulders to get the neck and airway in a neutral position (Fig. 2.4). If the mechanism suggests any chance of spinal injury, assume that the child's neck is injured and maintain spinal motion restriction throughout the assessment and management of the patient.

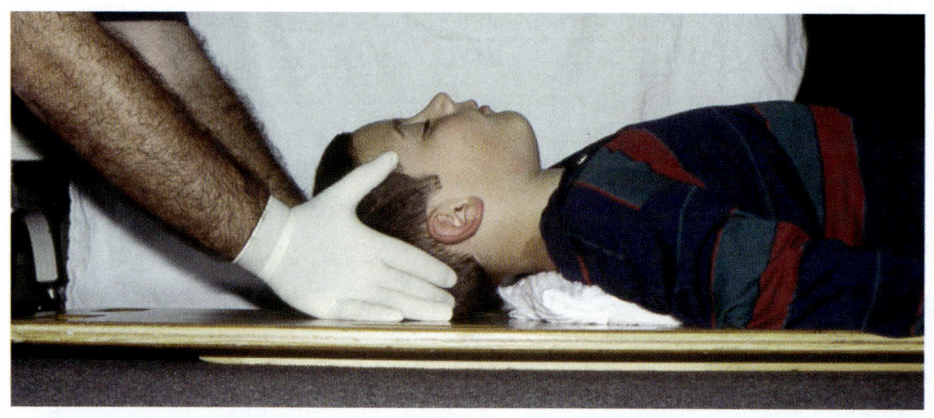

Figure 2.4 *Manually restrict motion of the cervical spine before assessing the airway. Padding under the shoulders may be necessary.*

After movement of the neck is manually restricted, assess the airway. Although a screaming child may be difficult to deal with, screaming usually indicates an open airway. Look for signs of upper airway occlusion, apnea, stridor, or agonal respirations. Listen carefully for air movement through the mouth. If the child is unconscious, open the airway using the modified jaw thrust maneuver. Listen carefully again. Be aware that children have a tendency to produce more secretions than adults. Have suction available and use it to clear the mouth of any blood or secretions. Have the second rescuer administer supplemental oxygen to the patient. *Always administer 100 percent oxygen.*

If the child is not breathing, is unresponsive, or is not exchanging air adequately, bag-valve-mask ventilation may be needed.

Breathing

Following the airway assessment, assess the child's breathing. Look at the child's respiratory rate, oxygenation, and breathing efforts. Compare the child's respiratory rate to the normal rate for the child's age listed on the card. Initially, when children are in respiratory distress, they breathe very quickly (tachypnea). As they have more difficulty breathing, the respiratory rate slows and periods of apnea may occur. Look at the color of the child's lips and nail beds. If they are not pink, the child may be hypoxic. Observe whether the child is having difficulty breathing. Note nostril flaring, retractions, and grunting. Look for the position of the trachea and jugular venous distention. Listen carefully to the child's lung fields, and assess how well they are moving air.

PEARLS

Develop your "street smarts." Approach the child in the same way each time: note the child's position, estimate the child's age, and note the child's general appearance. The more you use the same approach, the more skilled you will be at recognizing patterns.

PEARLS

Be aware that children may produce more secretions than adults. Have suction available and use it to clear the mouth of any blood or secretions.

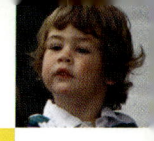

If the child is apneic or having severe respiratory distress, initiate ventilatory assistance by mouth-to-mask or bag-valve-mask ventilation (Fig. 2.5). A second rescuer should give 100 percent oxygen via an appropriately sized mask. While maintaining a good seal, ventilate at the rate the child would normally breathe. Watch the chest for rise and fall and listen carefully to the lungs for air exchange. It is preferable not to intubate the child on the scene. Intubation in the pediatric patient is often time-consuming and technically difficult. Studies have shown that in the prehospital setting, the pediatric patient outcomes of those ventilated with a bag-valve mask is just as good as those who are intubated. If the child can be effectively oxygenated and ventilated with a bag-valve mask, and the transport time is short, do not use precious time attempting intubation in the field. Maintain the child's airway with bag-valve-mask ventilation and remember to keep suction available for managing secretions. If the child cannot be oxygenated and ventilated with bag-valve-mask, then the child must be intubated at the scene.

If the child has evidence of a tension pneumothorax, (see Chapter 5), correct this problem rapidly or the child may progress to cardiopulmonary arrest. Treatment involves rapid transport and needle decompression performed in the manner described in the Airway and Chest Skill Station (see Chapter 6).

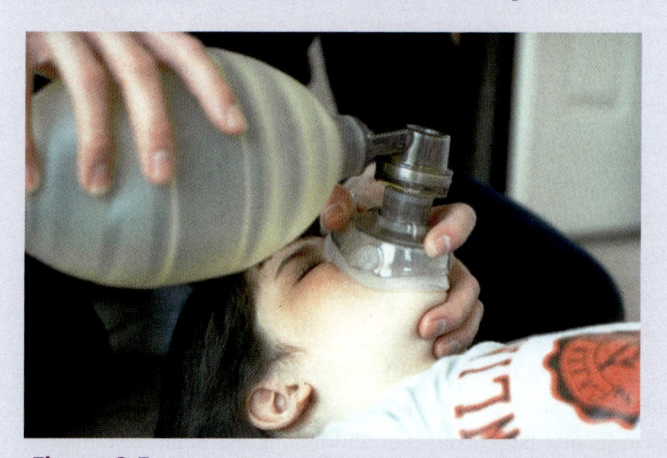

Figure 2.5 *Bag-valve-mask ventilation of a child.*

Circulation

Next, evaluate the child's circulation. Note the pulse; a well-perfused child should have a strong peripheral pulse (radial or dorsalis pedis). If this is absent, check for a central pulse (brachial, femoral, or carotid). The best indicators of shock in a child will be tachycardia, weak peripheral pulses, and prolonged central capillary refill (Fig. 2.6).

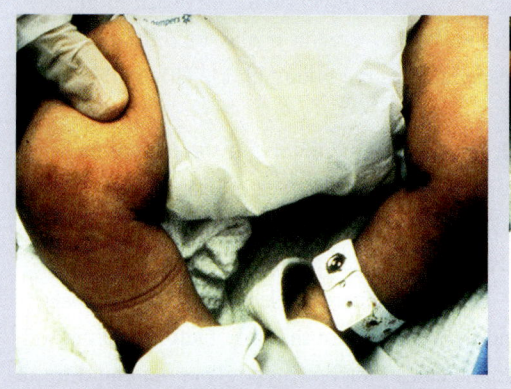

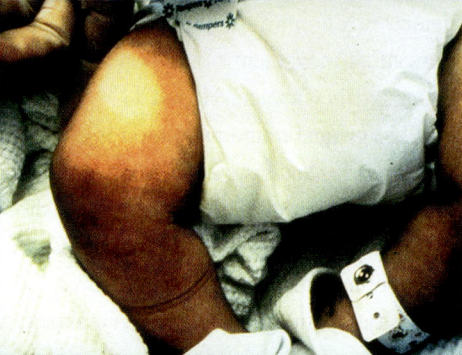

Figure 2.6 *Capilary refill demonstrated on an infant.*

Assessment of the Pediatric Patient

Infants sometimes will appear mottled. This may be a sign of poor perfusion or a result of being cold or scared. If there is time, and you have the appropriate equipment, a blood pressure reading may be obtained en route to the hospital. However, do not waste time, particularly in a severely injured child. *Remember that hypotension is a late finding in shock.* Immediate actions should include stopping all obvious bleeding and ensuring that the child is kept as warm as possible.

Rapid Trauma Survey or Focused Exam

Perform a rapid head-to-toe exam (Rapid Trauma Survey) on children who have been injured by a generalized mechanism (e.g., motor vehicle crash, auto–pedestrian collision, fall from a height, and so on). Children who have a focused injury (e.g., fall on outstretched arm and fractured wrist) or an insignificant injury (e.g., dropped rock on toe) may have a Focused Exam of the injured part only. Children with insignificant mechanisms of injury may not require an ITLS Secondary Survey.

Rapid Trauma Survey

The Rapid Trauma Survey is a quick examination of the head, neck, chest, abdomen, pelvis, and extremities. Also perform a neurological exam if there is altered mental status. Look for life-threatening injuries. By this time, the child should be adequately exposed to assess all the injuries, and all bleeding should be controlled. Parents may be able to assist with this since most children are taught not to allow strangers to disrobe them. *You can't assess what you can't see!*

Rapidly assess the child's head and neck for any bleeding, obvious injuries, or abnormalities. Look at, listen to, and feel the chest. Look for deformities, contusions, abrasions, perforations, burns, tenderness, lacerations, and swelling (DCAP BTLS). Listen to breath sounds on each side and note any abnormalities. Feel for tenderness, instability, or crepitus (TIC). If not already done, have one of your partners stabilize flail segments, seal open wounds, and decompress a tension pneumothorax.

Rapidly expose the abdomen. Gently palpate all four abdominal quadrants and note any contusions, abrasions, penetrations, or distention. If there is no complaint of pain in the pelvic area, gently palpate the pelvis noting any TIC. Quickly evaluate the lower extremities for obvious injury.

As soon as you finish the Rapid Trauma Survey, transfer the child to a spinal motion restriction device. Remember to log-roll the child the same way as you would an adult. This is the time to check the child's back carefully for any injuries. If an appropriate sized rigid collar is available, place it on the child and secure the collar and the child to the backboard. If an appropriate collar is not available, secure the child to the board in the neutral position using other methods to restrict spinal movement. It may be difficult to prevent all movement of the cervical spine, especially in the young child. This will be addressed in Chapters 10 and 11.

If a critical trauma situation is identified, transport immediately! If the patient has an altered mental status, perform a brief neurological exam to identify possible increased intracranial pressure (ICP). This exam should include the pupils, Modified (Pediatric) Glasgow Coma Score (GCS), and signs of Cushing's reflex. See Table 2.2 and Chapter 11 for more information about the Pediatric GCS. If no parents are present, look for medical identification devices. Head injury, shock, and hypoxia are not the only factors that cause altered mental status. Also consider nontraumatic causes such as hypoglycemia and drug or alcohol ingestion.

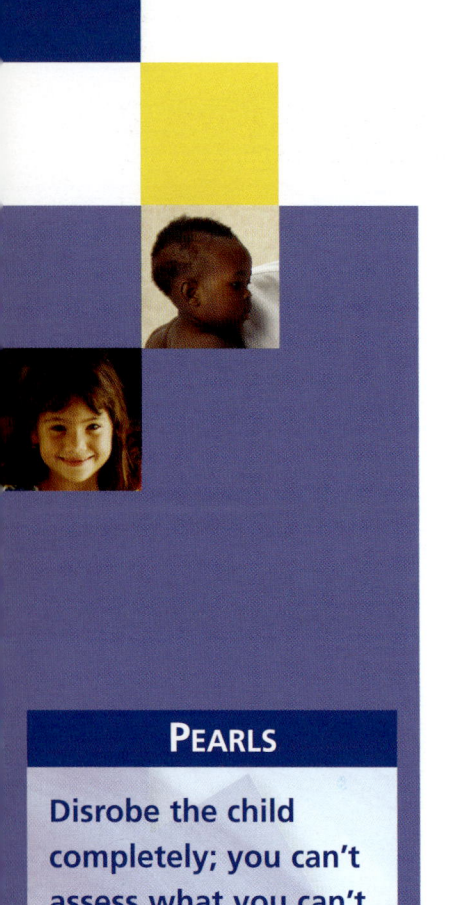

> **PEARLS**
>
> Disrobe the child completely; you can't assess what you can't see. As with adults, assess DCAP BTLS and TIC.

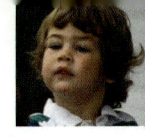

Table 2.2: Pediatric Glasgow Coma Scale

	Patient < 2 years	Patient > 2 years	
Eye Opening	Spontaneous	Spontaneous	4
	To speech	To voice	3
	To pain	To pain	2
	None	None	1
Verbal Response	Coos, babbles	Oriented	5
	Cries irritably	Confused	4
	Cries to pain	Inappropriate words	3
	Moans to pain	Incomprehensible	2
	None	None	1
Motor Response	Normal movements	Obeys commands	6
	Withdraws to touch	Localizes pain	5
	Withdrawal-pain	Withdrawal-pain	4
	Abnormal flexion	Flexion-pain	3
	Abnormal extension	Extension-pain	2
	None	None	1

Total = Eye + Verbal + Motor

SAMPLE History

While packaging the child, obtain as much history from the patient, parents, and family as possible. A "SAMPLE" history contains the following information:

- **S** Symptoms.
- **A** Allergies, particularly medications and immunization status.
- **M** Medications the child is taking or the parents have given the child.
- **P** Past illnesses, particularly bleeding disorders, congenital problems, heart disease, and birth history.
- **L** Last meal. Make a note of what the child had and what time it was eaten.
- **E** Events preceding the injury.

Critical Interventions and Transport Decisions

If you identify any of the following problems during the ITLS Primary Survey, the child should be considered a load-and-go patient. These patients should be packaged and transported as quickly as possible to a pediatric center.

1. Dangerous mechanism of injury
2. Unstable airway
3. Obvious respiratory difficulty
4. Shock or uncontrolled bleeding
5. Altered mental status
6. Poor general impression ("gut feeling")

Assessment of the Pediatric Patient

In these situations, rapid transport is critical. The decision about mode of transport should be guided by local protocol that takes into account the illness acuity and the time to the receiving hospital. Situations in which early arrival at a pediatric trauma center may make a significant difference in outcome include cold-water drowning, unstable airways, shock, severe head injuries, and multiple injuries. If the child is not identified as a priority patient as defined by load-and-go criteria, you may proceed to an ITLS Secondary Survey.

Critical Interventions at the Scene

Remember that you are spending minutes of the "Golden Hour" when you perform interventions at the scene. You should limit the on-scene interventions to those that can be performed by another team member while you are performing the ITLS Primary Survey or those interventions that are so critical that you cannot wait until you begin transport. Procedures that are usually performed at the scene include:

1. Initial airway management.
2. Administering high-flow, high-concentration oxygen.
3. Assisting ventilation.
4. Beginning CPR (team leader).
5. Controlling major external bleeding.
6. Sealing sucking chest wounds (team leader).
7. Decompressing tension pneumothorax if indicated (team leader).
8. Stabilizing impaled object.

Procedures that are not life saving—such as splinting, bandaging, inserting IV lines, or even emergency endotracheal intubation—must not delay transport if the patient is critical. If the patient is critical, call the hospital early so that preparations can be made for your arrival.

Critical Interventions During Transport

Orotracheal Intubation. If the child cannot be ventilated by bag-valve-mask ventilation, consider endotracheal (ET) intubation or the insertion of an alternative airway device. Quickly evaluate your ability to successfully intubate or place an alternative airway in order to not delay transportation. *Always maintain spinal motion restriction.* If the child is intubated, confirm that the ET tube is in the correct position and well-secured, and that motion of the child's head is restricted. Flexion of the neck will pull the tube out of the trachea and extension of the neck will move the ET tube down into the right mainstem bronchus. Once the airway is secured and correct placement of the ET or alternative airway device is confirmed (see Chapter 4), assess the child's respiratory status and support as necessary. As a standard of care, always use pulse oximetry and capnography to confirm and monitor tube position. If possible, all patients should have oxygen saturation readings greater than 95 percent. A reading of less than 95 percent may indicate early hypoxia and a need to look for the cause. A reading less than 90 percent is critical and requires immediate assessment and interventions as necessary to maintain adequate tissue oxygenation.

Decompression of a Tension Pneumothorax. If a child develops a tension pneumothorax in the field, you may have to decompress it in order to save the child. A tension pneumothorax is diagnosed by the combination of severe respiratory distress, decreased breath sounds on the side of the injury, and signs of circulatory collapse.

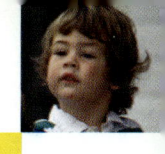

Distended neck veins, contralateral (opposite side) tracheal deviation, and ipsilateral (same side) hyperresonance to percussion are not usually present in pediatric cases. This will be discussed in more detail in Chapters 5 and 6.

Insertion of IV or IO Lines. IV access may be obtained en route, but if a prolonged extrication is required, it can be obtained at the scene. IV access may be difficult, especially if the patient has multisystem injury and is in shock. If IV access is obtained, give 20 mL/kg of normal saline or other medically approved crystalloid as a fluid bolus. After every bolus, recheck heart rate, pulses, and perfusion to evaluate progress. As soon as the heart rate and perfusion have returned to normal, run IV fluids at keep-open rates. This will prevent the child from becoming fluid overloaded. If local protocol allows, and you are unable to quickly obtain IV access, you may use an intraosseous infusion for the treatment of critically injured children. Do not attempt an intraosseous line unless the patient's airway and respiratory status have been stabilized (see Chapter 3). When you arrive at the hospital, inform the trauma team of the total amount of fluids the child has received.

Contacting Medical Direction

When you have a critical patient, it is extremely important to contact medical direction as early as possible. It takes time to get a trauma team in place, and the critical patient has no time to wait. Always notify the receiving facility of your estimated time of arrival (ETA), the condition of the patient, and any special needs on arrival.

ITLS Secondary Survey

The ITLS Secondary Survey is a comprehensive examination of the patient from head to toe. During this exam, look for all injuries, not just the life-threatening injuries. The acuity of the injuries and the time available prior to your arrival at the receiving institution determine how much of this you will complete.

Remember that the ITLS Primary Survey should be the first priority! In general, perform the ITLS Secondary Survey on a critical pediatric patient en route to the hospital, and on a stable pediatric patient at the scene. Early recognition and management of the ABCs is critical! Obtain complete vital signs and apply monitors, if not already done. Use the DCAP BTLS mnemonic (deformities, contusions, abrasions, penetrations, burns, tenderness, lacerations, or swelling) when examining for injuries while performing the ITLS Secondary Survey.

Proceed with the ITLS Secondary Survey as follows:

1. Repeat the Initial Assessment (and finish the SAMPLE history, if not already done).
2. Record level of consciousness (AVPU), airway, pulse, respiration, and blood pressure.
3. Consider using monitors (cardiac, pulse oximeter, capnometer). These are usually applied during transport.
4. Perform a neurological exam. If the child has an altered level of consciousness, record the pediatric GCS and exam of pupils (size, equality, reaction to light). Record motor function. (For example, is the child moving all extremities? Does the child have good muscle strength?). Record sensation. (Can the child feel you when you touch his fingers and toes? Does the unconscious child respond when you pinch his fingers and toes?)
5. Perform a Detailed (head-to-toe) Exam.

Assessment of the Pediatric Patient

a. **Head examination.** Perform a complete examination of the head; it is important to note cuts, bruises, hematomas, and depressions. If the child has an open fontanel, note whether it is flat or bulging. Note the presence of raccoon eyes and any fluid or blood from the nose (indicating anterior basilar skull fracture). Look for Battle's sign and any fluid or blood from the ear (indicating posterior basilar skull fracture). Check the pupils, noting whether they are equal and whether they react to light.
b. **Neck examination.** Note the external appearance of the neck. Note the position of the trachea and whether the neck veins are distended or flat. Often, this will be difficult in the young child or infant because the neck is short and fat.
c. **Chest examination.** Watch the chest rise and fall. Note symmetry and any bruises or crepitus. Listen carefully to the breath sounds.
d. **Abdominal examination.** Note any abdominal bruises or marks (e.g., seat belt). Also note if the patient has abdominal distention, tenderness, or guarding. Note pelvic stability.
e. **Extremity examination.** Note the location of any deformities and check the neurovascular status below the site of the injury. All active sites of bleeding should have been stopped during the Initial Assessment, but make sure the dressings are securely in place for transport. Carefully package any amputated parts.

ITLS Ongoing Exam

The ITLS Ongoing Exam is an abbreviated assessment to check for changes in the patient's condition (Fig. 2.7). In some critical cases with short transport times, this exam may take the place of the ITLS Secondary Survey.

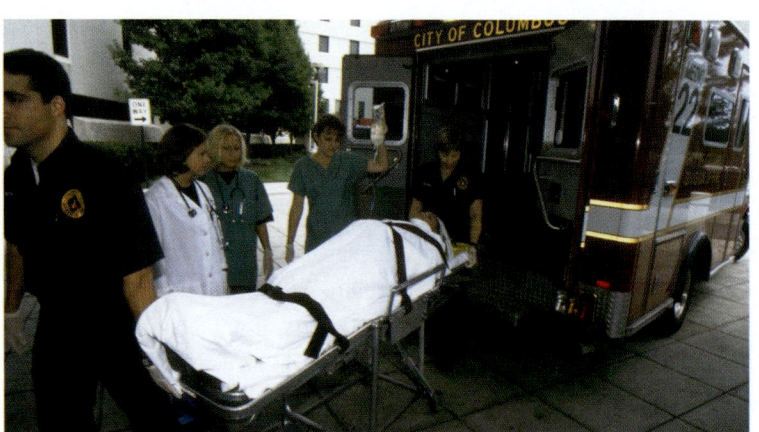

Figure 2.7 *The ITLS Ongoing Exam may be performed in the ambulance en route to the trauma center to find changes in the child's condition.*

The ITLS Ongoing Exam should be recorded every five minutes in critical pediatric patients and every 15 minutes in stable pediatric patients. Also perform the ITLS Ongoing Exam each time the child is moved, an intervention is performed, or his condition worsens. The purpose of this exam is to find any changes in the child's condition, so concentrate on reassessing those things that may change.

Perform the ITLS Ongoing Exam in the following order:

1. Ask the child about any changes in how he feels.
2. Reassess mental status (LOC and pupils, recheck GCS).

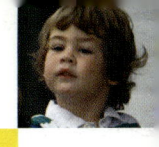

3. Reassess the ABCs.
    a. Reassess the airway.
        i. Recheck patency.
        ii. If the patient has suffered burns, assess for signs of inhalation injury.
    b. Reassess breathing and circulation.
        i. Recheck vital signs.
        ii. Note skin color, condition, and temperature.
        iii. Check the neck for jugular venous distention (JVD) and tracheal deviation. (If a collar has been applied, remove the front.)
        iv. Recheck the chest. Note the quality of breath sounds. If breath sounds are unequal, evaluate for splinting, pneumothorax, or hemothorax. Listen to the heart to see if the sounds have become muffled.
4. Reassess the abdomen if the mechanism suggests possible injury. Note the development of tenderness, distention, or rigidity.
5. Check each of the identified injuries (lacerations for bleeding, pulse, motor function and sensation [PMS] distal to all injured extremities; flails; pneumothorax; open chest wounds; and so on).
6. Check interventions:
    a. Check ET tube for patency and position.
    b. Check oxygen for flow rate.
    c. Check IVs for patency and rate of fluid.
    d. Check seals on sucking chest wounds.
    e. Check patency of tension pneumothorax decompression needle.
    f. Check splints and dressings.
    g. Check impaled objects to be sure they are well stabilized.
    h. Check all monitors (cardiac, pulse oximeter, and capnometer).

Accurately record what you see and what you do. Record changes in the patient's condition during transport. Record the time that interventions are performed. Record extenuating circumstances or significant details in the comments or remarks section of the written report.

Case Study *continued*

Susan, John, and Bob have been called to a home of an 18-month-old child who fell out of her crib. Their scene size-up revealed that the house was safe to enter. There they found the patient lying on her back and crying. The initial impression is good, as she was pink and crying to her

Assessment of the Pediatric Patient

mother, who was with her. Susan is acting as a team leader on this call. The team dons personal protective equipment, gathers the essential equipment and approaches the patient.

Susan begins her Initial Assessment by introducing the team to the patient and her mother. At the same time John stabilizes the patient's neck by holding her head. Bob explains to the child that he is going to put on a space man's mask and give her some magic gas to breathe. The patient allows Bob to give her the high-flow oxygen by mask. Bob then places a pediatric long backboard beside the patient. Susan proceeds with the Initial Assessment by checking breathing and circulation, as the level of consciousness and airway have been deemed satisfactory. The mother lifts her daughter's T-shirt up for Susan to assess the rate and quality of breathing. She then assesses the pulse rate and quality and capillary refill. All seemed fine.

Susan then performs a Rapid Trauma Survey, which reveals a bruise to the left side of the head. The neck has no obvious deformities; the neck veins are flat, and the trachea is in the midline. The chest has no external signs of injury. The patient complains that her left leg hurts. Breath sounds are present and equal. The heart sounds can be heard clearly and the rate is about 110 beats per minute. The patient does not cry or complain of pain when Susan examines her abdomen. The abdomen is not distended and soft. The pelvis feels stable.

Examination of extremities reveals an area of bruising and tenderness over the left thigh. Otherwise, the other limbs appear to be free from injury. Pulses, motor and sensory functions appear to be satisfactory.

Susan decides to log-roll the patient onto her left side to examine the back before placing her on a pediatric long board and splinting her left leg. She explains what and why they are doing things. The patient and her mother understand the reasons and cooperate.

Susan notifies medical direction that they have an 18-month-old with a probable fractured left femur and possible closed head injury from falling from a height. They move the patient to the ambulance for transport to hospital. The patient's mother accompanies her daughter and rides with the team.

En route, a SAMPLE history is taken from the mother, baseline vital signs are monitored, and an ITLS Secondary Survey is carried out. A venous cannula was inserted and intravenous analgesia is administered.

On arrival, the patient and her mother are handed over to the receiving hospital team.

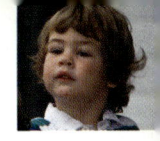

Further assessment and investigations confirmed that the patient had sustained a closed left femoral shaft fracture and a closed head injury with an underlying skull fracture. She was kept in hospital for further treatment under the care of the orthopedic and neurosurgical team. She was discharged from hospital several weeks later.

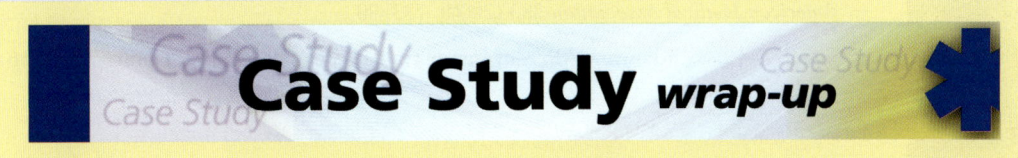

Case Study wrap-up

Toddlers are very adventurous and inquisitive. When not watched, they will climb and explore. The patient in this case fell from a height onto a hard surface, probably hitting her head and left thigh on the way down. Luckily, she suffered from injuries that were significant but not immediately life-threatening.

Susan and her team acted efficiently using the ITLS patient assessment skills to care for the patient and her mother before transporting her to an appropriate hospital for definitive treatment.

SUMMARY

1. Always consider the mechanism of injury and the child's size. If possible, prepare the correct equipment prior to arrival at the scene.
2. Stick with the basics: spinal motion restriction, airway, breathing, and circulation. Reassess the child continually.
3. If the child's condition changes, go back to the basics! Ensure an adequate airway, a stable respiratory status, and adequate circulation.
4. Continue to assess and reassess the child.
5. Rapid assessment, appropriate interventions, and transport to an appropriate facility are key to long-term pediatric patient survival.

Recommended Reading

Advanced Life Support Group. "The Seriously Injured Child." In *Pre-Hospital Paediatric Life Support: The Practical Approach*, 2nd ed. London: Blackwell BMJ Books, 2005.

American College of Surgeons. "The Extremes of Age." In *Advanced Trauma Life Support Program for Doctors*, 8th ed. Chicago: Author, 2008.

Bickley, Lynn S., and Peter G. Szilagyi, eds. *Bates' Guide to Physical Examination and History Taking*, 10th ed. Philadelphia: Lippincott, Williams and Wilkins, 2008.

Campbell, John Emory, ed. "Multicasualty Incidents and Triage," Appendix I. In *International Trauma Life Support for Prehospital Care Providers*, 6th ed., 400–407. Upper Saddle River, N.J.: Pearson/Prentice Hall, 2008.

Campbell, John Emory, ed. "Trauma in Children." In *International Trauma Life Support for Prehospital Care Providers*, 6th ed., 258–77. Upper Saddle River, N.J.: Pearson/Prentice Hall, 2008.

Engel, Joyce K. *Mosby's Pocket Guide to Pediatric Assessment*, 5th ed. St. Louis: Mosby, 2006.

European Resuscitation Council (UK). "The Injured Child." In *European Paediatric Life Support*, 2nd ed. Antwerp, Belguin: Author, 2006.

Gausche, Marianne., Roger J. Lewis, Samuel J. Stratton, et al. "Effect of Out-of-Hospital Pediatric Intubation on Survival and Neurological Outcome Controlled Clinical Trial." *Journal of the American Medical Association* 283 (2000): 783–90.

Salati, David S. "Know the ABCs of Caring for Children." *Nursing* 37 (spring 2007): 16–7.

3

CHAPTER 3
Patient Assessment Skills

John P. Crow, MD, FACS
Ann Hoffman, RN, CPN
Sherri Kovach, RN, EMT-B

Objectives

Upon completion of this Skills Chapter, you should be able to:

1. Correctly perform the ITLS Primary Survey.

2. Identify within 2 minutes which patients require load-and-go transport.

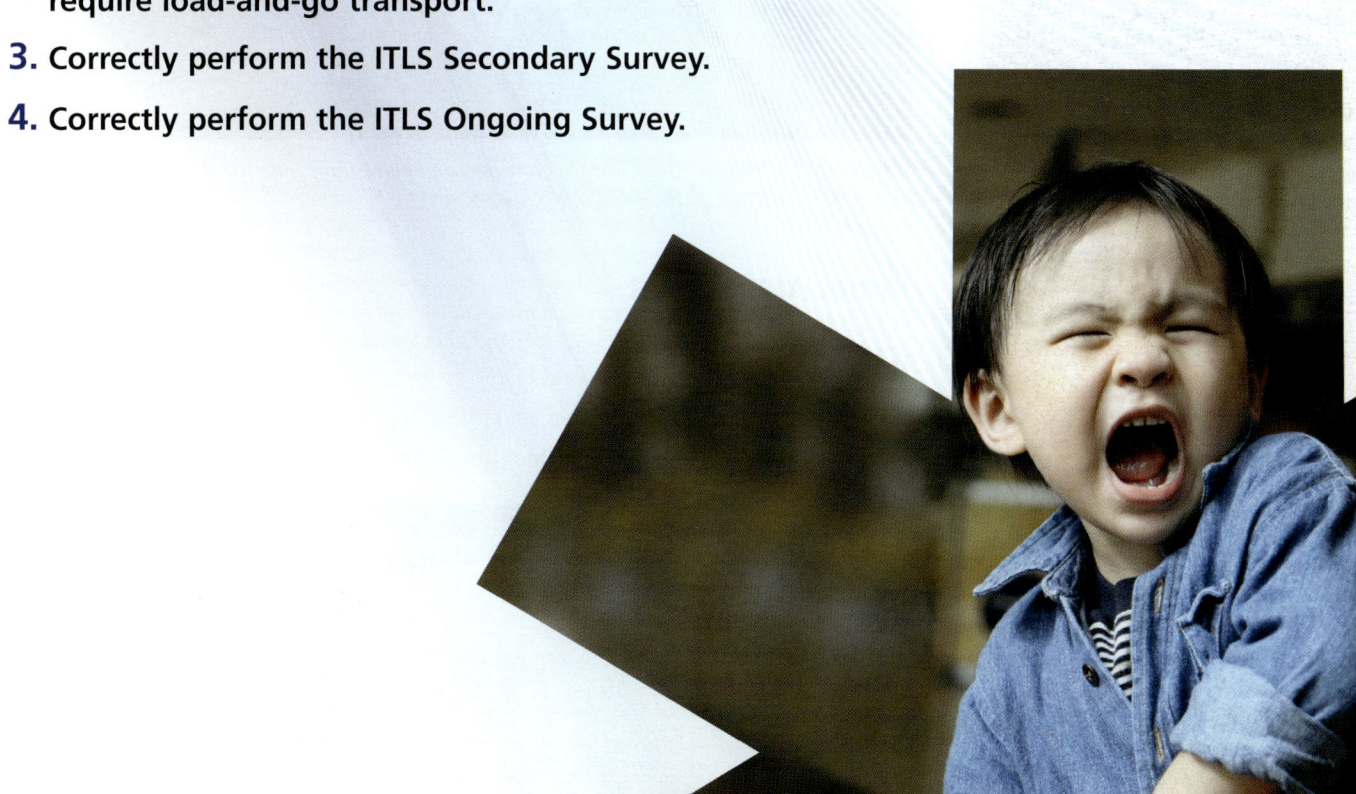

3. Correctly perform the ITLS Secondary Survey.

4. Correctly perform the ITLS Ongoing Survey.

ITLS PRIMARY SURVEY

The ITLS Primary Survey consists of Scene Size-Up; Initial Assessment of the child's level of consciousness, airway, breathing, and circulation; either a Rapid Trauma Survey (head-to-toe exam when the mechanism is generalized or the patient is unconscious) or Focused Exam (when the mechanism is very focused, e.g. single gunshot wound to leg); and a decision about the need for early transport.

Scene Size-Up

All rescuers must have proper personal protective equipment (PPE) available. Standard precautions must be observed (Fig. 3.1). Scan the area for dangers and for other victims. Call for more help or for special equipment necessary to complete the rescue. Consider the mechanism in relation to the size of the child. If a parent or guardian is at the scene, introduce yourself and present yourself in a very organized, efficient manner.

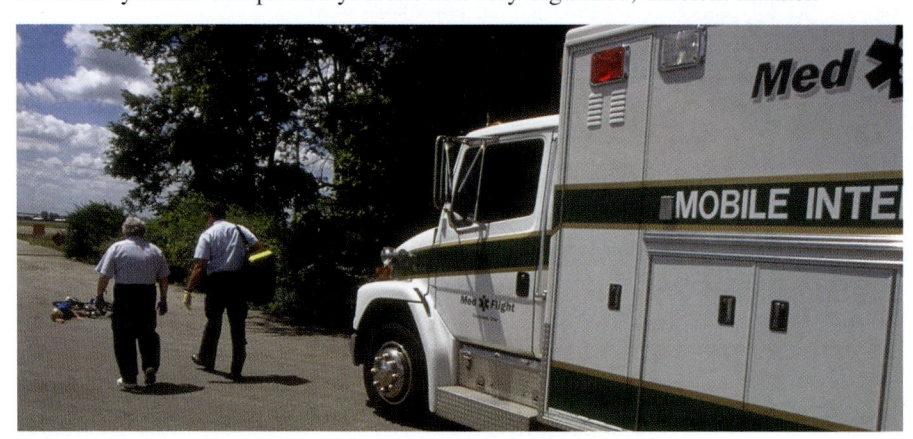

Figure 3.1 *Observe standard precautions and scan the scene for dangers and for other victims when performing the Scene Size-Up.*

Initial Assessment

General Impression

Form a general impression. As you begin your approach to the patient, note the child's position and general appearance, and estimate the child's age (Fig. 3.2).

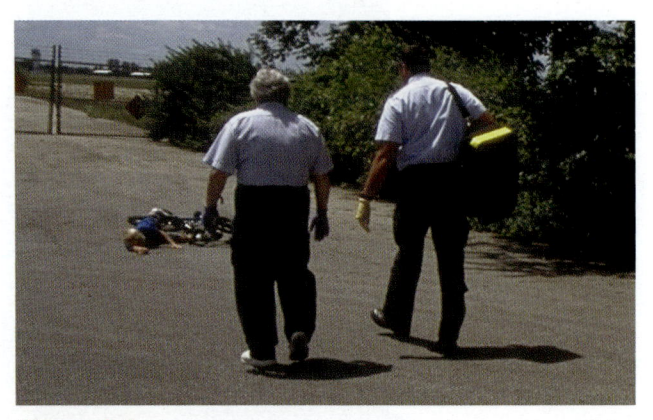

Figure 3.2 *As you approach the scene, form a general impression.*

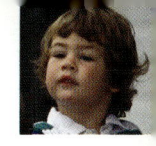

Level of Consciousness

Observe the child. Is he looking at you? Does he recognize his parents? Note whether the child is alert (A), responding to verbal command (V), responding only to pain (P), or is unresponsive (U). Continue to observe the child during the entire ITLS Primary Survey.

Airway and Cervical Spine

Assess the airway and upper torso while maintaining the cervical spine manually. Add padding under the shoulders to get the neck and airway in a neutral position. If the mechanism suggests any chance of neck injury, assume the child's neck is injured and maintain spinal motion restriction throughout the assessment and management of the patient. After the neck is manually restricted, assess the airway (Fig. 3.3). Look for signs of upper airway occlusion, apnea, or agonal respiration. Listen carefully for air movement through the mouth. If the child is unconscious, open the airway using the modified jaw thrust maneuver. Listen carefully again. Have suction available and use it to clear the mouth of any blood or secretions. If an assistant is available, have this rescuer place 100 percent oxygen on the patient (Fig. 3.4).

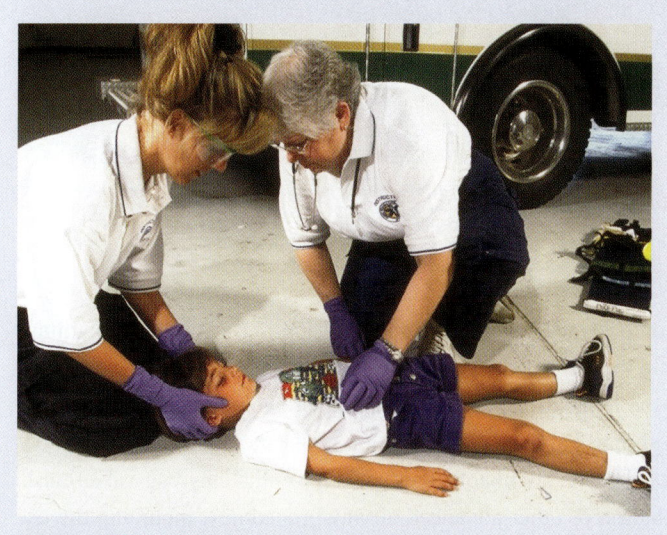

Figure 3.3 *Maintain manual spinal motion restriction before assessing the airway.*

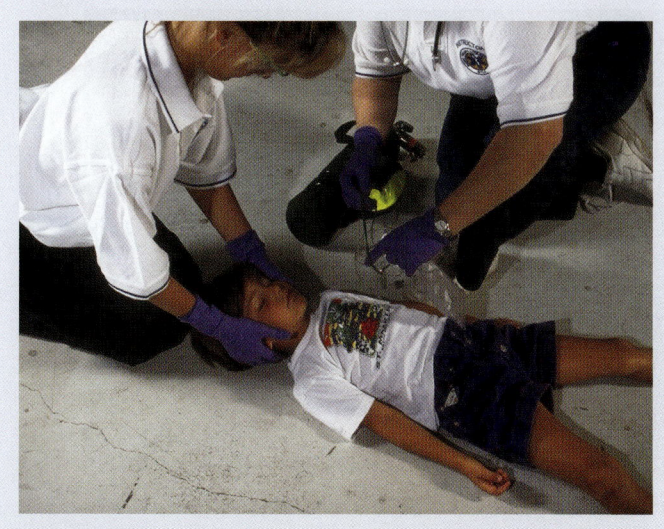

Figure 3.4 *Administer 100 percent oxygen using an appropriately sized mask.*

Patient Assessment Skills

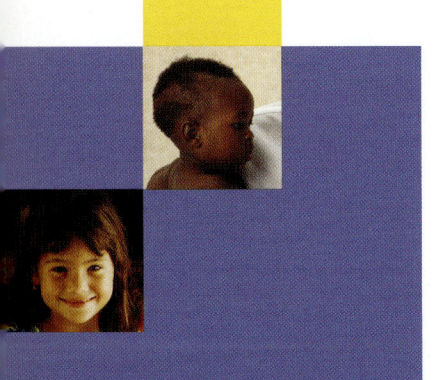

Breathing

Following the assessment of the airway, assess the child's breathing (Fig. 3.5). Look at the patient's respiratory rate, oxygenation, and efforts to breathe. Compare the child's respiratory rate to the normal rate listed on the card for the age of the child. Look at the color of the child's lips and nail beds. They should be pink. If they are not, the child is likely hypoxic. Observe how hard the child is working to breathe. Note nostril flaring, retractions, and grunting. Look for the position of the trachea and jugular venous distention. Listen carefully to the child's lung fields; assess how well he is moving air.

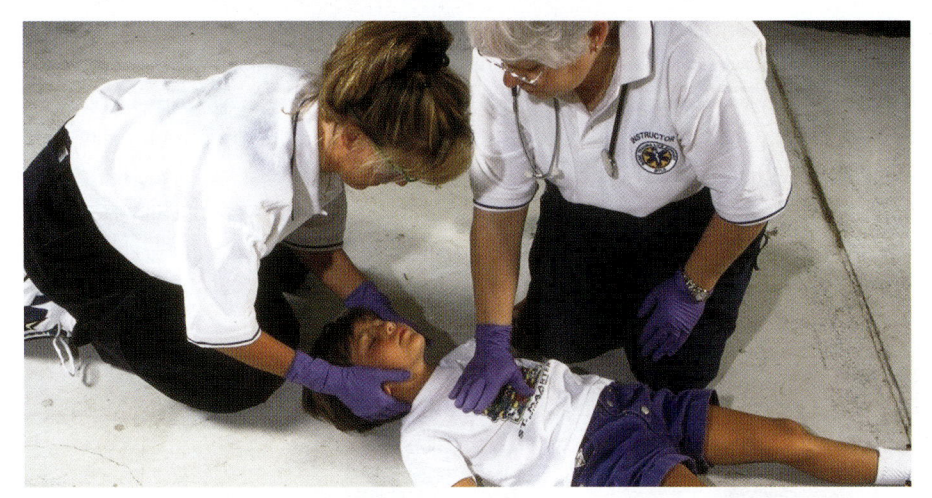

Figure 3.5 *Assess the child's breathing, including respiratory rate, oxygenation, and efforts to breathe.*

If the child is apneic or having severe respiratory distress, initiate ventilatory assistance using mouth-to-mask ventilation or bag-valve-mask ventilation (Fig. 3.6). While maintaining a good seal, ventilate at the rate the child would normally breathe. Watch the chest for rise and fall and listen carefully to the lungs for air exchange. If you are able to do so effectively, maintain the child's airway with bag-valve-mask ventilation and remember to keep suction available for managing secretions. If you are unable to effectively ventilate by bag-valve-mask ventilation, then perform intubation or other advanced airway procedures, including the use of a Blind Insertion Airway Device (BIAD).

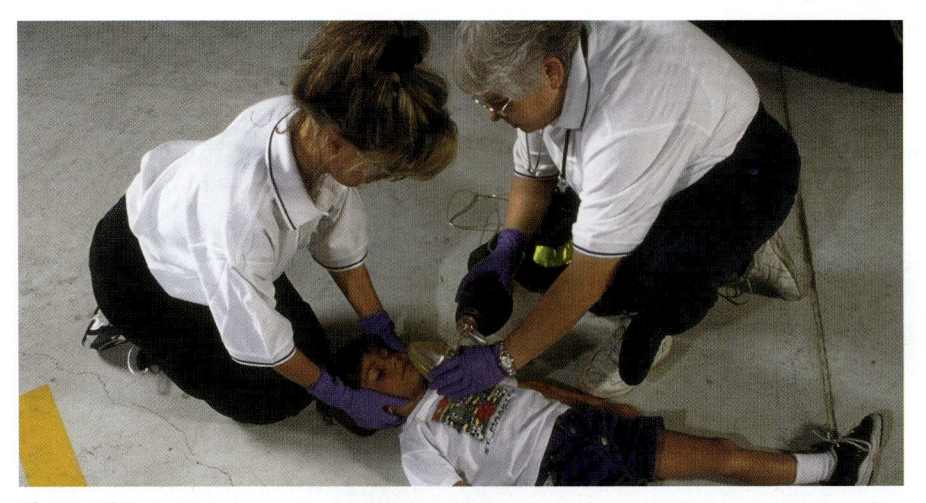

Figure 3.6 *Initiate bag-valve-mask ventilation if needed, ventilating at the rate the child would normally breathe.*

Pediatric Trauma Life Support

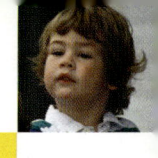

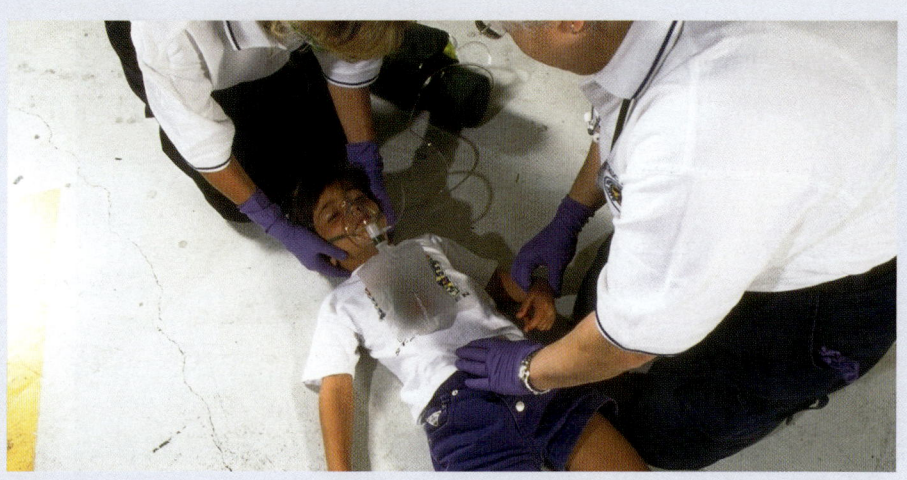

Figure 3.7 *Check the pulse as part of your assessment of the child's circulation.*

Circulation

Next, evaluate the child's circulation. Note the pulse (radial or dorsalis pedis) (Fig. 3.7). If this is absent, check for a central pulse (brachial, femoral, or carotid). Count the pulse and check your card to see if this is normal for the child's age. Stop all obvious bleeding and ensure that the child is kept as warm as possible (Fig. 3.8).

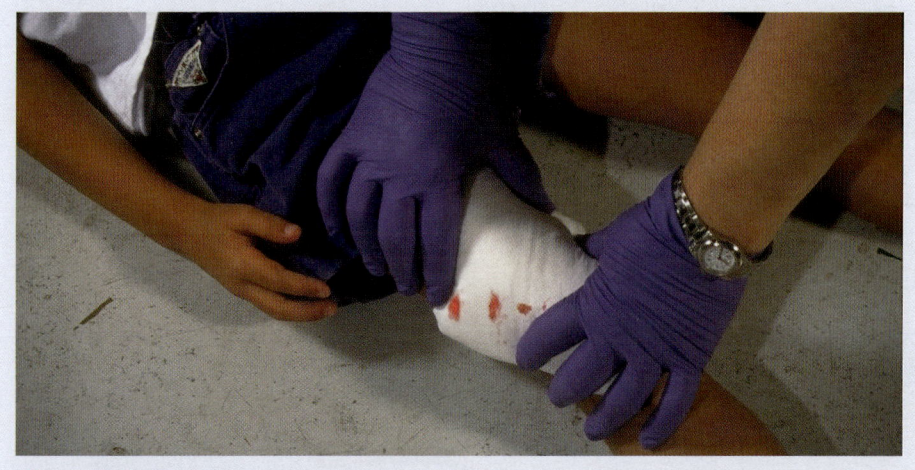

Figure 3.8 *Stop all obvious bleeding.*

Rapid Trauma Survey or Focused Exam

Rapid Trauma Survey

During this time, expose the child adequately to assess all the injuries (Fig. 3.9). Parents may be able to assist with this, since most children are taught not to allow strangers to disrobe them

Rapidly assess the child's head and neck for any bleeding, obvious injuries, or abnormalities. Look at, listen to, and feel the chest. Look for asymmetric or paradoxical movement of the chest and signs of blunt or penetrating trauma. Listen to breath sounds on each side and note any abnormalities. Feel for tenderness, instability, or crepitus (TIC). If not already done, have one of your partners stabilize flail segments, seal open wounds, and needle-decompress any tension pneumothorax.

Rapidly expose the abdomen. Gently palpate all four abdominal quadrants and note for DCAP BTLS and distention. If there is no complaint of pain in the pelvic area, gently palpate the pelvis, noting any TIC. Quickly evaluate the lower extremities for obvious injury.

Patient Assessment Skills

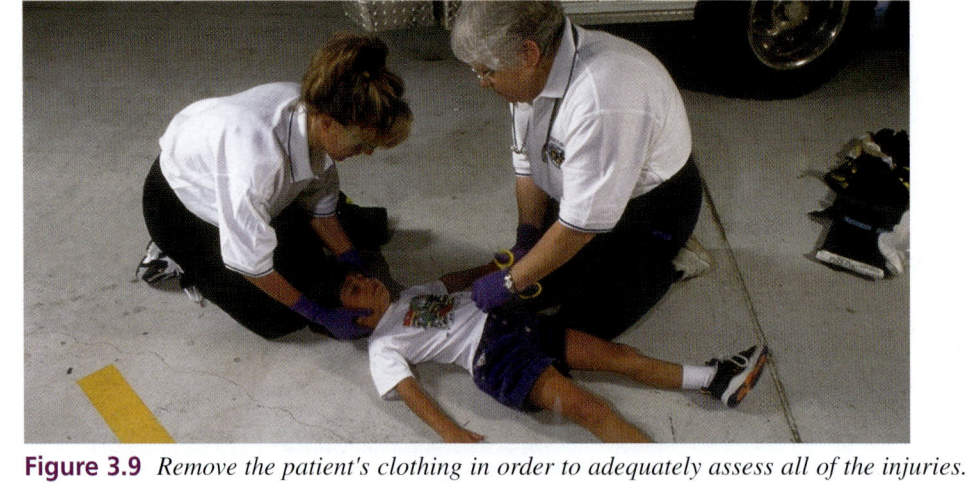

Figure 3.9 *Remove the patient's clothing in order to adequately assess all of the injuries.*

As soon as you finish the Rapid Trauma Survey, transfer the child to a spinal motion restriction device. Log-roll the child and check his back carefully for any injuries. Place a cervical collar on the patient and secure the collar and the patient to the backboard. If an appropriate collar is not available, secure the patient to the board in the neutral position using other methods to immobilize the spine

If there is a critical trauma situation identified, transport immediately! If the patient has an altered mental status, do a brief neurological exam to identify signs of possible increased intracranial pressure (ICP) and record the Glasgow Coma Scale (GCS) score or the modified GCS score for children younger than two years of age. If no parents are present, look for medical identification devices.

Focused Exam

Perform a Focused Exam of an injured area if a specific injury is identified (Fig. 3.10). Check for DCAP BTLS. Accomplish bleeding control and splinting if indicated.

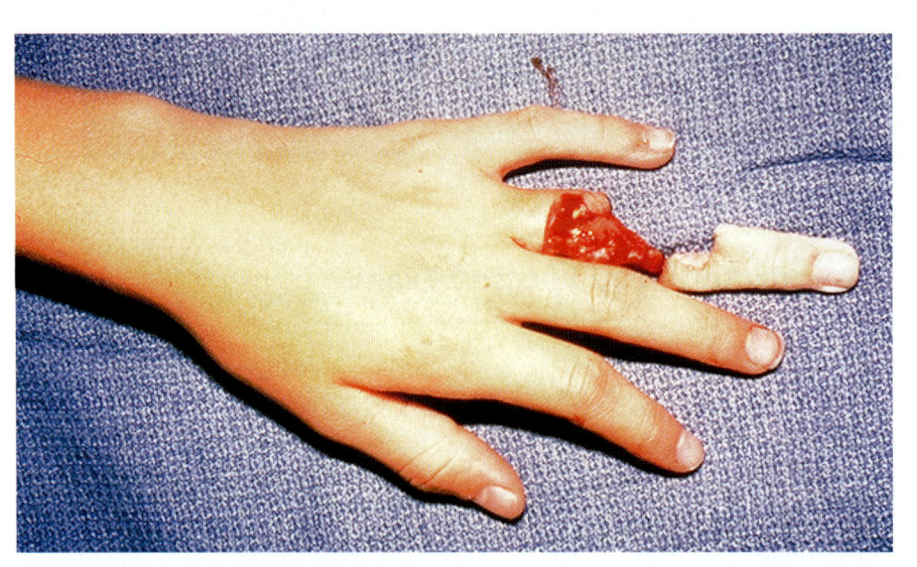

Figure 3.10 *A Focused Exam should be performed if a specific injury, such as a finger avulsion, is identified.*

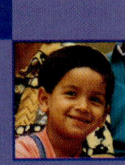

Pediatric Trauma Life Support

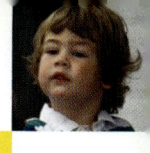

SAMPLE History

While packaging the patient, obtain as much history from the patient, parents, and family as possible. A "SAMPLE" history contains the following information:

- **S** Symptoms.
- **A** Allergies, particularly medications and immunization status.
- **M** Medications the child is taking or the parents have given.
- **P** Past illnesses, particularly bleeding disorders, congenital problems, heart disease, and birth history.
- **L** Last meal. Make a note of what the child had and what time it was eaten.
- **E** Events preceding the injury.

Critical Interventions and Transport Decisions

If you identify any of the following problems during the ITLS Primary Survey, the child should be considered a load-and-go patient. Package and transport these patients as quickly as possible to a pediatric center.

1. A significant mechanism of injury and/or poor general health of the patient
2. Unstable airway
3. Obvious respiratory difficulty
4. Shock or uncontrolled bleeding
5. Altered mental status
6. Poor general impression ("gut feeling")

If the patent is not identified as a load-and-go patient, you may proceed to an ITLS Secondary Survey.

Critical Interventions at the Scene

The following procedures are usually performed at the scene:

1. Perform initial airway management.
2. Administer high-flow, high-concentration oxygen.
3. Assist ventilation.
4. Begin CPR (team leader).
5. Control major external bleeding.
6. Seal sucking chest wounds.
7. Needle-decompress tension pneumothorax if indicated.
8. Stabilize impaled object.

Critical Interventions During Transport

The following interventions can be performed during transport of the pediatric patient:

1. Perform advanced airway procedure.
2. Decompress a tension pneumothorax if not already performed.
3. Insert IV or IO lines.
4. Splint and bandage.

Patient Assessment Skills

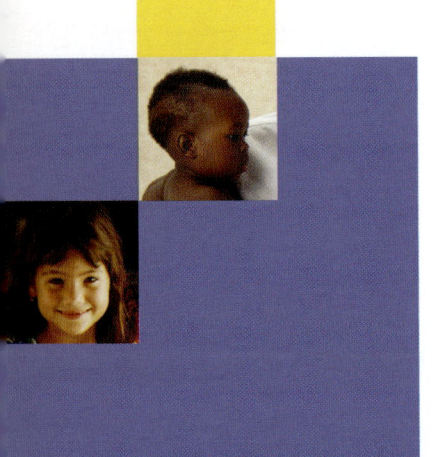

Contacting Medical Direction

Notify the receiving facility of your estimated time of arrival, the condition of the child, and any special needs on arrival (Fig. 3.11).

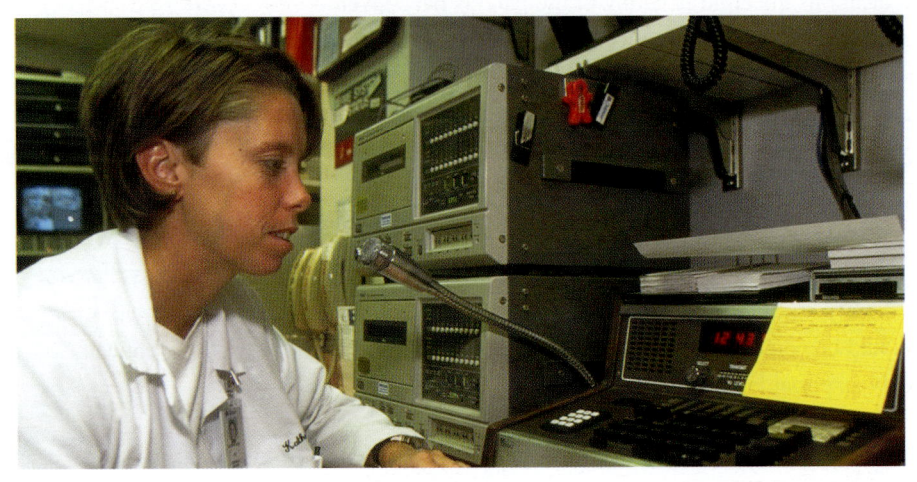

Figure 3.11 *Contact medical direction to alert them to the condition of the child and your estimated time of arrival.*

ITLS SECONDARY SURVEY

Proceed with the ITLS Secondary Survey as follows:

1. Repeat the Initial Assessment (and finish the SAMPLE history if not already done).
2. Record level of consciousness (AVPU), airway, pulse, respiration, and blood pressure.
3. Consider using monitors (cardiac, pulse oximeter, capnometer). These are usually applied during transport.
4. Perform a neurological exam. If the child has an altered level of consciousness, record the pediatric GCS score, and record exam of pupils (size, equality, reaction to light). Record motor function. (For example, is the patient moving all extremities? Does the child have good muscle strength?) Record sensation. Can the child feel you when you touch his fingers and toes? Does the unconscious child respond when you pinch his fingers and toes?
5. Perform a detailed head-to-toe exam.
   a. **Head examination.** Examine the head, noting cuts, bruises, hematomas, and depressions. If the child has an open fontanel, note whether it is flat or bulging. Note any fluid or blood from the nose and ears. Look for raccoon eyes and postauricular or mastoid ecchymosis (Battle's sign). Check the pupils and note whether they are equal and whether they react to light. Check the mouth and teeth (Fig. 3.12).
   b. **Neck examination.** Note the external appearance of the neck. Note the position of the trachea and if the neck veins are distended or flat.
   c. **Chest examination.** Watch the chest rise and fall. Note symmetry and any bruises or crepitus (Fig. 3.13). Listen carefully to the breath sounds.

Pediatric Trauma Life Support

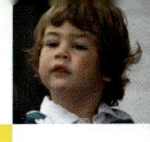

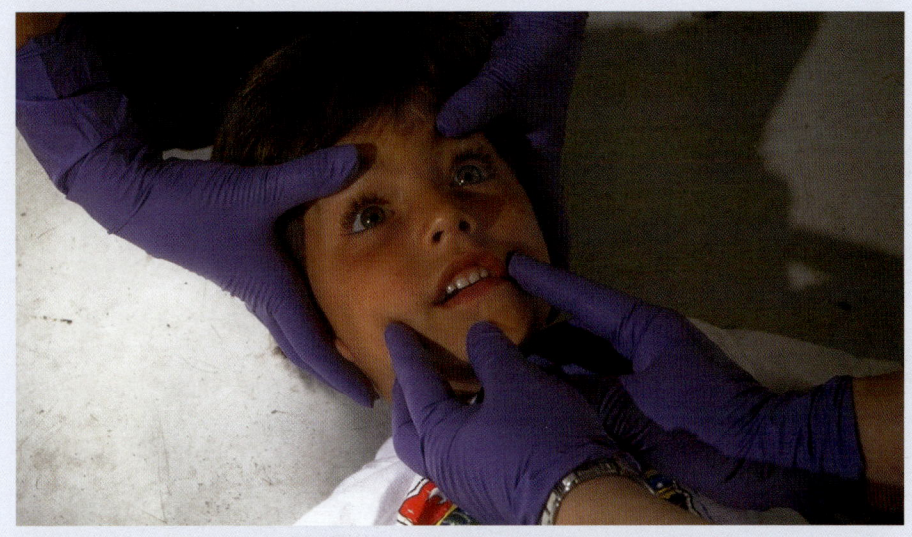

Figure 3.12 *When examining the head, check the pupils, noting whether they are equal and reactive to light. Don't forget to check the mouth and teeth.*

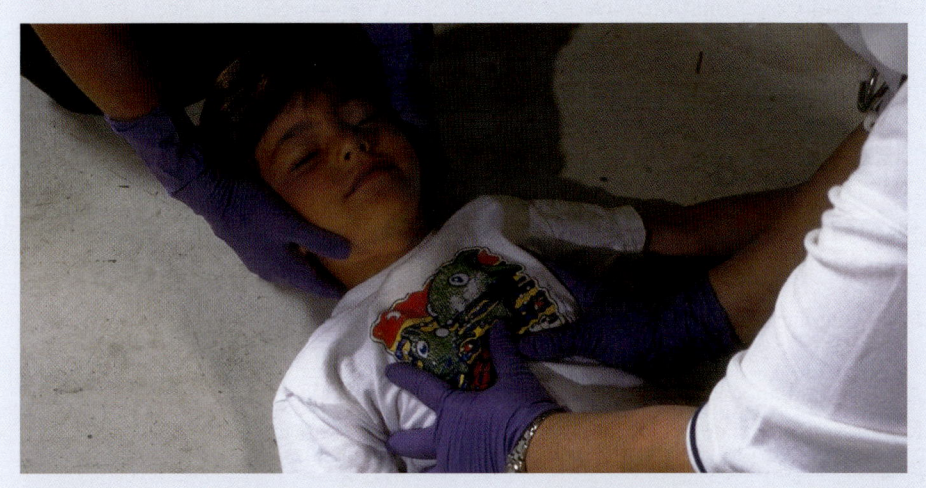

Figure 3.13 *Note symmetry of the chest and any bruises or crepitus.*

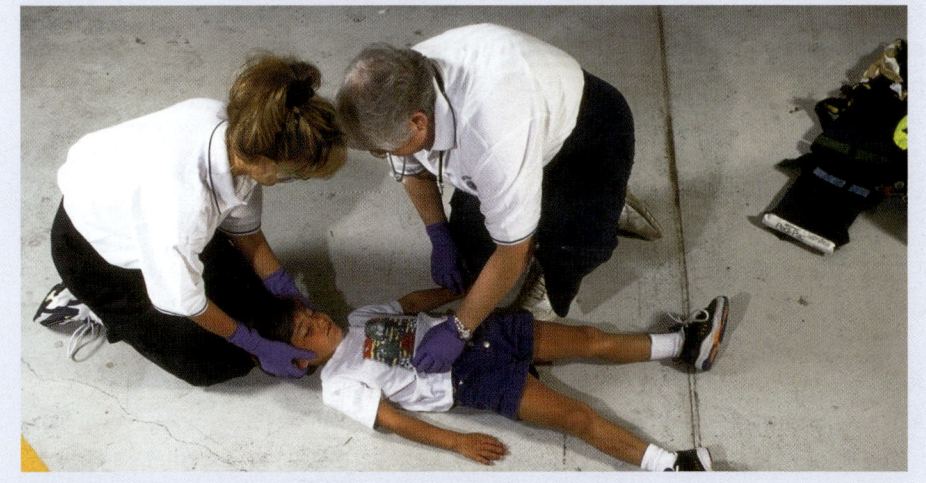

Figure 3.14 *Examine the abdomen for bruising or marks, distention, tenderness, or guarding.*

    d. Abdominal examination. Note any abdominal bruises or marks (e.g., seat belt). Also note if the patient has abdominal distention, tenderness, or guarding (Fig. 3.14). Note pelvic stability.

Patient Assessment Skills   47

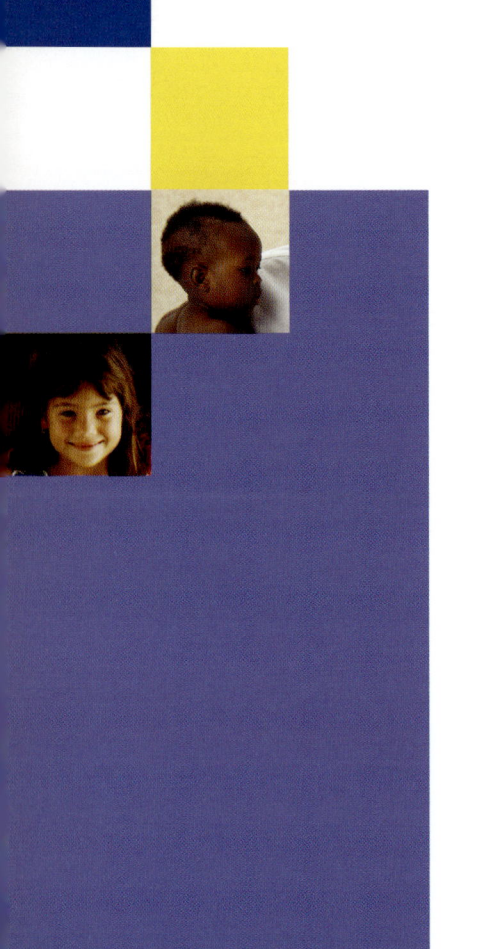

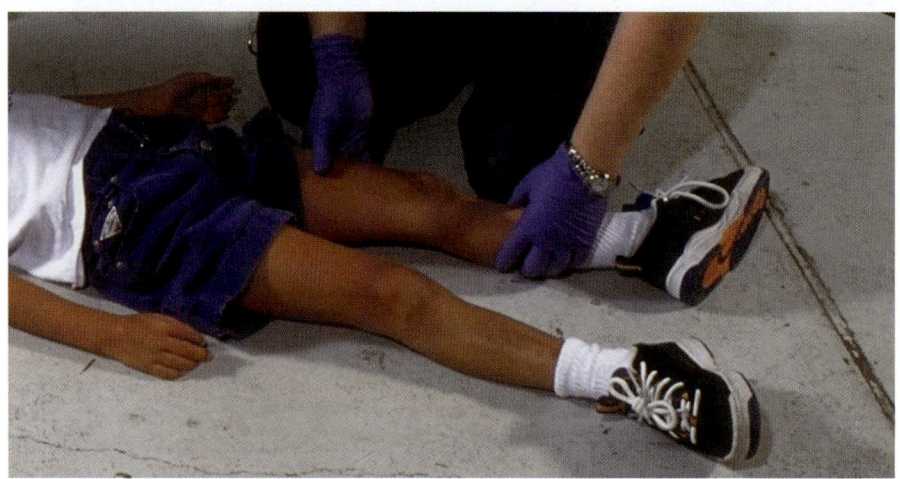

Figure 3.15 *Examine the extremities for any deformities.*

e. **Extremity examination.** Note the location of any deformities and check the neurovascular status below the site of the injury (Fig. 3.15). All active sites of bleeding should have been stopped during the ITLS Primary Survey, but make sure the dressings are securely in place for transport. Carefully package any amputated parts (see Chapter 13).

ITLS ONGOING EXAM

The ITLS Ongoing Exam should be performed in the following order:

1. Ask the child about any changes in how he feels.
2. Reassess mental status (LOC and pupils, recheck GCS score).
3. Reassess the ABCs.
    a. Reassess the airway:
4. Recheck patency.
    a. If burn patient, assess for signs of inhalation injury.
    b. Reassess breathing and circulation:
        i. Recheck vital signs.
        ii. Note skin color, condition, and temperature.
        iii. Check the neck for jugular venous distention (JVD) and tracheal deviation. (If a collar has been applied, remove the front.)
        iv. Recheck the chest. Note the quality of breath sounds. If breath sounds are unequal, evaluate for splinting, pneumothorax, or hemothorax. Listen to the heart to see if the sounds have become muffled.
5. Reassess the abdomen for tenderness, distention, or rigidity.
    a. Check each of the identified injuries (lacerations for bleeding; pulse, motor functions, and sensation [PMS] distal to all injured extremities; flails; pneumothorax; open chest wounds; and so on).
6. Check interventions:
    a. Check airway device for patency and position.
    b. Check oxygen for flow rate.
    c. Check IVs for patency and rate of fluid.
    d. Check seals on sucking chest wounds.

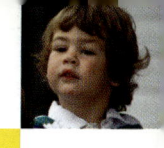

- e. Check patency of tension pneumothorax decompression needle.
- f. Check splints and dressings.
- g. Check impaled objects to be sure they are well stabilized.
- h. Check cardiac monitor and pulse oximeter.
- i. Check capnograph, if intubated

Accurately record what you see and what you do. Record changes in the child's condition during transport. Record the time that interventions are performed. Record extenuating circumstances or significant details in the comments or remarks section of the written report.

PATIENT ASSESSMENT AND MANAGEMENT

Short written trauma scenarios will be used along with a model (to act as the patient). You will be divided into teams to practice the management of simulated trauma situations using the principles and techniques taught in the course. You will be evaluated in the same manner on the second day of the course. You will be expected to use all the principles and techniques taught in this course while managing these simulated patients. To familiarize yourself with the evaluation procedure, you will be given a copy of a scenario and a grade sheet. Review Chapter 2 and the previous surveys in this chapter.

GROUND RULES FOR TEACHING AND EVALUATION

1. You will be allowed to stay together in three-member groups (different-sized groups are optional) throughout the practice and evaluation stations.
2. You will have three practice scenarios. This allows each member of the team to be the team leader once.
3. You will be evaluated as the team leader once.
4. You will assist as a member of the rescue team during two scenarios in which another member of your team is being evaluated as team leader. You may assist, but the team leader must do all assessments. This gives you a total of six scenarios from which to learn: three practices, one evaluation, and two assists while others are evaluated.
5. Wait outside the door until the instructor comes out and gives you your scenario.
6. You will be allowed to look over your equipment before you start your exam.
7. Be sure to ask about scene safety if not provided in the scenario.
8. Be sure to apply your personal protective gear.
9. If you have a live model for a patient, you must talk to that person just as you would a real patient. It is best to explain what you are doing as you examine the patient. Be confident and reassuring.
10. You must ask your instructor for things you cannot find out from your patient. Examples are blood pressure, pulse, and breath sounds.
11. Wounds and fractures must be dressed or splinted just as if they were real. Procedures must be done correctly (such as blood pressure, log-rolling, strapping, and splinting).
12. If you need a piece of equipment that is not available, ask your instructor. They may allow you to simulate the equipment.
13. During practice and evaluation, you may be allowed to go (or may be directed) to any station, but you cannot go to the same station twice.

Patient Assessment Skills

You will be graded on the following:

1. Assessment of the scene
2. Assessment of the patient
3. Management of the patient
4. Efficient use of time
5. Leadership
6. Judgment
7. Problem-solving ability
8. Patient interaction

When you finish your testing scenario, there is to be no discussion of the case. If you have any questions, they will be answered after the faculty meeting at the end of the course.

4

CHAPTER 4
The Pediatric Airway

Ann Marie Dietrich, MD, FACEP, FAAP
Michael J. Stoner, MD

Objectives
Upon completion of this chapter, you should be able to:

1. Discuss why early recognition and management of pediatric airway compromise is critical.

2. Describe how the pediatric airway differs from the adult airway.

3. Describe the common causes and signs of respiratory distress.

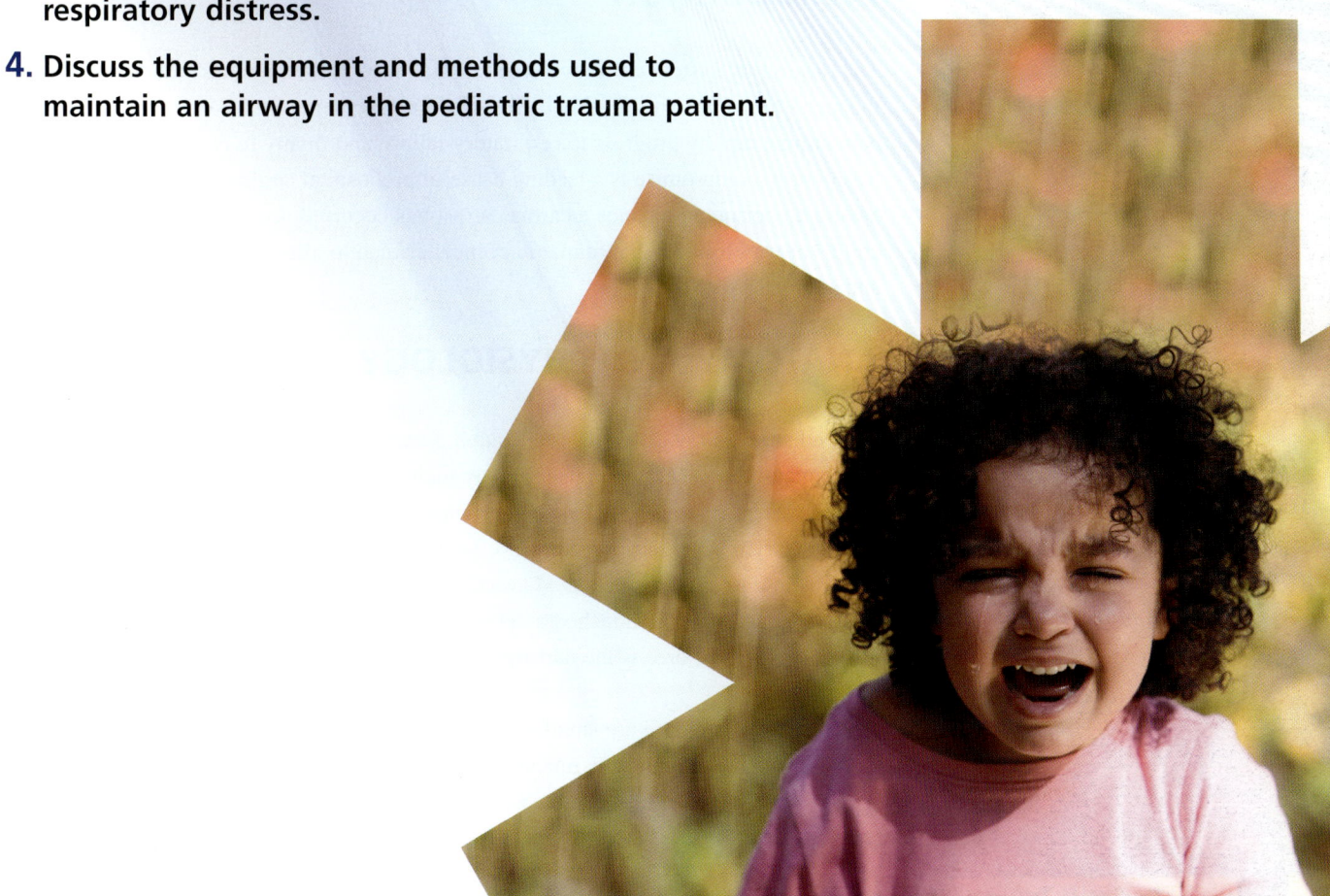

4. Discuss the equipment and methods used to maintain an airway in the pediatric trauma patient.

Case Study

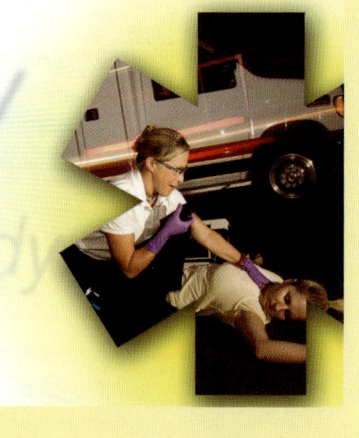

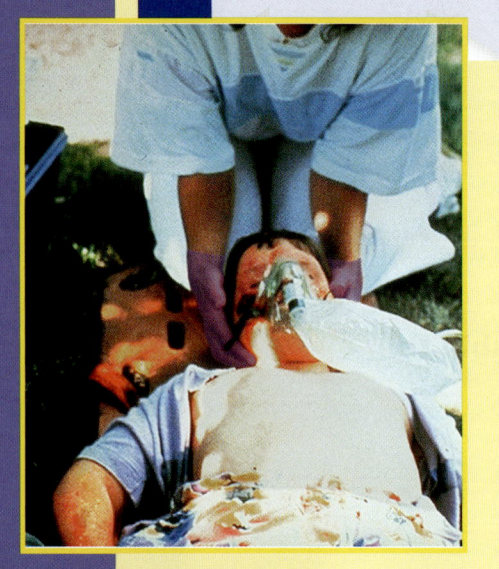

Bob, Susan and John of the Emergency Transport System (ETS) have been called to attend to a trailer home fire. They are told that a 4-year-old male in was found trapped in the bedroom in which a gas heater caused a fire and had been rescued by the fire department. He reportedly is in severe respiratory distress. How should the team approach this patient? What is the mechanism of injury? What type of assessment should they perform? What should they do first? Is this a load-and-go situation? Keep these questions in mind as you read the chapter. Then, at the end of the chapter, find out how the rescuers completed this call.

INTRODUCTION

The respiratory system delivers oxygen to the blood and eliminates carbon dioxide. Inadequate function (respiratory distress) or management of this system in the pediatric patient may rapidly progress to respiratory failure and finally to cardiopulmonary arrest. Respiratory compromise is a leading cause of prehospital cardiac arrest, with most children having a poor outcome once a cardiac arrest has occurred. Early management of the child's airway following a traumatic event is critical to allow for adequate oxygenation and ventilation.

ANATOMY AND PHYSIOLOGY

The pediatric airway differs from the adult airway in several important ways (Fig. 4.1). Anatomic differences of the upper airway include the following:
1. The tongue is relatively larger in proportion to the rest of the oral cavity.
2. The larynx is higher in the neck (C3–4) compared with that of the adult (C4–5).
3. The infant epiglottis is angled away from the long axis of the trachea.
4. The vocal folds are attached anteriorly at a lower level rather than posteriorly.
5. The subglottic area is the narrowest portion of the infant larynx.

The airways of children are smaller, and the supporting cartilage is less developed. Because of their smaller size, mucus, blood, or edema can easily obstruct them (Fig. 4.2). Airway obstruction results in increased resistance. Mechanically, children have problems compensating for respiratory difficulties. In young children, the ribs are very pliable and

PEARLS

Because respiratory compromise is a leading cause of prehospital arrest in children, early recognition and management of the airway is crucial.

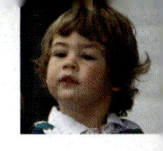

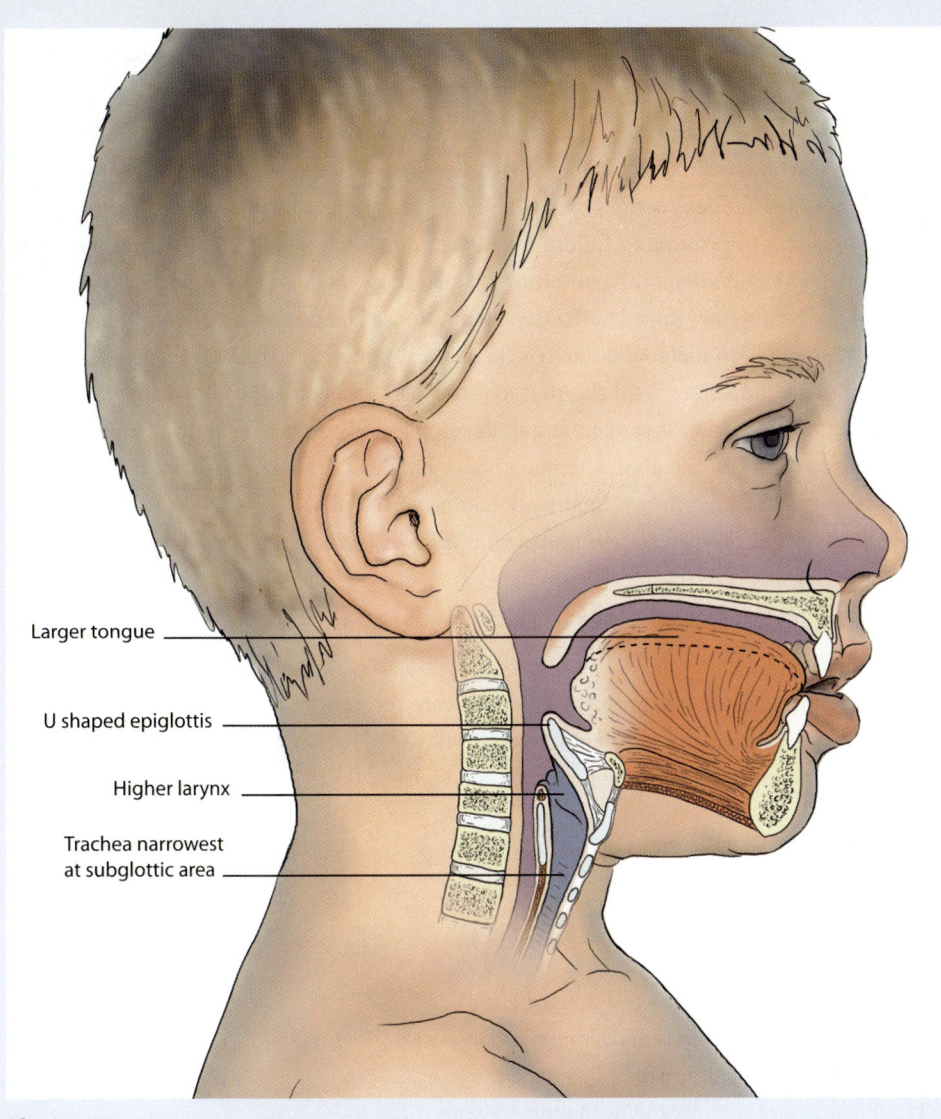

Figure 4.1 *Anatomic differences in the pediatric airway*

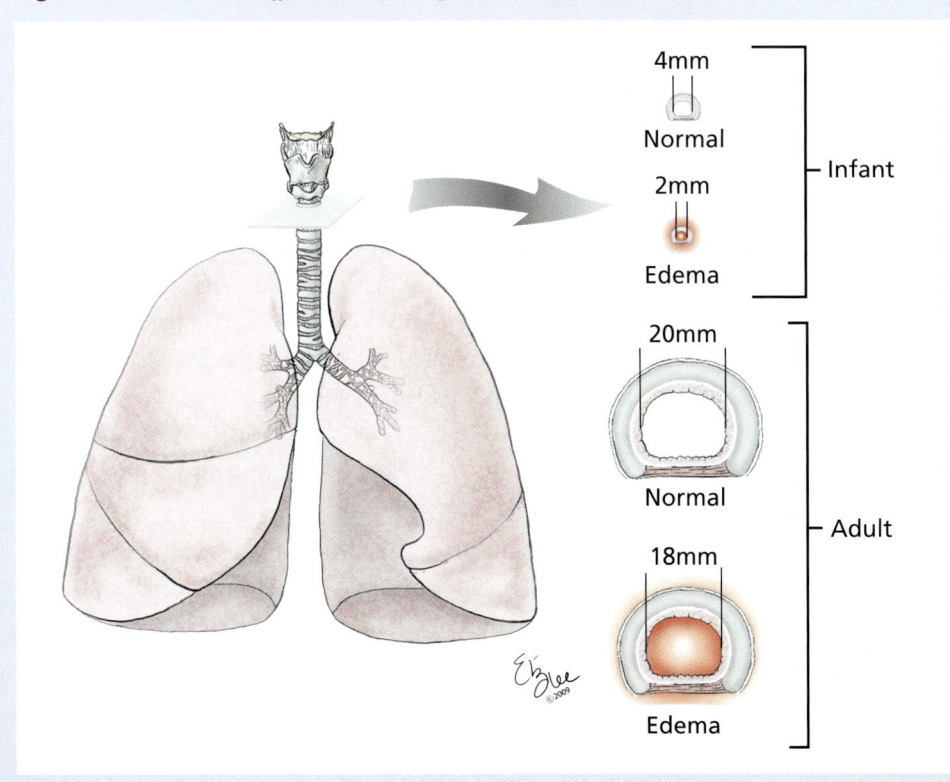

Figure 4.2 Edema can easily obstruct the smaller airway of an infant or child.

The Pediatric Airway

fail to support the lungs. This may lead to paradoxical movement of the chest (sternal and intercostal retractions) when respiratory difficulty occurs. Because children have poorly developed muscles and less compensatory reserve than adults, the progression from respiratory distress to respiratory failure may occur quickly. In addition, the child's tidal volume is dependent on diaphragmatic function and movement. Therefore, gastric or abdominal distention may impede effective respirations. The pediatric patient is further compromised by a high metabolic rate (oxygen consumption is 6 mL/kg/min to 8 mL/kg/min in a child versus 3 mL/kg/min to 4 mL/kg/min in an adult). When inadequate respirations or apnea occur, hypoxemia will develop rapidly. Other conditions, such as hypothermia, overdoses, metabolic derangements, and head trauma may also result in airway compromise or aggravate an already compromised airway. *The goal of emergency airway management is early recognition and rapid intervention.*

PATIENT ASSESSMENT

Airway assessment is the most critical aspect of care for a pediatric trauma patient. Failure to identify an airway problem in a child may lead to further patient compromise and cardiopulmonary arrest. Maintaining an open airway is critical.

Follow the standard approach to patient assessment:
1. ITLS Primary Survey
   A. Scene Size-Up
   B. Initial Assessment
   C. Rapid Trauma Survey or Focused Exam
   D. Critical Interventions and Transport Decisions
   E. Contact medical direction as needed.
2. ITLS Secondary Survey and/or Ongoing Exam

ITLS Primary Survey

Scene Size-Up
The Scene Size-Up should be handled as taught in the ITLS course. Establish the safety of the environment and gain as much information as possible regarding the mechanism of injury to aid the child's assessment and stabilization. Carefully evaluate the scene for clues to the mechanism of injury, such as evidence of fire or damage to the vehicle. Whenever possible, note restraining devices used and how the child was positioned in them. Placing small children in adult restraining devices may result in an injury. For example, a shoulder strap that crosses the child's trachea may cause injury to that area.

Initial Assessment
Airway
As described in Chapter 2, all pediatric trauma patients who have been subjected to a mechanism of injury that could injure the spine or an unknown mechanism of injury should have spinal motion restriction instituted (Fig. 4.3). As manual control of the neck is taken, determine whether the child has an open airway.

PEARLS

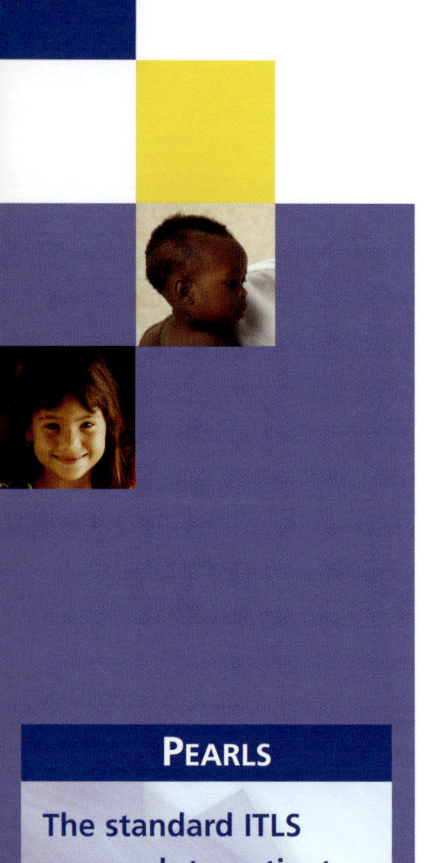

The standard ITLS approach to patient assessment should be used for pediatric patients, remembering that the goal of emergency airway therapy is early recognition and rapid intervention.

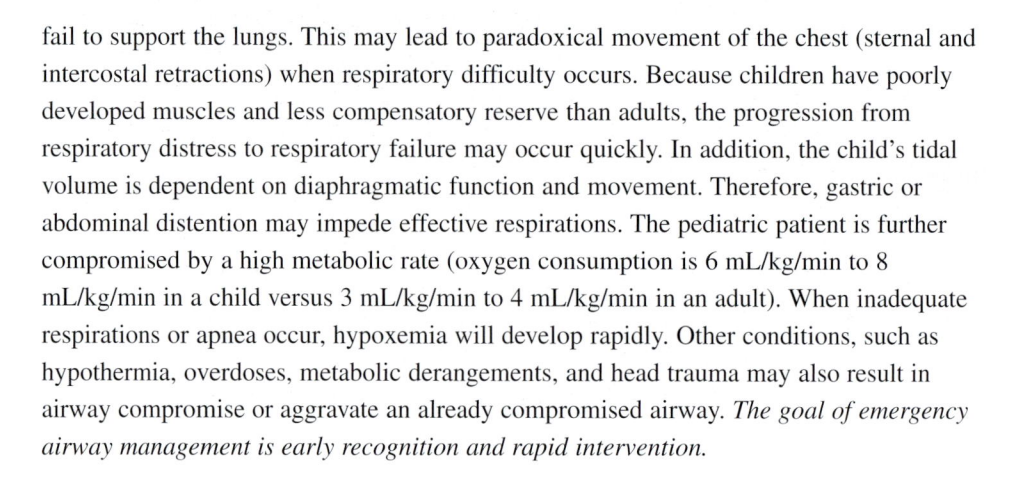

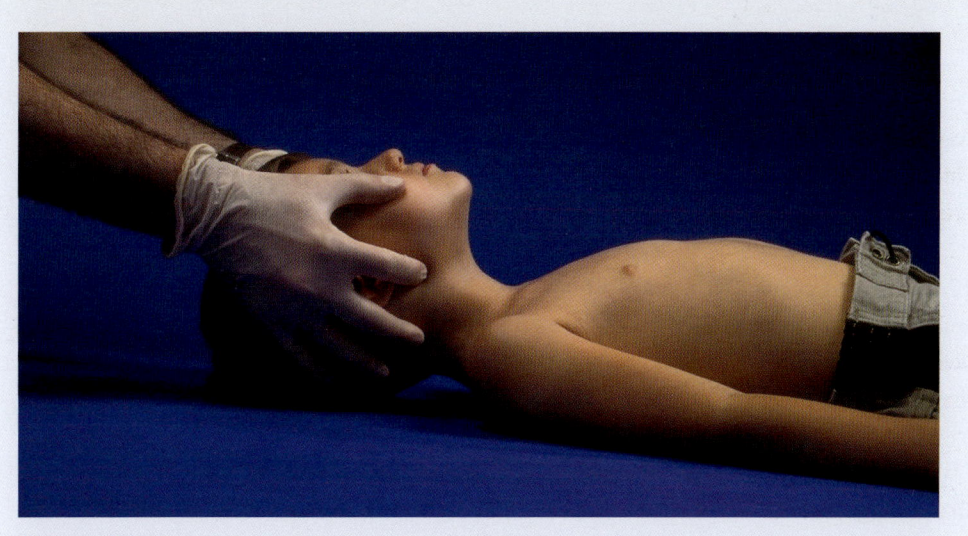

Figure 4.3 *Manual restriction of the head and neck is the first step to assessing the pediatric airway.*

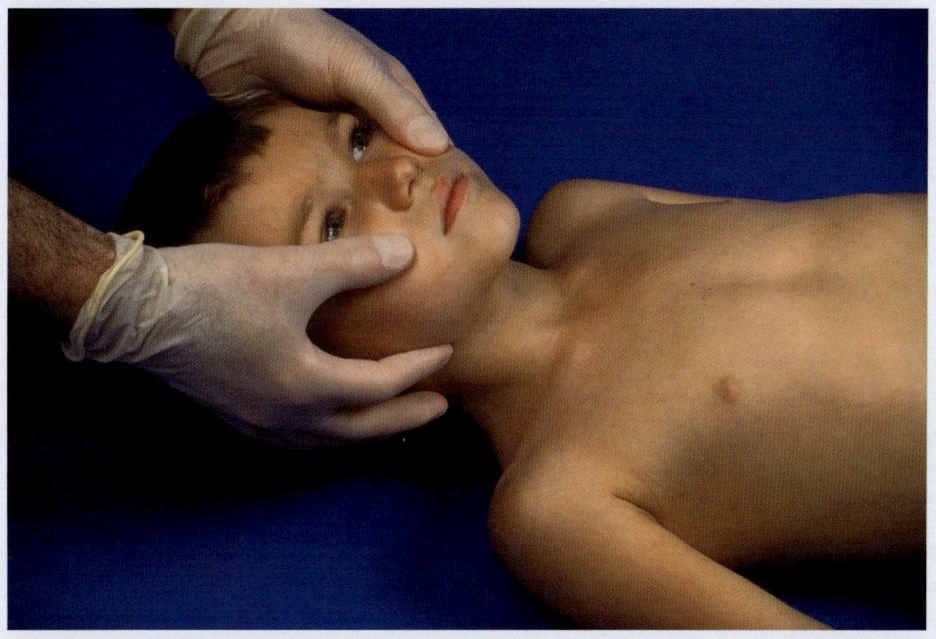

Figure 4.4 *Open the airway with a modified jaw thrust maneuver if the child is not breathing or showing signs of airway obstruction.*

> **PEARLS**
>
> The correct use of a bag-valve mask is a skill that all providers must master. Basic airway management in the pediatric patient is essential.

If the child is not breathing or is showing signs of an obstructed airway, open the airway with a modified jaw thrust maneuver (Fig. 4.4). If the airway is obstructed, consider a foreign body, as children are always placing things in their mouths. Reposition again and begin bag-valve-mask ventilation. If you are having difficulty providing effective bag-valve-mask ventilation, your partner may need to help you achieve a good seal with the mask. Always use 100 percent oxygen and make sure that there is chest movement with each administered breath. The volume of each ventilation given should be 10 mL/kg. So, a 20-kg child should receive 200 mL of tidal volume per breath. As shown in Chapter 6, mask size should be based on achieving a tight seal over the face with the mask extending from the bridge of the nose to the cleft of the chin. The correct use of a bag-valve mask is a skill that all providers must master.

An oropharyngeal airway may be inserted in an unconscious child to assist with maintaining an open airway. A nasal trumpet may be used to assist ventilation as long as there is no evidence of nasal or facial trauma. If a child cannot be ventilated with a

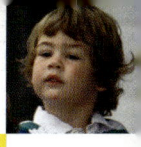

The Pediatric Airway

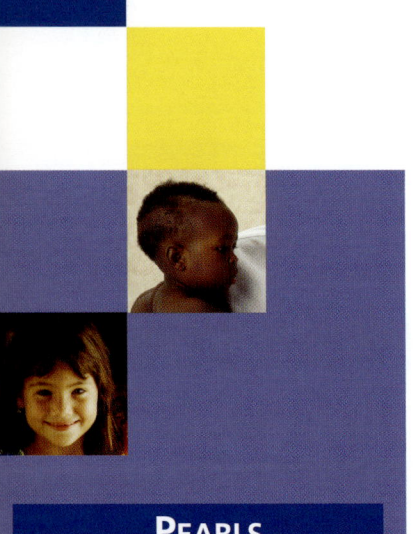

bag-valve mask, he should be intubated while maintaining spinal motion restriction. In children with a complete obstruction of the upper airway due to a foreign body, severe oropharyngeal injuries, or a laryngeal fracture, a cricothyroidotomy may be required.

There are two approaches: needle and surgical cricothyroidotomy. For children under 12 years old, a needle cricothyroidotomy is preferred to surgical cricothyroidotomy. Both techniques can be used in the adolescent (> 12 years), but the surgical technique allows better protection of the airway. Surgical cricothyroidotomy is contradicted in children less than 5 years; a needle technique may be used in an emergency.

The needle cricothyroidotomy technique is discussed in Chapter 6.

Breathing

If the child is breathing, determine the effectiveness of the ventilations. One sign of an upper airway obstruction is stridor. Stridor is an inspiratory high-pitched sound originating from a narrowing in the upper airway. This may be caused by a congenital abnormality, foreign body, infection, trauma, or swelling in the upper airway. If the child is adequately maintaining his airway, stabilize the spine and transport. Any visible foreign objects should be removed. Most children will have a patent airway when the head is placed in a neutral position. When assessing pediatric breath sounds, it is important to listen to both lung fields and to determine the child's "work" of breathing. Because children have such a thin chest wall, breath sounds are easily transmitted and may be misleading. For example, in children with a pneumothorax, the breath sounds may not be absent. Wheezing or a prolonged expiratory phase may be present if the child has aspirated, has a lower respiratory infection, or has a preexisting problem with asthma. Whether the respiratory problem involves the upper airway or the lower airway, you must decide if the child's oxygenation and ventilation are adequate. Signs of respiratory distress include tachypnea (fast breathing), nasal flaring, retractions, use of accessory muscles, or grunting. Grunting is a sound produced by premature glottic closure accompanying chest wall contraction and is the child's attempt to increase airway pressure and keep the airway open.

First assess the child's respiratory rate and compare it with the normal respiratory rate for that age. Nasal flaring and retractions indicate increased work of breathing. Retractions involve the child's use of accessory muscles (intercostal, subcostal, and suprasternal) to assist with adequate oxygen delivery and ventilation (Fig. 4.5). Grunting is the child's attempt to increase airway pressure and keep the airway open. When a child is showing signs of respiratory distress, it is very important to determine the etiology and make the appropriate intervention to prevent the progression to respiratory failure. The airway should be assessed to be sure it is open, and the chest should be assessed for evidence of a pneumothorax, hemothorax, or bony injury (i.e., rib fracture). All children should receive 100 percent oxygen.

Respiratory failure is a condition characterized by inadequate oxygenation and/or ventilation. It should be anticipated in any child who shows an increased respiratory rate and then begins to show signs of fatigue, or has an altered level of consciousness, poor muscle tone, or cyanosis. Children usually progress very quickly from respiratory distress to failure; therefore, early intervention is crucial.

Chapter 5 focuses on specific injuries that may cause breathing problems in the child and their appropriate management.

PEARLS

Stridor, a high-pitched inspiratory sound originating from a narrowing in the upper airway, should be assumed to be a sign of an upper airway obstruction.

PEARLS

Position child's airway in neutral position; listen to both lung fields and assess "work of breathing"; protect the C-spine; deliver 100% oxygen.

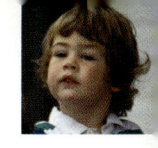

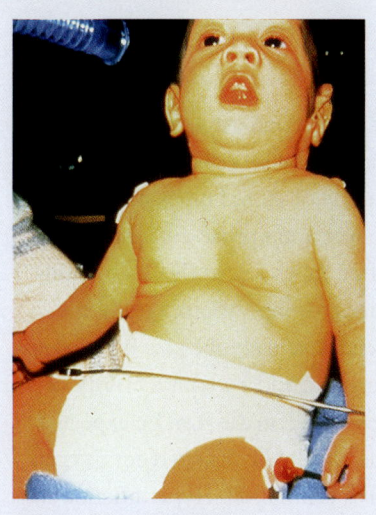

Figure 4.5 *Retractions involve the use of accessory muscles to assist with ventilation.*

Circulation
Assess the circulation, as discussed in Chapter 2. Assess pulse rate and quality and the presence of peripheral pulses. The most common cause of bradycardia (slow heart rate) in children is hypoxia.

Rapid Trauma Survey
Perform a rapid head-to-toe survey as described in Chapter 2.

Brief Neurological Assessment
Hypoxia may lead to changes in the child's behavior. All children with mental status changes should have early, aggressive airway management. It is critical that children with an abnormal mental status be well oxygenated.

Critical Interventions and Transport Decisions
All children with an unstable airway, respiratory insufficiency, or an altered mental status must be packaged rapidly and transported to an appropriate institution (load-and-go).

It is critical that the airway be managed as early as possible. Maintain adequate oxygenation and ventilation to ensure a good outcome for the child.

Airway
Spinal motion restriction should be maintained throughout any airway manipulations, particularly intubation attempts, if there is any possibility of trauma. Studies have shown that in the prehospital setting, the outcome of pediatric patients ventilated with a bag-valve mask is just as good as those who are intubated. If the patient is effectively ventilated with a bag-valve mask, and the anticipated transport time is short, intubation should not be performed in the field. The exception to this is the child whom you can ventilate with a bag-valve mask, but is in danger of losing his airway to upper airway swelling (airway burns). In this case, it is important to intubate as soon as possible, before there is too much swelling. If you cannot ventilate the child with a bag-valve mask, proceed with endotracheal intubation. If intubation is required, have all the necessary equipment prepared prior to the intubation attempt (Fig. 4.6). Suction should be easily accessible. Do not prolong suction attempts, as this may result in bradycardia from stimulation of the vagus nerve, particularly in children less than 6 months old.

> **PEARLS**
>
> **Manage the airway as early as possible. Adequate oxygenation and ventilation ensures a better outcome for the child.**

The Pediatric Airway

PEARLS

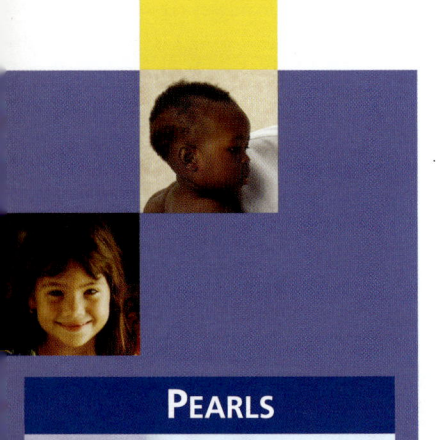

Recommendations for pediatric intubation vary depending on transport time and local policy.

Make available endotracheal tubes that are one half-size smaller and one half-size larger than appropriate for the age and size of the child. Currently, all children less than eight years old should receive an uncuffed tube, but new data shows that the use of cuffed tubes may be helpful in certain situations. Controversy exists as to the most appropriate cuff pressure to minimize damage to the child's trachea. Therefore, cuffed tubes are, at this time, only for the in-hospital setting. Place a card with the correct sizes for the various ages in the intubation box (Table 4.1). A quick way to estimate the endotracheal tube size is to use the child's external nares or the size of the child's smallest finger. Children with a history of previous intubations, stridor, or a history of malformations of the airway can be expected to need a smaller size endotracheal tube. Preoxygenate the child with 100 percent oxygen prior to intubation attempts, making sure to avoid excessive ventilation. Hyperinflation has been shown to impede venous return to the heart, and, therefore, cardiac output. It also increases the chance of filling the stomach with air, causing vomiting and aspiration.

The most skilled provider available should perform all pediatric intubations. If the child is easily oxygenated and ventilated with a bag-valve mask, and there is a short transport time, do not intubate the child prior to arrival at the hospital. Multiple intubation attempts may damage the airway and delay transport to a trauma center. As a rule, any individual should make no more than two attempts. During the intubation, the Sellick maneuver, gentle pressure on the cricoid cartilage, may be used to close the esophagus to minimize the child's risk of aspiration (Fig. 4.7). If there is any danger of cervical spine injury, careful motion restriction must be maintained. A detailed discussion of the procedure of endotracheal intubation is discussed in Chapter 6.

Table 4.1: Equipment Size by Age Group

Age	Endotracheal Tube Size (mm)	Suction Catheter Size (F)	Entrotracheal Tube Depth
Premature	2.5	5	For all infants <1 yr,
Newborn	3.0–3.5	6–8	use the following formula to calculate:
1-6 mo	3.5–4.0	8	7 + (child's weight in kg) = _____ cm depth
7-12 mo	4.0–4.5	8–10	
18 mo	4.0–4.5	8–10	For all children > 1 yr,
3 yr	4.5–5.0	10	use one of the following formulas to calculate:
6 yr	5.0	10	12 + ? (child's age in years) = _____ cm depth
8 yr	5.5–6.0	10	OR
10 yr	5.5–6.0	10	3 x ETT Size (in mm) = ____ mm depth
12 yr	6.5–6.5	10	
15 yr	6.5–8.0	10–14	

58 Pediatric Trauma Life Support

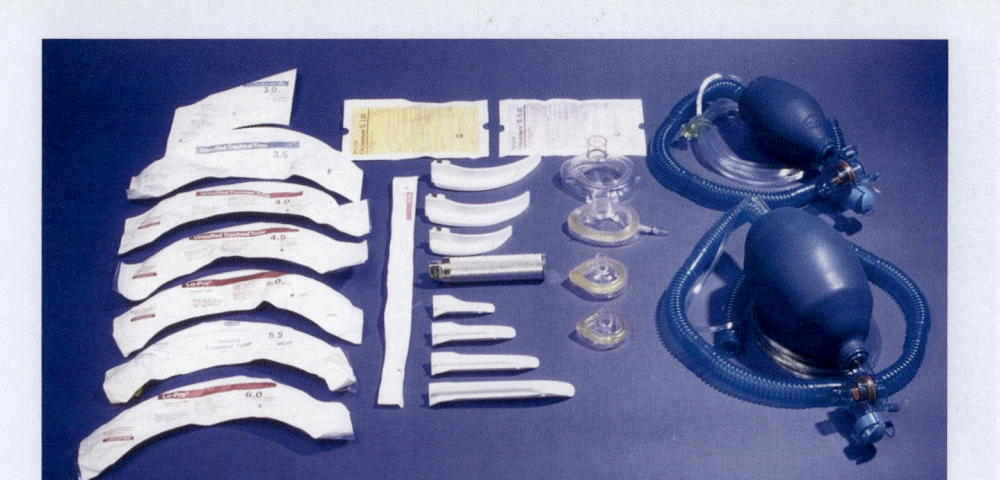

Figure 4.6 *Endotracheal intubation equipment is available in several sizes for pediatric patients.*

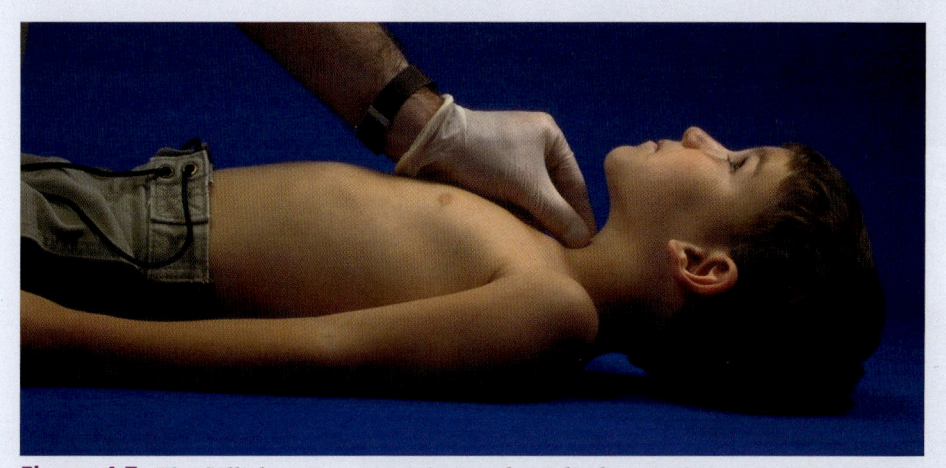

Figure 4.7 *The Sellick maneuver minimizes the risk of aspiration.*

Pulse oximetry is important in the assessment of the oxygenation of a child. Place the probe on a well-perfused area, usually a finger, toe, or earlobe, and observe the monitor. If the monitor is receiving a pulse oximetry reading correctly, the patient's pulse will correlate with the pulse seen on the monitor. All pediatric trauma patients should have a pulse oximetry reading of greater than 95 percent; less than 90 percent is unacceptable because this correlates with an arterial PO_2 of 56 to 60 mmHg (too low). Factors that may interfere with an accurate pulse oximetry reading include: a cold finger or toe, poor perfusion (shock), incorrect probe placement, or nail polish. If the pulse oximetry reading does not match the way the child appears clinically, reassess the patient and move the probe to a warm site and recheck the reading.

Blind insertion airway devices (BIADs) are now available for the pediatric population (Fig. 4.8). Studies show that they can be used by prehospital providers to manage pediatric airways, especially in the older pediatric population. Difficulties include choosing the appropriate size, risk of overventilating with resulting insufflation of air into the stomach, and the inability of the devices to prevent aspiration. This is offset by the ease of use and ease of skill maintenance. As with adult patients, these devices will likely play a greater role in field airway management for pediatric patients in the future.

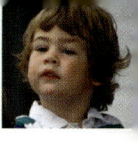

> **PEARLS**
>
> Assure ET tube placement by assessing rise and fall of the chest, equal breath sounds. Secondary confirmation using the appropriately sized end-tidal CO_2 detector or capnography is essential.

The Pediatric Airway

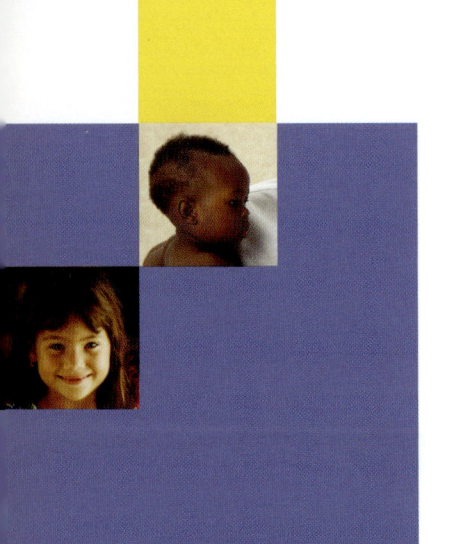

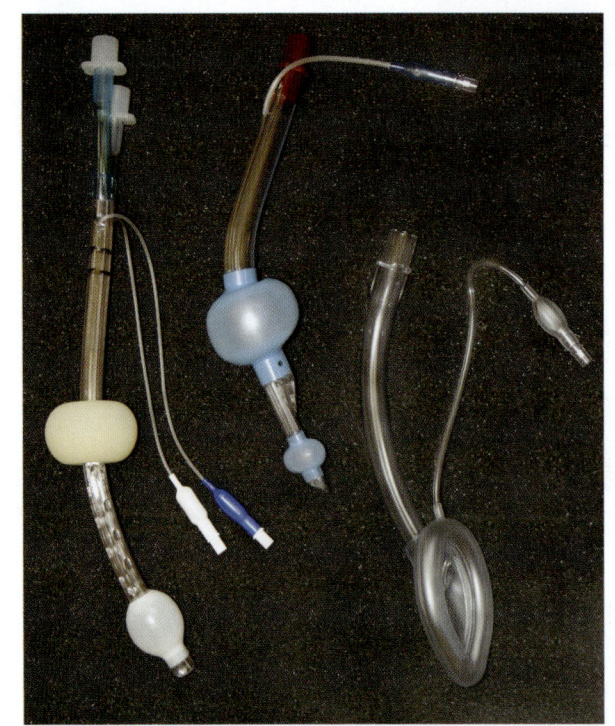

Figure 4.8 BIADs such as the Combitube (left), KING LT-D airway (center), and laryngeal mask airway (LMA) are available in smaller sizes for pediatric patients.

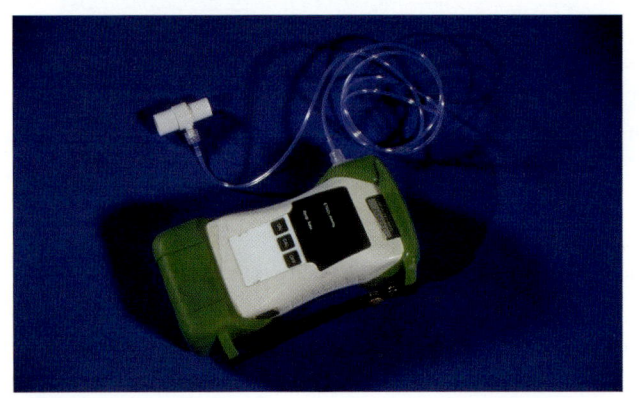

Figure 4.9 A capnometer can confirm the placement of the ET tube.

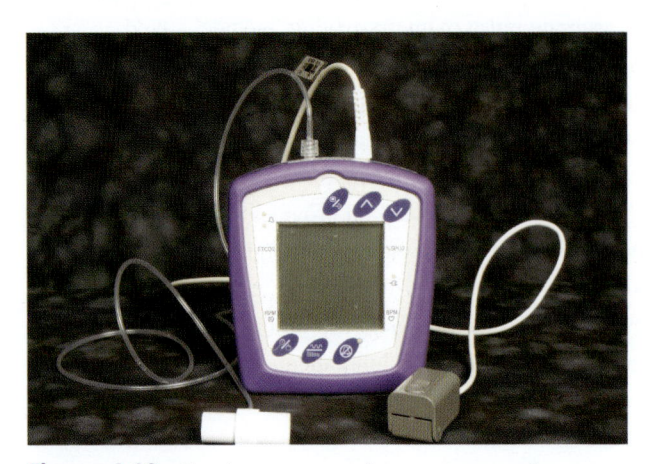

Figure 4.10 Continuous wave-form capnography provides breath-to-breath feedback of tube confirmation and adequacy of ventilations.

Pediatric Trauma Life Support

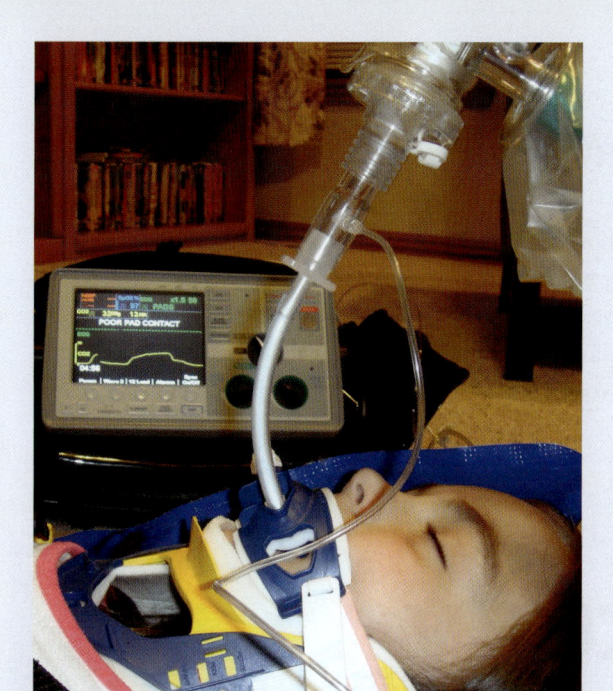

Figure 4.11 *Capnography on the intubated child maintains "airway tube vigilance" as seen with continuous wave-form monitoring.*

Breathing
All children should be maintained on 100 percent oxygen during transport. If the child is intubated, carefully assess endotracheal tube placement. Symmetric rise and fall of the chest, equal breath sounds bilaterally, vapor in the tube, and acceptable pulse oximetry readings all suggest that the tube is correctly positioned. A secondary confirmation is necessary to further ensure that the endotracheal tube is in the trachea. An exhaled CO_2 device works well (Fig. 4.9). Even better is continuous waveform capnography (Figs. 4.10, 4.11). If the abdomen is distended, consider placing an orogastric tube to allow deflation of the stomach. Chapter 5 discusses specific chest injuries that may be discovered.

Circulation
If time permits, IV access may be obtained during transport on all patients with respiratory compromise. If the child has signs and symptoms of shock, fluid resuscitation should be initiated. If the patient is stable, fluid administration should be kept to a minimum so that pulmonary edema does not occur.

Medications
Occasionally, sedation may be necessary to allow for maintaining the endotracheal tube. Short-acting nonparalytic medications may be used if they are part of the agency's established protocol or approved by medical direction. Benzodiazepines, such as midazolam, produce amnesia and sedation with minimal hemodynamic depression and are frequently used to sedate an intubated patient.

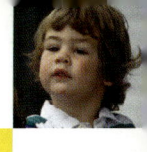

The Pediatric Airway

ITLS SECONDARY SURVEY

During the ITLS Secondary Survey, note any facial injuries, abrasions, bruises, or fractures. Also record any swelling or bruises to the neck. Document any fluid that is draining from the ears or nose. As discussed in Chapter 5, carefully document any bruises or injuries to the child's chest. Any child with altered mental status should have a fingerstick blood sugar check to rule out hypoglycemia during the ITLS Secondary Survey.

Case Study *continued*

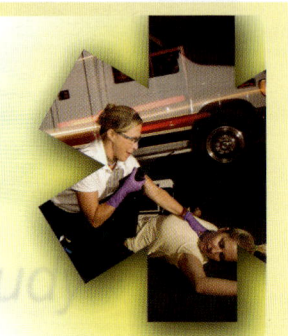

Bob, Susan, and John of the Emergency Transport System (ETS) have been called to attend to a trailer home fire. Upon arrival, the scene size-up reveals that the fire service had rescued the boy from the trailer home and placed him in a shaded area upwind from the trailer home. They find a 4-year-old male in severe respiratory distress.

Susan acts as team leader and she begins the Initial Assessment; her general impression is poor. The patient is awake but appears very anxious. He has blistering of his lips, nose, mouth, and some on his arms and legs. He was wearing shorts and a short-sleeved shirt and his clothes did not catch on fire. There was no explosion.

The team acts quickly. John stabilizes the patient's neck while Susan begins the exam. The boy reports that his mother was at a nearby grocery store. His respiratory rate is fast and stridorous. Bob administers oxygen by a nonrebreather mask while Susan finishes the Initial Assessment. She notes that his radial pulse is rapid and fast. Capillary refill is 3 seconds.

A Focused Exam is performed in view of the given mechanism of injury (no explosion). Blistering to his lips, nose and mouth in conjunction with soot on his face makes Susan think of a possible inhalational injury to his airway. Trachea is midline. On auscultation of his chest, breath sounds are present bilaterally; there is some inspiratory and expiratory wheezing as well as stridor. The child has a rapid heart rate of 160 bpm. Bob places the child on a pulse oximetry monitor, which reads 92 percent on 100 percent oxygen. The team decides this is a load-and-go situation.

Pediatric Trauma Life Support

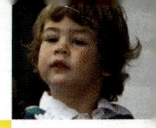

They provide 100 percent oxygen and because of continued stridor and a long transport time to the burn center, choose to sedate the child and insert an endotracheal tube by the oral route. They take verbal consent from the patient's mother, who has now returned from the store. They are informed the child has no allergies, takes no medications, has no history of medical problems (no asthma), and last ate about four hours ago. Using appropriate drugs and equipment, the procedure goes well. The child is loaded on to the ambulance and the mother accompanies them.

Susan notifies medical direction of their findings and intervention. She performs an ITLS Secondary Survey en route and notes that the child's condition improved after rapid control of the unstable airway.

The hospital trauma team was waiting upon the ambulance arrival to receive the patient with burns and inhalation injury. The child eventually recovers.

Case Study wrap-up

This is an example of the exception to the rule that you avoid intubation of a child in the field if he can be oxygenated and ventilated with bag-valve-mask ventilation. The reason early intubation is necessary is that this child has a high likelihood of pulmonary involvement, which could cause continued swelling and obstruction of the airway. It may be impossible to intubate later because of edema of the airway, and it is important to gain control while it is still possible. In this situation, the child has a gag reflex and you may need to sedate and/or paralyze the child in order to insert the oral endotracheal tube. Unlike in an awake adult in whom you might first try nasotracheal intubation, in a small child, this is contraindicated because the anatomy is too small. This child likely has poisoning from carbon monoxide or other toxic gases, so continued administration of 100 percent oxygen is very important.

The Pediatric Airway

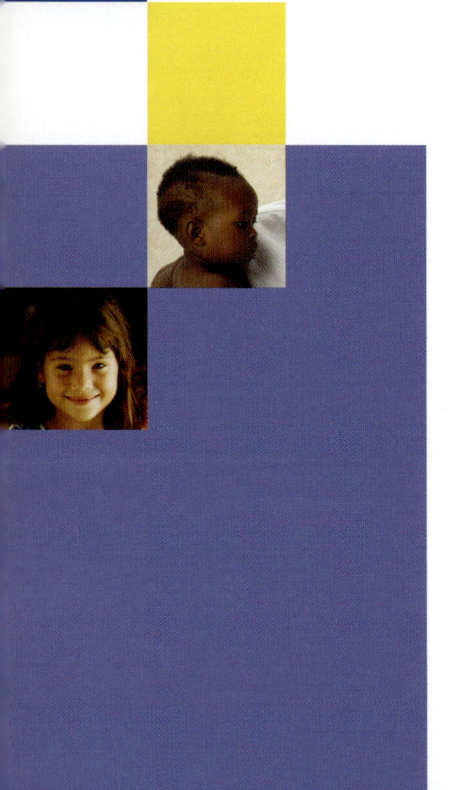

SUMMARY

1. The pediatric airway anatomy and physiology is different from the adult.
2. Identify early signs and symptoms of respiratory distress rapidly and manage them aggressively.
3. The most common cause of cardiopulmonary arrest in the child is respiratory arrest.
4. The most important intervention in the critical pediatric trauma patient is maintaining an open airway.

Recommended Reading

Advanced Life Support Group. "Procedures: Airway and Breathing." In *Pre-Hospital Paediatric Life Support: The Practical Approach*, 2nd ed. London: Blackwell BMJ Books, 2005.

American College of Surgeons. "Airway and Ventilatory Management." In *Advanced Trauma Life Support for Doctors*, 8th ed. Chicago: Author, 2008.

American Heart Association (AHA). "2005 Guidelines for Cardiopulmonary Resuscitation (CPR) and Emergency Cardiovascular Care (ECC) of Pediatric and Neonatal Patients: Pediatric Basic Life Support." *Pediatrics* 117 (May 2006): e989–e1004 (doi:10.1542/peds.2006-0219).

Bledsoe, Gregory H. and Stephen M. Schexnayder. "Pediatric Rapid Sequence Intubation: A Review." *Pediatric Emergency Care* 20 (May 2004): 339–44.

Campbell, John Emory, ed. "Initial Airway Management." In *International Trauma Life Support for Prehospital Care Providers*, 6th ed., 58–77. Upper Saddle River, N.J.: Pearson/Prentice Hall, 2008.

Dunford, James V., et al. "Incidence of Transient Hypoxia and Pulse Rate Reactivity During Paramedic Rapid Sequence Intubation." *Annals of Emergency Medicine* 42 (December 2003): 721–28.

European Resuscitation Council (UK). "The Injured Child." In *European Paediatric Life Support*, 2nd ed. Antwerp, Belguin: Author, 2006.

Fleisher, Gary R., Stephen Ludwig, Fred M. Henretig, Richard M. Ruddy, and Benjamin K. Silverman, eds. *Textbook of Pediatric Emergency Medicine*, 5th ed. Philadelphia: Lippincott Williams and Wilkins, 2005.

Gausche, Marianne, Roger J. Lewis, Samuel J. Stratton, et al. "Effect of Out-of-Hospital Pediatric Intubation on Survival and Neurological Outcome: A Controlled Clinical Trial." *Journal of the American Medical Association* 283 (2000): 783–90.

Gausche-Hill, Marianne, et al. *Pediatric Airway Management for the Pre-Hospital Professional*. Sudbury, M.A.: Jones & Bartlett, 2004.

Guyette, Francis X, Kimberly R. Roth, David C. LaCovey, and Jon C. Rittenberger. "Feasibility of Laryngeal Mask Airway Use by Prehospital Personnel in Simulated Pediatric Respiratory Arrest." *Prehospital Emergency Care* 11 (2007): 245–49.

Luten, Robert. "Accurate Endotracheal Tube Placement in Children: Depth of Insertion is Part of the Process." *Pediatric Critical Care Medicine* 6 (September 2005): 606–8.

Perkin, Ronald M. "Pitfalls in Pediatric Airway Management." *Pediatric Emergency Medicine Reports* 2 (1997).

Todres, David. "Pediatric Airway Control and Ventilation." *Annals of Emergency Medicine* 22 (1993): 440.

Von Goedecke, Achim. "Field Airway Management Disasters." *Anesthesia and Analgesia* 104 (March 2007): 481–83.

5

CHAPTER 5
Pediatric Thoracic Trauma

Robert E. Falcone, MD, FACS
Holly Herron, RN, MS, CNS, EMT-P

Objectives
Upon completion of this chapter, you should be able to:

1. Describe the major signs and symptoms of pediatric thoracic trauma.

2. Discuss the pathophysiology and initial management of pediatric thoracic trauma.

3. Compare the clinical presentation of massive hemothorax and tension pneumothorax.

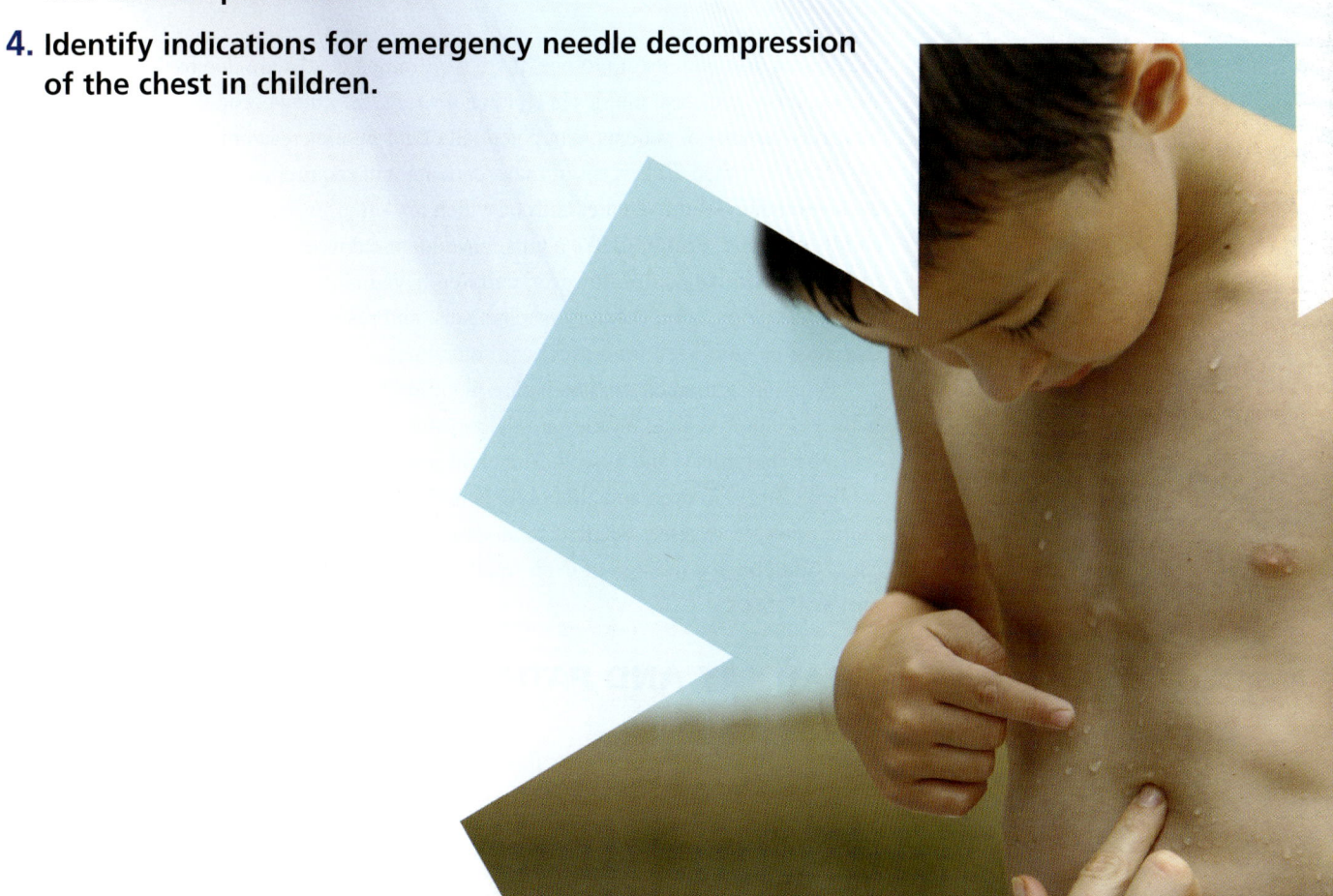

4. Identify indications for emergency needle decompression of the chest in children.

Case Study

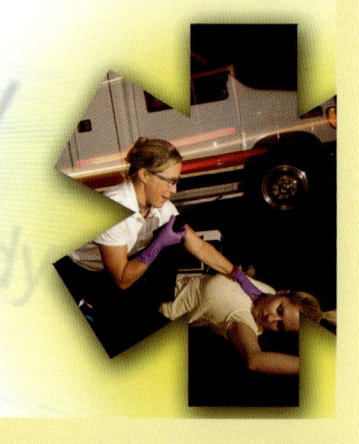

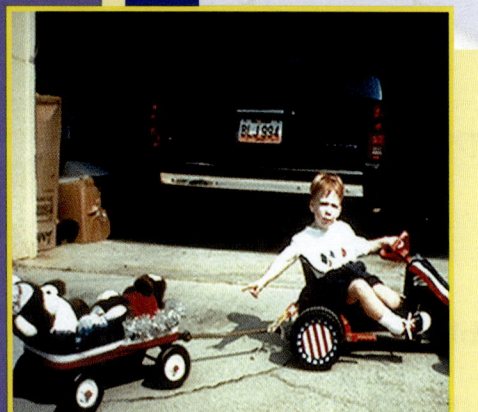

John, Susan, and Bob of the Emergency Transport System (ETS) have been called to a residential area. An 18-month-old child was backed over by the family car while leaving the driveway. As the father was slowly moving in reverse, he felt the rear wheel "run over" an object; he immediately stopped the car and found the child under the car.

What sort of injuries should they expect from this mechanism? How does evaluation and treatment of an 18-month-old differ from an adult? Keep these questions in mind as you read the chapter. Then, at the end of the chapter, find out how the rescuers completed the call.

PEARLS

Because of strong compensatory mechanisms, children have the ability to maintain normal or near-normal blood pressure even as they slip into severe shock. Monitor the child carefully for early signs of shock including increased respiratory and/or heart rates, or any change in mental status.

INTRODUCTION

In children, as in adults, up to one quarter of trauma deaths are due to thoracic injury. Although isolated chest injuries in children are rare, they may occur as part of a multisystem injury. Two-thirds of patients with potentially fatal injuries reach the emergency department alive, and less than 20 percent of these patients will require surgery. Expedient initial evaluation and definitive care, both of which are often initiated in the field, determine the child's outcome. Children, like adults, have identical treatment priorities and management techniques. Unlike adults, however, children have unique mechanisms of injury, anatomy, pathophysiology, compensatory mechanisms, and resuscitative and psychosocial concerns that must be addressed for a successful outcome.

Penetrating thoracic trauma is rare in children, especially in the preadolescent years. Falls and motor vehicle injuries are the most common mechanisms of injury, followed by sports-related injury, and assault. The child provides a smaller target for the focus of applied energy, so even an automobile bumper that strikes the thorax of a small child can injure multiple systems; whereas in an adult that same bumper may injure only the rib cage. Additionally, the loss of even small amounts of blood can place a young child in profound shock.

ANATOMY AND PATHOPHYSIOLOGY

Compared to an adult, the child's thoracic cage, like the rest of the child's skeleton, is incompletely calcified and provides less protection for the internal organs. In children, multisystem involvement is the rule rather than the exception, and serious injury without external evidence of injury is quite common. This places great importance on the mechanism of injury as a sign of significant injury in the child. Until proven otherwise, there must be a high index of suspicion of an injury in a child who has sustained a significant mechanism of injury.

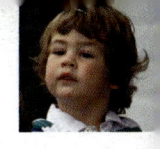

The thorax of a child extends from the base of the neck to the umbilicus. The bony cavity is formed by 12 pairs of incompletely calcified ribs that join along the spine posteriorly and with the sternum anteriorly. There is an intercostal bundle of nerve, artery, and vein that runs along the inferior border of each rib. The thoracic cavity and its contents are lined with a thin membrane called the pleura. There is a potential space between the visceral pleura on the lungs and the parietal pleura on the chest wall. This space can become filled with air (pneumothorax) or blood (hemothorax). The adult space can hold up to 3 liters of fluid. In the child, it is proportional to the child's size.

Figure 5.1 is an illustration of the child's thoracic cavity and its contents. Each side of the chest contains a lung separated in the middle by the mediastinum, which contains (in order from front to back) the heart, tracheobronchial tree, superior and inferior vena cava, esophagus, aorta, and posterior spine. The chest and abdomen are separated by a muscular and ligamentous structure called the diaphragm. The level of the diaphragm changes with inspiration and expiration, and, in general, any injury below the level of the nipples is considered not only a thoracic injury but potentially an intra-abdominal injury as well. Figure 5.2 shows the intrathoracic abdominal contents.

> **PEARLS**
>
> **Because a child's thoracic cage is incompletely calcified and provides less protection for internal organs, suspect serious injury without external evidence of injury. Carefully assess the mechanism of injury and assume significant injury until proven otherwise.**

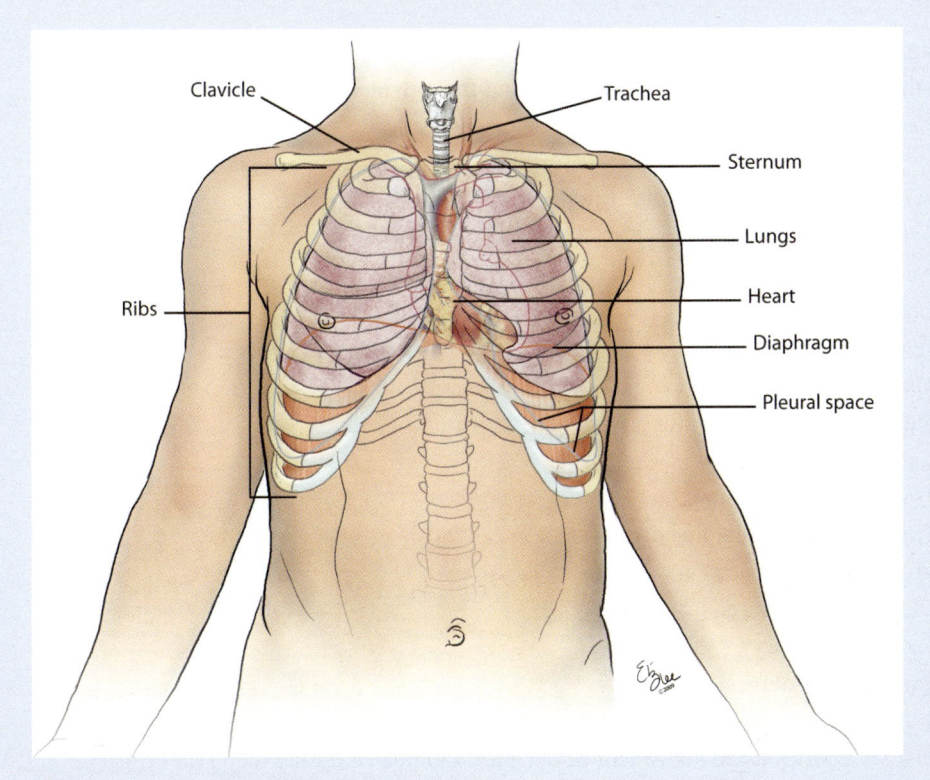

Figure 5.1 *The thoracic cavity of a child.*

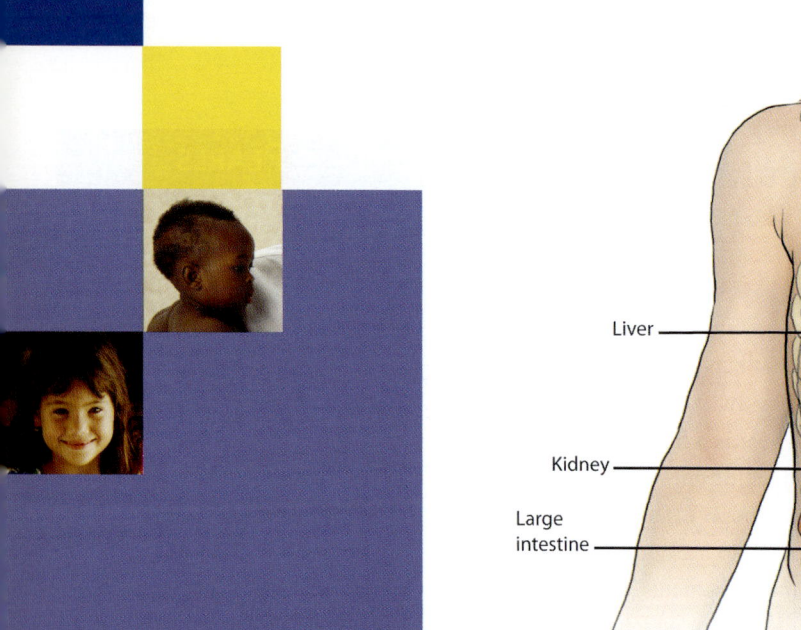

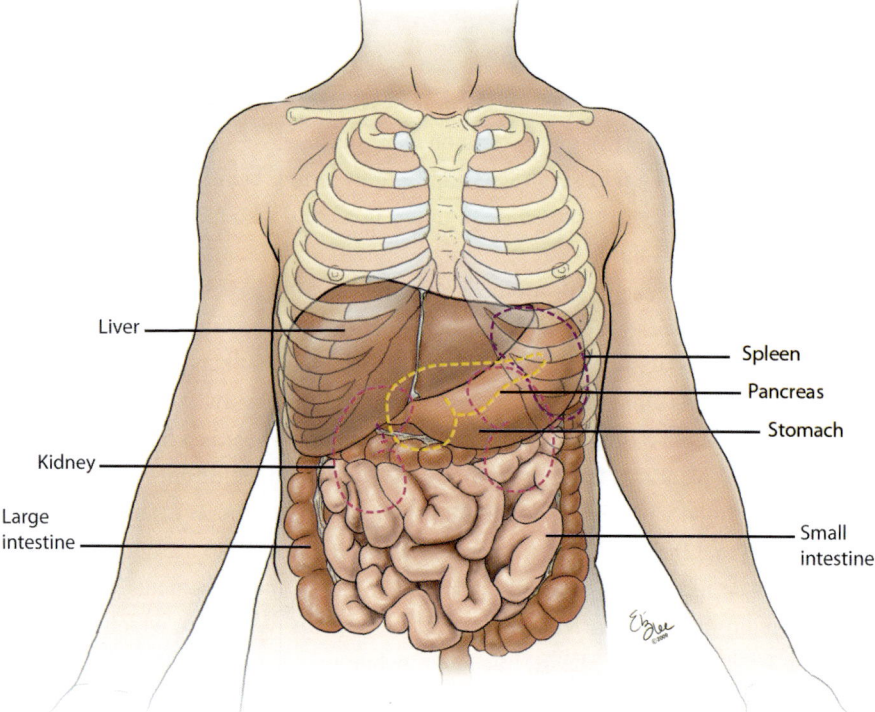

Liver
Spleen
Pancreas
Stomach
Kidney
Large intestine
Small intestine

Figure 5.2 *The intrathoracic abdominal contents of a child.*

PATIENT ASSESSMENT

The signs and symptoms of significant intrathoracic injury in a child are similar to those of an adult, but clinical findings may be subtle and the provider should have a high index of suspicion to make an accurate and timely diagnosis.

Following are the "Deadly Dozen" life-threatening thoracic injuries:

1. Airway obstruction
2. Open pneumothorax
3. Tension pneumothorax
4. Massive hemothorax
5. Flail chest and rib fractures
6. Cardiac tamponade
7. Traumatic aortic rupture
8. Tracheal or bronchial tree disruption
9. Myocardial contusion
10. Diaphragmatic tear
11. Esophageal injury
12. Pulmonary contusion

The first six injuries listed above will be detected and treated during the ITLS Primary Survey. The last six injuries listed above are more likely to be detected during the ITLS Secondary Survey or during hospital evaluation.

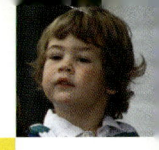

Follow the standard approach for assessment of the pediatric trauma patient:

1. ITLS Primary Survey
   A. Scene Size-Up
   B. Initial Assessment
   C. Rapid Trauma Survey or Focused Exam
   D. Critical Interventions and Transport Decisions
   E. Contact medical direction as needed.
2. ITLS Secondary Survey and/or Ongoing Exam

ITLS Primary Survey

Scene Size-Up
The child with a significant mechanism of injury has a significant injury until proven otherwise.

Initial Assessment
Airway and Cervical Spine
After careful application of spinal motion restriction of the child's cervical spine, open the child's airway. Airway management is the first priority in the care of an injured child and is addressed in Chapter 4.

Breathing
In addition to the findings of tachypnea, flaring, retracting, grunting, and apnea, the child with a chest injury may present with shortness of breath and/or pain. A small child may not be able to verbalize these complaints. If the child's airway is open and the child shows signs of respiratory distress, perform a rapid evaluation of the chest. This should include an evaluation of the patient's overall condition and color. Are the lips and mucous membranes pink or blue? Carefully inspect the chest for external evidence of injury. Observe the motion of the chest. Is it symmetric or not? Is there a flail segment? Palpate the position of the trachea and observe the neck veins for distention. The chest should be auscultated for breath sounds. Remember that the chest wall in children is thin, so sometimes it is difficult to appreciate subtle differences in breath sounds. All children with a suspected chest injury should receive 100 percent oxygen and have their ventilation assisted as necessary regardless of the specific thoracic injury suspected (Fig. 5.3) If available, pulse oximetry should be used to monitor the patient's oxygen saturation and capnography used to monitor the patient's CO_2 level.

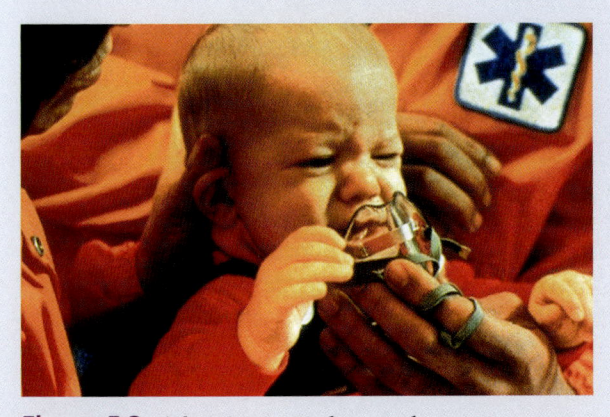

Figure 5.3 *Administer supplemental oxygen to any pediatric patient with a suspected chest injury.*

> **PEARLS**
>
> A small child may not be able to verbalize respiratory complaints. If the child's airway is open and the child shows signs of respiratory distress, perform a rapid evaluation of the chest to include color, "work of breathing," and symmetry.

> **PEARLS**
>
> All children with a suspected chest injury should receive 100 percent oxygen with assisted ventilation as necessary regardless of the specific thoracic injury suspected.

Pediatric Thoracic Trauma

Chest injuries that require immediate action include open pneumothorax, tension pneumothorax, and flail chest.

Open Pneumothorax Open pneumothorax, a "sucking" chest wound, is due to penetrating thoracic injury and is unusual in the preadolescent child. The signs and symptoms are proportionate to the chest wall defect. Normally, with each respiration, a negative pressure develops in the thoracic cavity by the contracting diaphragm and expanding chest wall. Air is drawn through the upper respiratory tree and the lungs expand. A large defect in the chest wall creates a path of lesser resistance for airflow, which results in the air entering the pleural space rather than the respiratory tree, making ventilation and oxygenation difficult. Closing the chest wall defect prevents air from sucking into the thoracic cavity on inspiration, but this closure must allow air to exit on expiration in order to prevent the development of a tension pneumothorax. This may be accomplished safely by using any available pad, then making that pad nonocclusive by taping it on three sides (Fig. 5.4). A commercial chest seal is available (Asherman Chest Seal®) that has a flutter valve to prevent development of tension pneumothorax (Fig. 5.5).

Tension Pneumothorax A tension pneumothorax results when a lung leak due to blunt or penetrating trauma fails to seal (Fig. 5.6). A one-way valve effect may be produced, leading to air buildup in the pleural space with each breath. This can result in the mediastinum shifting to the side opposite the tension pneumothorax with rapidly progressive dyspnea, cyanosis, and death. In young children, this may be particularly problematic, as their mobile mediastinum can create a rapid compromise of pulmonary and cardiac function. Early diagnosis is critical.

Clinically, breath sounds are generally diminished on the side of the pneumothorax. However, breath sounds may be misleading in the young child. Their presence or absence should not be the sole criterion for diagnosis. Percussion may reveal hyperresonance, although this is very unreliable in the pediatric population. Hypotension, distended neck veins, and tracheal deviation—which are best appreciated by palpating the neck—occur as the process progresses. These are much more reliable, but often late, findings in a child.

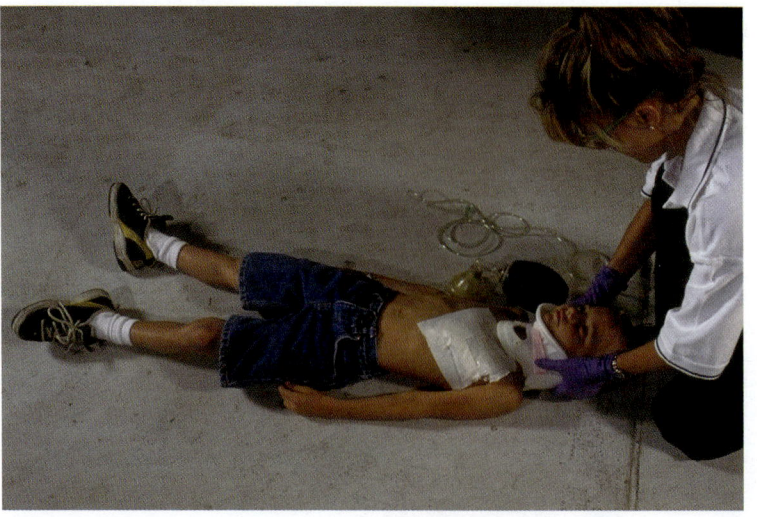

Figure 5.4 *Close any sucking chest wounds by using any available pad and taping it on three sides to make it nonocclusive.*

Pediatric Trauma Life Support

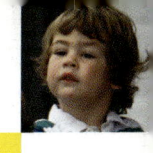

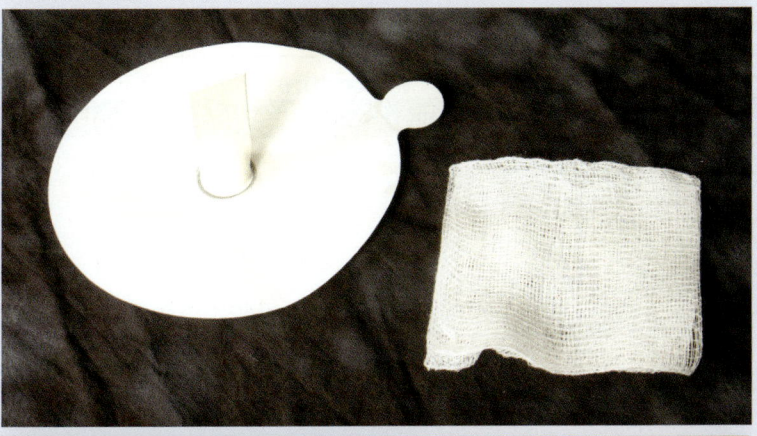

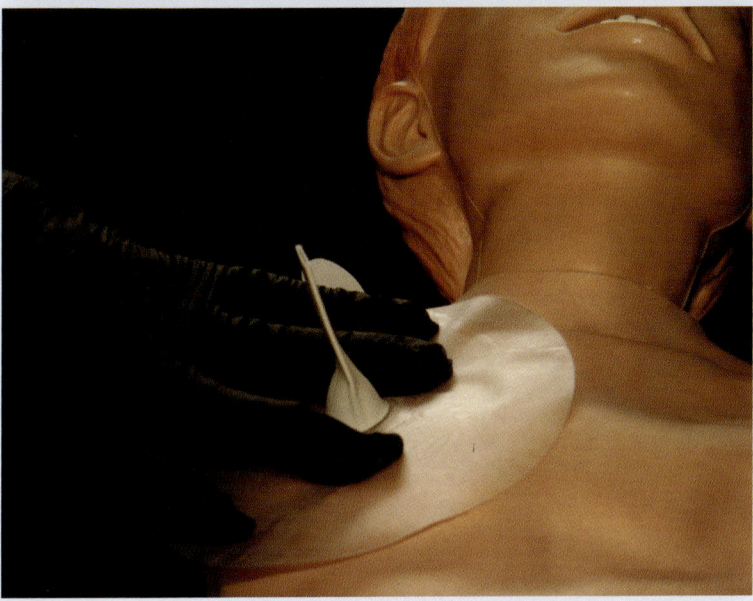

Figure 5.5 *The Asherman Chest Seal has a flutter valve to prevent development of a tension pneumothorax.*

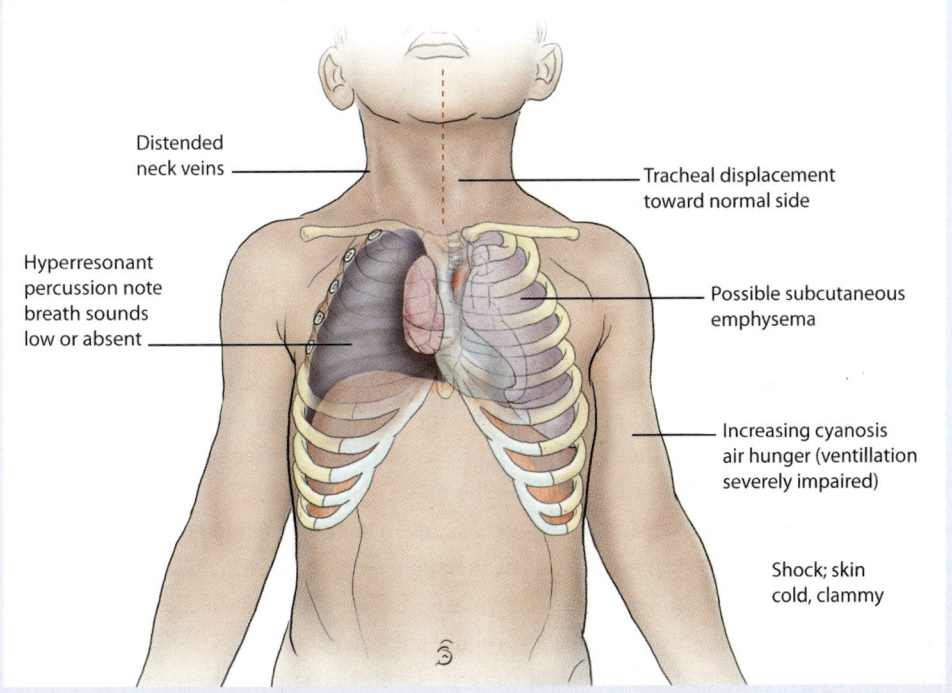

Figure 5.6 *Tension pneumothorax results from a build-up of air in the pleural space due to a lung leak that fails to seal.*

Pediatric Thoracic Trauma

Table 5.1: Age-appropriate Catheters

Age (Yr)	Size (kg)	Procedure IV	Needle Decompression
<1	<10	24–20g	20–16g
1–5	10–20	20–18g	16–14g
5–12	20–40	18–16g	16–14g
>12	>40	18–14g	16–14g

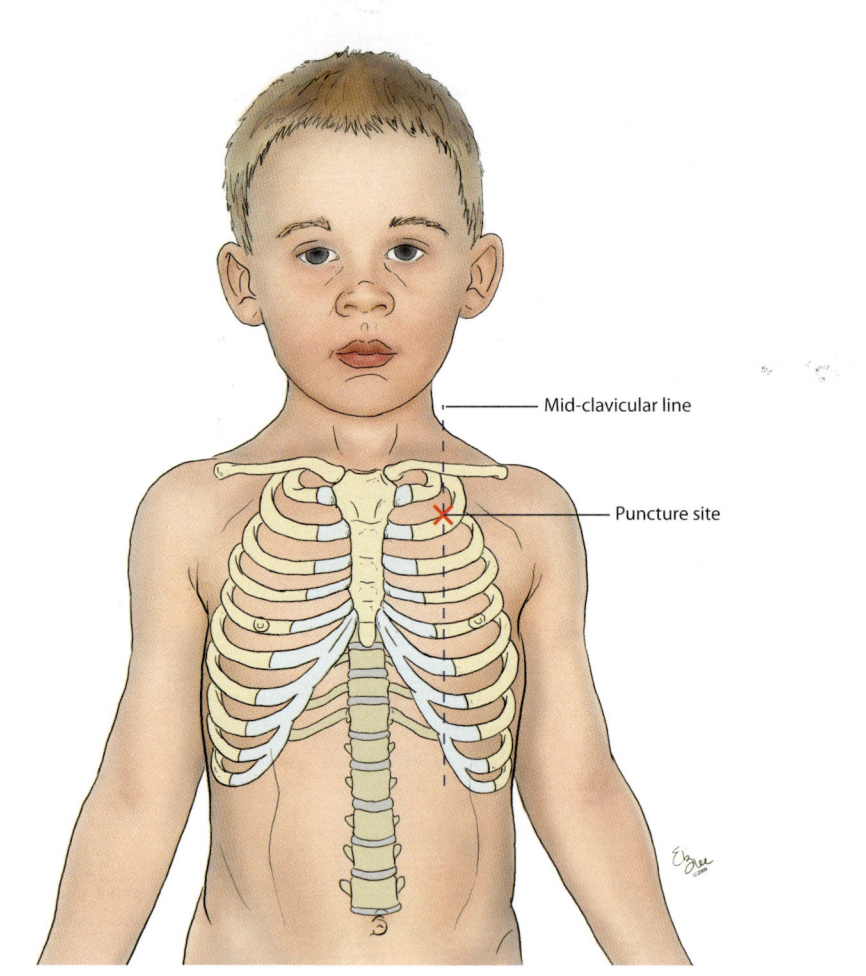

Figure 5.7 *A catheter should be inserted over the top of the second or third rib in the midclavicular line to decompress a tension pneumothorax.*

If a symptomatic tension pneumothorax is diagnosed, the chest must be decompressed by inserting an appropriately sized plastic catheter (Table 5.1) over the top of the second or third rib in the midclavicular line (Fig. 5.7). An acceptable alternative method is to insert the catheter over the fourth or fifth rib along the midaxillary line. If the catheter is left open to air, this converts a tension pneumothorax into a simple pneumothorax. Indications to perform an emergency decompression of a tension pneumothorax include loss of consciousness, severe respiratory distress, cyanosis, and traumatic cardiorespiratory arrest with evidence of chest injury. If protocols prohibit chest decompression, the patient must be immediately transported to the nearest facility. Needle decompression is a temporary option; if it is performed, it must be replaced with a chest tube as soon as possible.

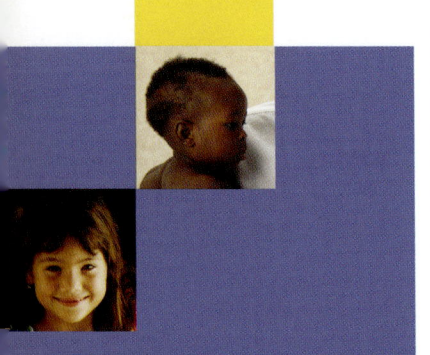

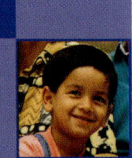

Pediatric Trauma Life Support

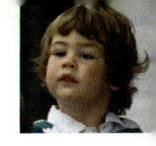

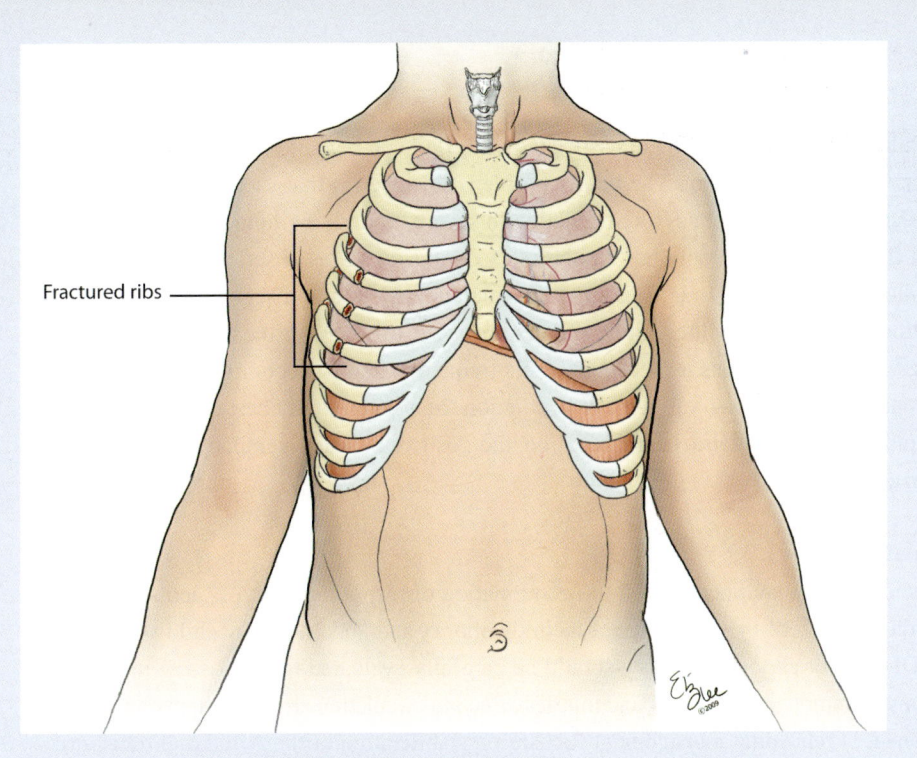

Figure 5.8a *Anatomy of a flail chest in a child.*

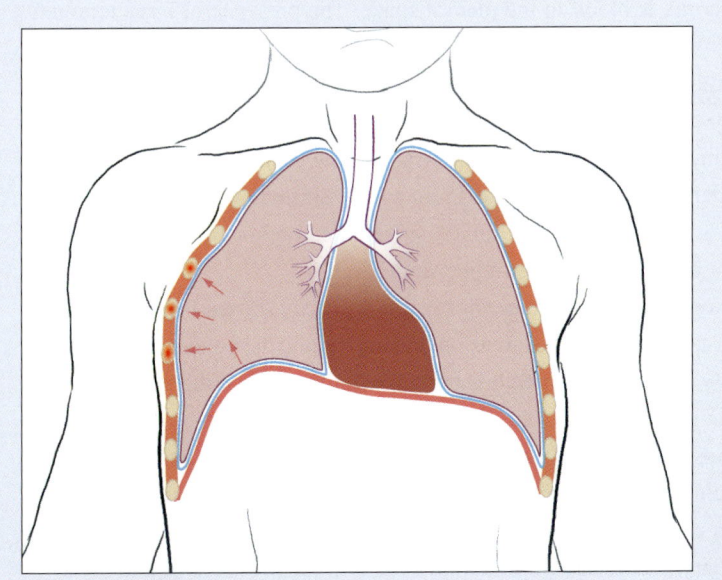

Figure 5.8b *Flail chest on inspiration*

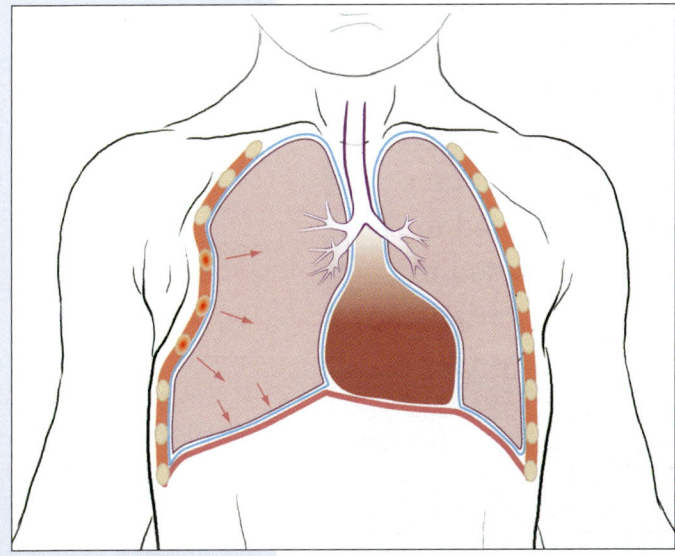

Figure 5.8c *Flail chest on expiration*

Flail Chest By definition, a flail chest occurs when three or more adjacent ribs are fractured in at least two places. This results in a segment of chest wall that is no longer mechanically contiguous with the rest of the thorax. The flail can occur laterally or anteriorly and typically produces a paradoxical motion such that on inspiration, while the rest of the chest expands, the flail sucks in; on expiration, when the rest of the chest contracts, the flail flutters out (Fig. 5.8). It is unusual, because of the flexible nature of a child's ribs, for a "true" flail chest to occur. However, when rib fractures do occur, any number of rib fractures—not necessarily two contiguous ribs—may result in paradoxical movement of the chest. Frequently, in an adult, the paradoxical motion associated with a flail segment is not of significance. Although this injury is unusual

Pediatric Thoracic Trauma

Pearls

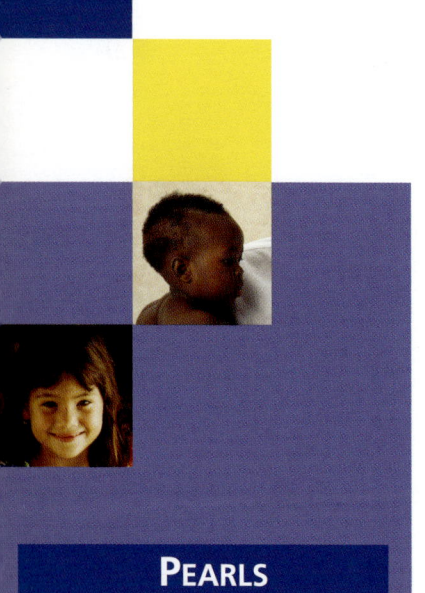

Three thoracic injuries are life-threatening and require immediate intervention: open pneumothorax, tension pneumothorax, and flail chest. Provide 100 percent oxygen and be prepared to use the skills needed to immediately intervene.

in a child, paradoxical movement associated with flail can be quite debilitating and may mandate assisted ventilation. The bigger problem, however, is that such serious injury to the chest wall is almost always associated with severe, underlying lung injury. A patient with a flail segment generally has a pulmonary contusion and is at serious risk for a hemothorax or pneumothorax. Findings may include a visible flail segment, tenderness to palpation of the chest wall, crepitus, and respiratory distress. After the airway has been secured, assist ventilations as necessary. This frequently can be accomplished effectively in a young child with bag-valve-mask ventilation. In a severe flail chest condition, the best stabilization is endotracheal intubation and positive pressure ventilation (internal stabilization).

Circulation

Thoracic trauma may present with the combination of respiratory distress and shock. In addition, because of the proximity of a child's thorax and abdomen, any child with an isolated chest or abdominal injury should be carefully evaluated for coexisting injury. The two most common pediatric thoracic injuries affecting circulation are hemothorax and cardiac tamponade. Prehospital management focuses on stabilization of the ABCs and transport.

Hemothorax A hemothorax is blood in the pleural space. The presence of large amounts of blood involving up to one half or more of one thoracic cavity is considered a massive hemothorax. Massive hemothorax, which is most often caused by penetrating rather than blunt trauma, is generally caused by disruption of a major pulmonary or systemic vessel. Blood accumulating within a pleural space compresses the lung on the affected side. If blood accumulates under pressure, the mediastinum can be shifted away from the hemothorax, resulting in a "tension" effect. Unlike tension pneumothorax, though, this cannot be adequately relieved by needle decompression.

The signs and symptoms of massive hemothorax are primarily those of hypovolemia and respiratory compromise (Fig. 5.9). Like a tension pneumothorax, the patient is generally hypotensive, in respiratory distress, and breath sounds are diminished on the affected side. However, unlike a tension pneumothorax, the chest may be dull to percussion (unreliable in children), the neck veins are generally flat, and the trachea is almost always in the midline. In the young child with a very mobile mediastinum, the neck veins may become distended and the trachea can be shifted. In this situation, it is reasonable to attempt a midclavicular or midaxillary needle decompression to rule out the presence of a tension pneumothorax. Table 5.2 provides a comparison between tension pneumothorax and massive hemothorax. Monitor the child very closely when treating him for a massive hemothorax. After the airway and breathing have been appropriately addressed, shock must be managed, following the guidelines in Chapter 7.

Cardiac Tamponade Cardiac tamponade is usually due to penetrating injury and is unusual in preadolescent children. The heart is surrounded by the pericardial sac, which is an inelastic membrane. If the potential space between the heart and the pericardium fills with air, blood, or fluid, this disrupts normal cardiac mechanics and may cause severe hemodynamic derangement. As this space fills with fluid, the heart is compressed, which limits diastolic filling. This then limits cardiac output and may result in poor perfusion and hypotension. Signs and symptoms include the diagnostic triad of hypotension, distended neck veins, and muffled heart tones. A patient also may have a paradoxical pulse, which

Pediatric Trauma Life Support

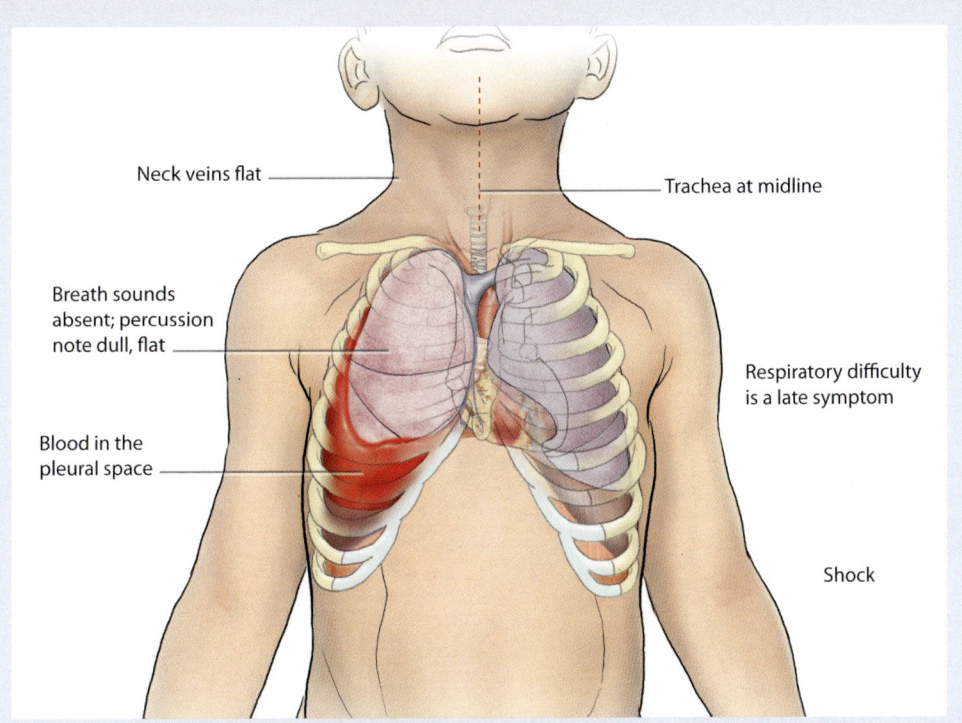

Figure 5.9 *Massive hemothorax is indicated by the presence of a large amount of blood involving one half of one thoracic cavity or more.*

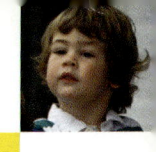

PEARLS

Hemothorax and cardiac tamponade are less common in children; prehospital management focuses on stabilization of the ABCs and transport.

Table 5.2: Tension Pneumothorax, Massive Hemothorax, and Cardiac Tamponade

Signs/Symptoms	Tension Pneumothorax	Massive Hemothorax	Cardiac Tamponade
Respiratory distress	Yes	No[1]	No[1]
Shock	Yes	Yes	Yes
JVD	Yes	No	Yes
Tracheal shift	Yes	No[2]	No
Breath sounds	Decreased	Decreased	Normal
Resonance	Increased	Decreased	Normal

1 Respiratory distress may occur late in the process
2 Tracheal shift may occur late in the process

can be evidenced by the loss of peripheral pulse during inspiration. Cardiac tamponade is sometimes difficult to distinguish from a tension pneumothorax (Table 5.2). Stabilize the ABCs and prepare to transport the patient. This injury is rapidly fatal and cannot be readily treated in the prehospital setting. Quick package and transport are crucial. Figure 5.10 summarizes the pathophysiology and physical findings of cardiac tamponade.

Rapid Trauma Survey

A rapid head-to-toe survey is necessary to rule out other life-threatening injuries. The energy necessary to cause injuries to the thorax may be enough to cause injury to other regions of the body such as the head or abdomen.

Pediatric Thoracic Trauma

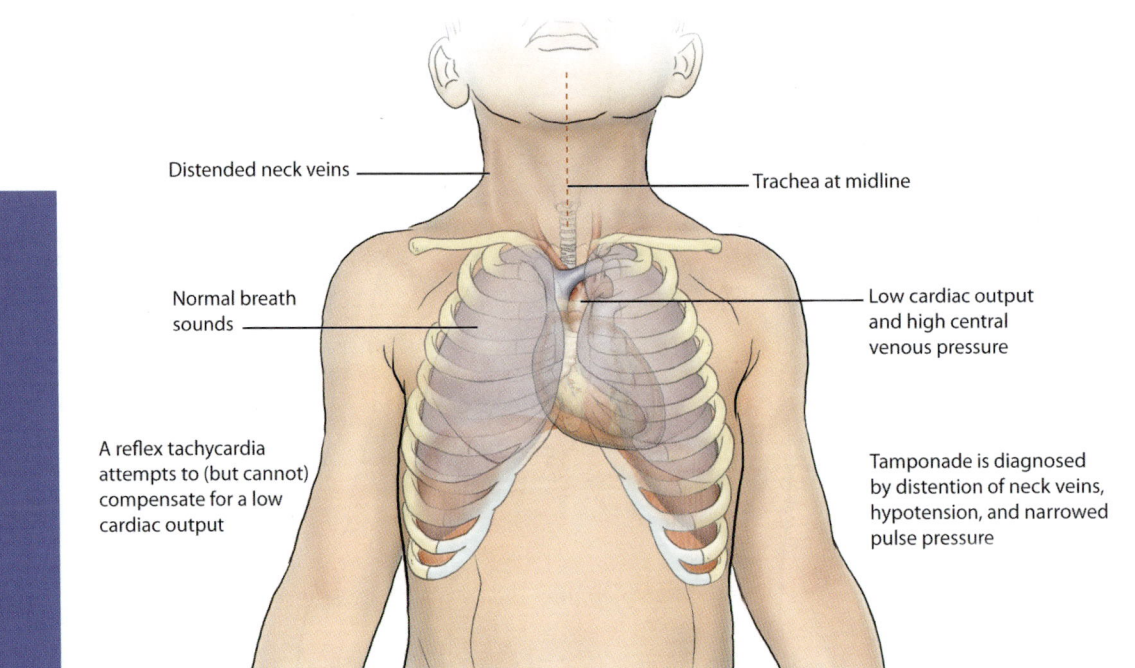

Figure 5.10a *Cardiac tamponade occurs when the space between the heart and pericardium fills with air, blood, or fluid.*

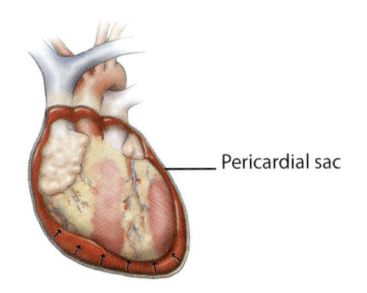

Labels: Distended neck veins; Trachea at midline; Normal breath sounds; Low cardiac output and high central venous pressure; A reflex tachycardia attempts to (but cannot) compensate for a low cardiac output; Tamponade is diagnosed by distention of neck veins, hypotension, and narrowed pulse pressure.

Pericardial sac

Blood in the pericardial sac compresses the heart and impaires ventricular filling

Figure 5.10b *A detailed view of the heart in a patient with a cardiac tamponade.*

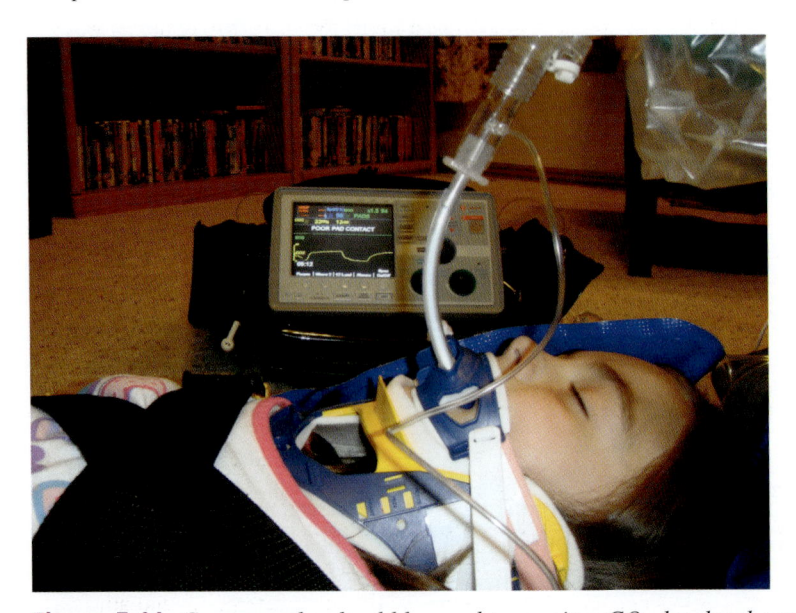

Figure 5.11 *Capnography should be used to monitor CO_2 levels whenever available.*

Pediatric Trauma Life Support

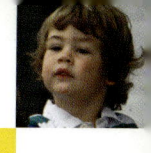

Critical Interventions and Transport Decisions

Any child with an unstable injury, insufficient respiration, shock, or an altered mental status should be a load-and-go patient and therefore rapidly packaged and transported. If the child has an open pneumothorax, tension pneumothorax, hemothorax, or flail chest, extra care should be taken to expedite transport. The child should be rapidly and appropriately packaged for transport. Any child who has a chest injury should be monitored with a cardiac monitor (possible injury to the heart), and pulse oximetry. All children should be on 100 percent oxygen to maintain oxygen saturation above 95 percent. If available, capnography should be used to monitor CO_2 level (Fig. 5.11).

Airway and Cervical Spine

Most airways can be stabilized with bag-valve-mask ventilation. If the child cannot be effectively bag-valve-mask ventilated, then endotracheal intubation should be performed prior to transport to the receiving facility. It is rare for a child to require endotracheal intubation.

Breathing

If a child with multiple injuries is being ventilated with bag-valve-mask ventilation, you should be vigilant for a decrease in lung compliance revealed by difficulty in squeezing the bag. Children are especially prone to barotrauma, and you should be alert to the possibility of the development of a tension pneumothorax in anyone receiving assisted ventilation. Pulse oximetry and capnography will provide a continual assessment of the patient's oxygen saturation and CO_2 level.

Circulation

All children with a chest injury should have continuous cardiac monitoring. Although uncommon in pediatric patients, children with a chest injury occasionally will have an associated cardiac injury and may develop dysrhythmias. If time allows, IV access may be established en route to the hospital. If the child has signs or symptoms of shock, appropriate fluid resuscitation, as discussed in Chapter 7, should be instituted. The use of the pneumatic antishock garment (PASG) is not appropriate in a thoracic injury and should not be used for the child with a suspected chest injury because it may increase intrathoracic bleeding to a lethal level. Inflation of the abdominal compartment also may further compromise the respiratory status of the child.

ITLS Secondary Survey

Complete a detailed assessment if time allows. Some children with thoracic trauma need to have their injuries identified in the field, but the majority of their management will occur at the hospital. A comprehensive list of potential thoracic injuries follows.

Traumatic Aortic Rupture

Traumatic aortic rupture is the most common cause of sudden death in motor vehicle collisions or falls from heights in adults. It is very uncommon in young children because of their elastic and mobile aortas. However, when it does occur in a child, it is almost always fatal. For survivors, salvage is possible with prompt diagnosis and surgery. Signs and physical findings in the prehospital setting are not specific and an advanced diagnostic test such as a CT scan is usually required for diagnosis. As long as you follow the usual management of thoracic trauma (100 percent oxygen, cardiac monitor, and rapid transport), you will give your patient the best chance of survival.

Tracheal or Bronchial Tree Injury

This injury may result from either blunt or penetrating trauma and is relatively rare, even more so in young children than in adults. Definitive management is difficult in the prehospital setting, and a high index of suspicion will allow for early diagnosis and treatment once the appropriate facility is reached. Disruption of the trachea or bronchus often results in subcutaneous emphysema and tension pneumothorax. Treatment in the field should be aimed at managing these entities. Again, the focus should be on the rapid package and transport of the patient after securing the airway and administration of 100 percent oxygen. The patient should be monitored carefully for the development of a tension pneumothorax and dysrhythmias.

Myocardial Contusion

This is an unusual and much over-diagnosed entity in adults. In children, it is also unusual, but more often under-diagnosed. It should be a consideration in any patient suffering blunt chest injury. Blunt injury to the central chest can result in a bruise or contusion to the heart. Abnormalities can range from mild tachycardia to cardiovascular collapse. Symptoms may be absent or include chest pain and shortness of breath. Findings may include external evidence of injury, tachycardia, or abnormalities on ECG. Assess and treat the patient's ABCs and remember to monitor for development of dysrhythmias. Be prepared to treat dysrhythmias as they occur. Use ACLS/PALS protocols.

Diaphragmatic Injury

Traumatic diaphragmatic injury can occur in thoracoabdominal penetrating injury or from any severe blunt injury to the thorax or abdomen that results in a sudden increase in intra-abdominal pressure. This may include seatbelt injuries, kicks to the abdomen, falls, or crush injuries. A blunt or penetrating force leads to a tear in the diaphragm. Intra-abdominal pressure, which is generally positive, overcomes intrapleural pressure, which is generally negative, forcing intra-abdominal contents into the chest. This can compromise blood supply to the intra-abdominal contents and diminish ventilatory capacity of the affected lung. Ruptures tend to occur more often on the left side than the right side and are difficult to diagnose in the prehospital setting. Symptoms may include chest or abdominal pain and shortness of breath (very nonspecific). Findings may include external evidence of thoracoabdominal penetrating or blunt injury, abnormalities in chest wall excursion or ventilatory rate, diminished breath sounds in the chest, or bowel sounds heard in the chest. The abdomen on occasion appears scaphoid if a large quantity of the abdominal content has entered the chest. Like traumatic aortic rupture, this injury usually requires advanced hospital diagnostic tests to confirm. After addressing the ABCs, rapidly package and transport the patient. Placement of a nasogastric tube en route to the receiving facility may be considered if time and protocols allow.

Esophageal Injury

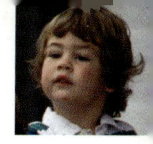

Esophageal injury is rare and almost always due to penetrating injury. Its diagnosis in the prehospital setting is not generally possible, and management should be limited to the associated trauma.

Pulmonary Contusion

Pulmonary contusion is the most common form of chest injury following blunt trauma and, in the child, may occur with no external evidence of injury. It should be diagnosed based on a high index of suspicion and treated in the prehospital setting with supportive care. Special attention should be given to maintaining oxygen saturation above 95 percent.

Rib Fractures

Rib fractures in the child, even when isolated, carry a very high mortality rate and should be treated as a sign of serious injury. Because of the flexibility of a child's chest, a rib fracture indicates that the child has received a focused injury with a high degree of force. This extreme force almost always results in underlying lung damage. Fractures of the first and second ribs can be associated with vascular injury. Fractures of the fifth through twelfth ribs can be associated with intra-abdominal injury. The management should be to provide supportive care and to realize that rib fractures are a strong indicator of severe trauma in the child. Unexplained rib fractures are suggestive of child abuse.

Other Injuries

Other thoracic injuries in the child may include impalement injuries, traumatic asphyxia, thoracic spine injury, sternal fracture, and simple pneumothorax.

Impalement injuries should be treated as impalement injuries anywhere, i.e., the impaled object should be left in place and stabilized. Associated abnormalities should be dealt with as appropriate. It is important to remember that, depending on the object and the location, there is a potential for development of any of the injuries previously mentioned.

Traumatic asphyxia is a physical finding and a misnomer because the condition is not caused by asphyxia. The syndrome results from a severe compression injury to the chest, such as compression under a heavy object. The sudden pressure on the heart and mediastinum transmits this force to the capillaries of the head and neck and results in confluent petecchial hemorrhages above the level of the compression with swelling of the head and neck, capillary hemorrhage, and discoloration. Traumatic asphyxia indicates that the patient has suffered severe blunt injury and should be an indication that significant underlying trauma may be present.

Thoracic spine and sternal fractures are also indications that the patient has suffered severe injury and should be treated as such. In addition, the potential for thoracic spine injury should be dealt with by appropriate spinal motion restriction. Sternal fractures are associated with myocardial contusions, so monitor the patient for dysrhythmias en route to the hospital.

Simple pneumothorax, which is generally well tolerated by adults, may not be so easily tolerated by children. A simple pneumothorax should be suspected if breath sounds are diminished and the child is in respiratory distress. Increased resonance is an unreliable indicator in pediatric patients. Patients with a simple pneumothorax should be prepared for emergency needle decompression during transport if a tension pneumothorax develops.

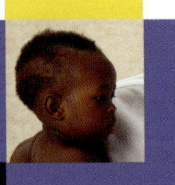

Case Study *continued*

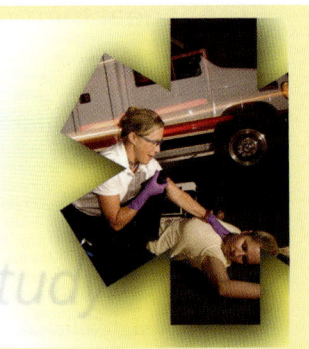

John, Susan, and Bob of the Emergency Transport System (ETS) have been called to a residential area. An 18-month-old child was backed over by the family car while leaving the driveway. As the father was slowly moving in reverse, he felt the rear wheel "run over" an object; he immediately stopped the car and found the child under the car. The scene is safe, and both parents are with the child.

Susan acts as the team leader. Her general impression is poor. Upon arrival, the child is unresponsive with rapid, shallow, labored respirations at a fast rate. Carotid pulses were present and faintly palpable at a fast rate. No radial pulses were palpable. Susan decides this is a priority patient and a load-and-go situation. Bob stabilizes the neck, and John immediately opens the airway and gives assisted ventilation with a bag-valve mask and high-concentration oxygen.

In performing a Rapid Trauma Survey, tire marks are noted on the left chest, which extend to the sternum. Crepitus is noted on the left upper chest, but no subcutaneous emphysema is present upon palpation. Breath sounds are very diminished in the left lung field. The trachea is midline with neck veins flat. John is not happy with the response from bag-valve-mask ventilation with high-flow, high-concentration oxygen. Spinal motion restriction is maintained. Because of the inability to ventilate the child by use of a bag-valve mask and a persistent pulse oximetry reading of <90 percent, the child is intubated in the field.

With the assistance of the parents, the child is placed on a pediatric long board and transported to the ambulance. Medical direction is notified. Two large-bore IVs are initiated en route and two fluid boluses of 20 mL/kg are administered for tachycardia and poor perfusion. Reassessment of the ABCs in the ITLS Ongoing Exam indicates a patent and secured airway via endotracheal tube. Assisted ventilations are easy to deliver and result in a pulse oximetry reading of 95 percent. The child's heart rate decreases to about 130 bpm with volume resuscitation.

Upon arrival at the receiving facility, the child has strong carotid and radial pulses. The child was admitted to the hospital with a hemothorax and pulmonary contusion. He was discharged home 21 days later.

Pediatric Trauma Life Support

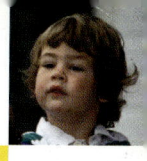

Case Study *wrap-up*

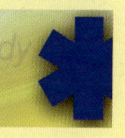

In this case, as you approach the child, you should recognize that this mechanism of injury is very likely to result in life-threatening injuries. Care must be taken to open the airway while maintaining spinal motion restriction. Achieve airway management and assist breathing without delay. The presentation of profound shock must be quickly addressed. Immediate IV access and fluid bolus during transport is required. The diagnosis of hemothorax is uncommon in children but can rapidly become life-threatening due to the limited circulating blood volume present in a small child. The loss of even small amounts of blood can place a young child in profound shock. Tachycardia and poor perfusion are early indicators of shock; hypotension is a very late finding. Because of strong compensatory mechanisms, children have the ability to maintain normal or near-normal blood pressure in compensated shock. The absence of breath sounds and the presence of shock should suggest hemothorax or tension pneumothorax, which may be associated with a coexisting abdominal injury.

SUMMARY

1. The presence of chest injuries often accompanies multisystem trauma.
2. Underlying injuries may be difficult as relatively minimal external evidence of trauma may be present.
3. Completion of the ITLS Primary Assessment and early identification of tension pneumothorax, cardiac tamponade and flail chest are essential to facilitate appropriate interventions.
4. Airway management, ventilatory support and maintenance of adequate perfusion remain paramount for a positive outcome of your pediatric patient.

Recommended Reading

American College of Surgeons. "Thoracic Trauma." In *Advanced Trauma Life Support for Doctors*, 8th ed. Chicago: Author, 2008.

Bliss, David and Mark Silen. "Pediatric Thoracic Trauma." *Critical Care Medicine* 30 (2002): s409–15.

Campbell, John Emory, ed. "Thoracic Trauma." In *International Trauma Life Support for Prehospital Care Providers*, 6th ed., 94–113. Upper Saddle River, N.J.: Pearson/Prentice Hall, 2008.

Garcia, Victor F., Catherine S. Gotschall, et al. "Rib Fractures in Children: A Marker of Severe Trauma." *Journal of Trauma* 30 (1990): 695.

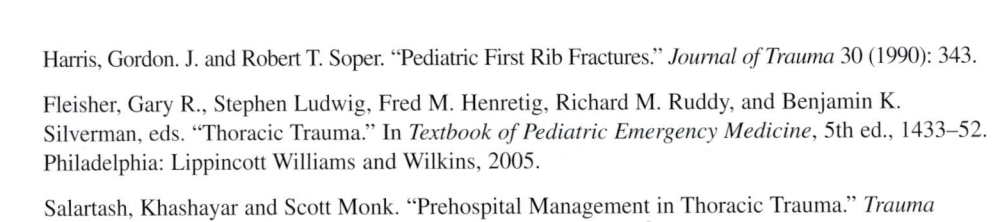

Harris, Gordon. J. and Robert T. Soper. "Pediatric First Rib Fractures." *Journal of Trauma* 30 (1990): 343.

Fleisher, Gary R., Stephen Ludwig, Fred M. Henretig, Richard M. Ruddy, and Benjamin K. Silverman, eds. "Thoracic Trauma." In *Textbook of Pediatric Emergency Medicine*, 5th ed., 1433–52. Philadelphia: Lippincott Williams and Wilkins, 2005.

Salartash, Khashayar and Scott Monk. "Prehospital Management in Thoracic Trauma." *Trauma Quarterly* 14 (1998): 161–66.

6

CHAPTER 6

Airway Management and Thoracic Trauma Skills

John P. Crow, MD, FACS
Ann Hoffman, RN, CPN
Sherri Kovach, RN, EMT-B

Objectives

On completion of this skill station, you should be able to:

BASIC AIRWAY MANAGEMENT

1. Perform a pediatric airway assessment.
2. Identify indications and contraindications for airway management devices including oropharyngeal airways, nasopharyngeal airways, and bag-valve-mask ventilation.
3. Manage the pediatric airway using devices appropriate to patient presentations and treatment protocols.

ADVANCED AIRWAY MANAGEMENT

1. Perform an endotracheal intubation using in-line spinal motion restriction.
2. Discuss the indications for needle cricothyroidotomy.
3. Discuss the indications for needle decompression of the chest.

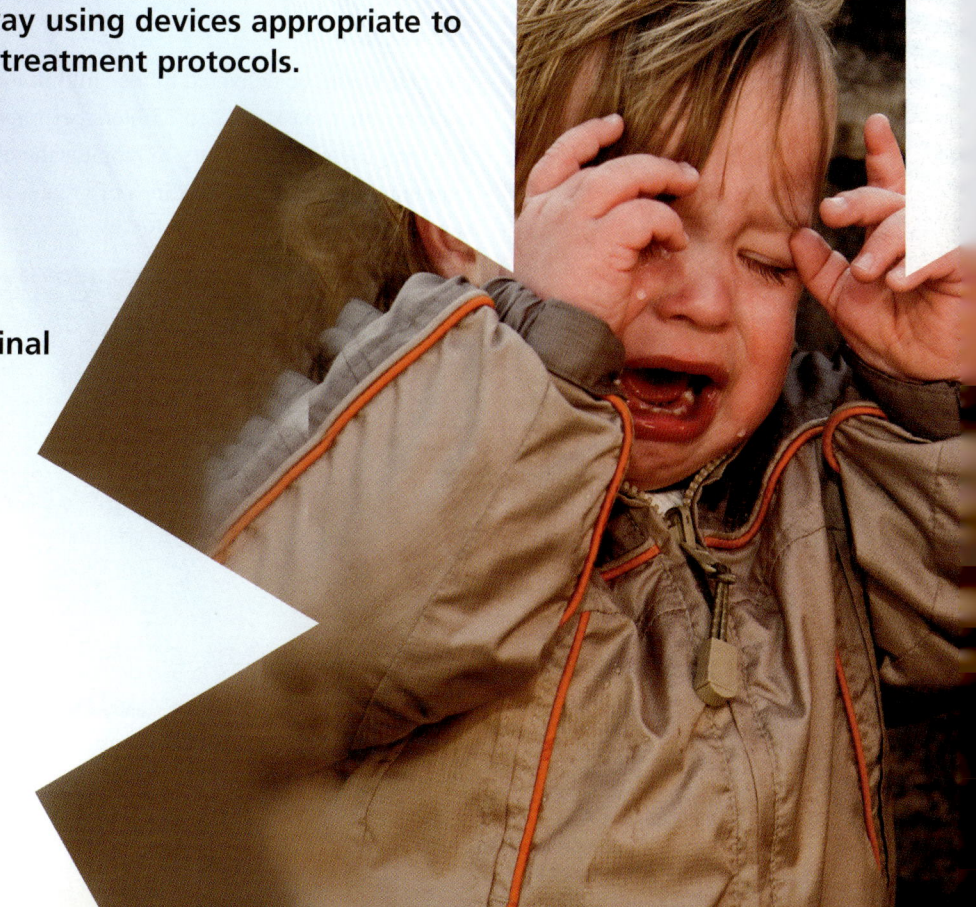

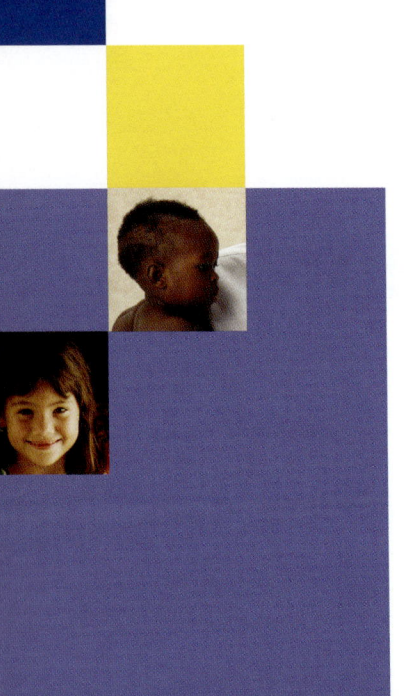

BASIC AIRWAY MANAGEMENT

Airway Assessment

After completing the Scene Size-Up, approach the pediatric patient and initiate the ITLS Primary Survey beginning with obtaining a general impression. As you apply spinal motion restriction, proceed with determining the level of consciousness. In assessing the airway, if the oropharynx is without evidence of secretions, blood, foreign body, or anatomical deformity and the child can speak in a clear voice or has a normal cry, monitor the child's ability to maintain a clear airway. This does not ensure that the child will always be able to maintain that airway, so continue reassessing and monitoring the child's airway on an ongoing basis.

Immediately address any evidence of foreign objects, bleeding, or loose teeth by removal and oropharynx suctioning. If the child does not respond verbally, open the airway using the modified jaw thrust. If the child's level of consciousness remains diminished and there is no gag reflex, you may need to utilize an airway adjunct and initiate bag-valve-mask ventilation.

Supplemental Oxygen

Indications
Always administer supplemental oxygen (Fig. 6.1).

Contraindications
None.

Procedure
Oxygen should be delivered to the child in the highest concentration possible. A pediatric nonrebreather mask at 12 to 15 liters per minute of oxygen should be placed on the child. You may use pulse oximetry to monitor the child's oxygenation (Fig. 6.2). The goal is to maintain pulse oximetry readings of greater than 95 percent. Remember that poor perfusion may also compromise pulse oximetry readings.

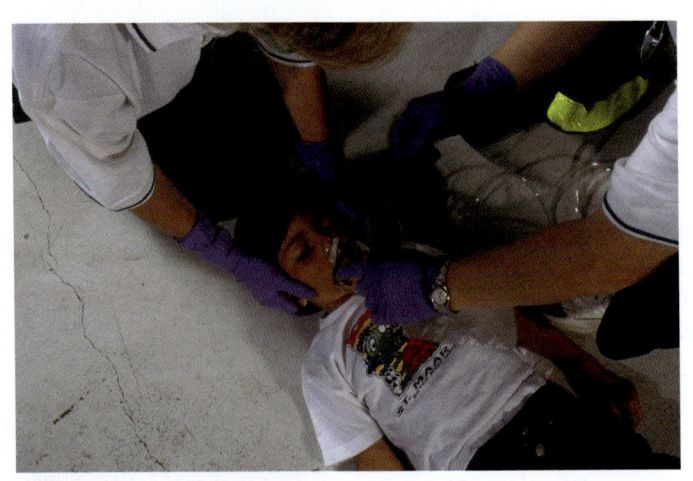

Figure 6.1 *Administer supplemental 100 percent oxygen to pediatric patients.*

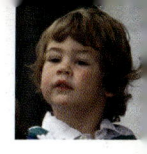

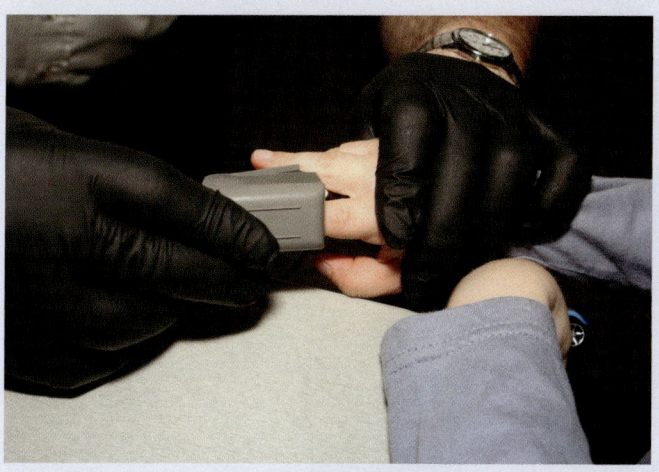

Figure 6.2 *Use a pulse oximeter to monitor the child's oxygenation, maintaining readings of 95 percent or greater.*

Oropharyngeal Airway

Indications

In children who are unconscious and unable to maintain their own airway, you may use an artificial airway such as an oropharyngeal airway. Normally, nasopharyngeal airways are not used due to the small size of the nares and because small children are mouth breathers.

Contraindications

Do not use an oropharyngeal airway on children who have a gag reflex, because the device may stimulate vomiting.

Procedure

Correct insertion is critical. Estimate the correct size as shown in Figure 6.3. The base should be at the level of the incisors and the tip at the angle of the jaw. It may be helpful to use a tongue blade to depress the tongue and insert the oropharyngeal airway (Fig. 6.4). In children, it is not recommended to insert the oropharyngeal airway upside down and rotate into place. This may result in soft tissue trauma and possible hemorrhage. Have suction available, as a patient who tolerates an oral airway still has a diminished gag reflex and is at risk for aspiration.

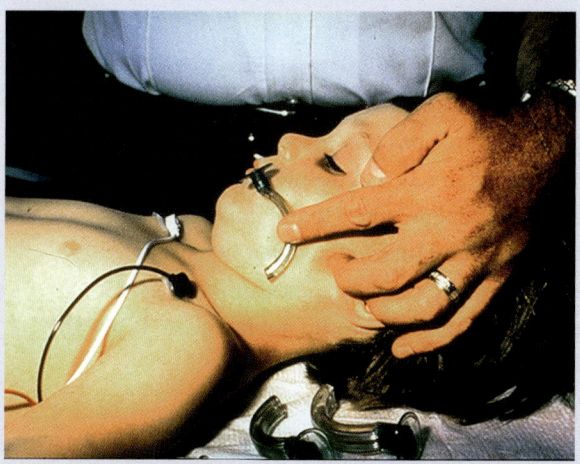

Figure 6.3 *Estimate the size of the oropharyngeal airway by measuring the base of it against the level of the child's incisors and the tip at the angle of the child's jaw.*

Airway Management and Thoracic Trauma Skills

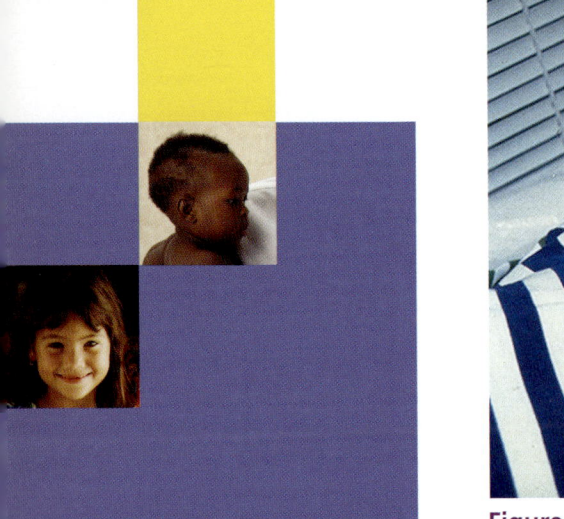

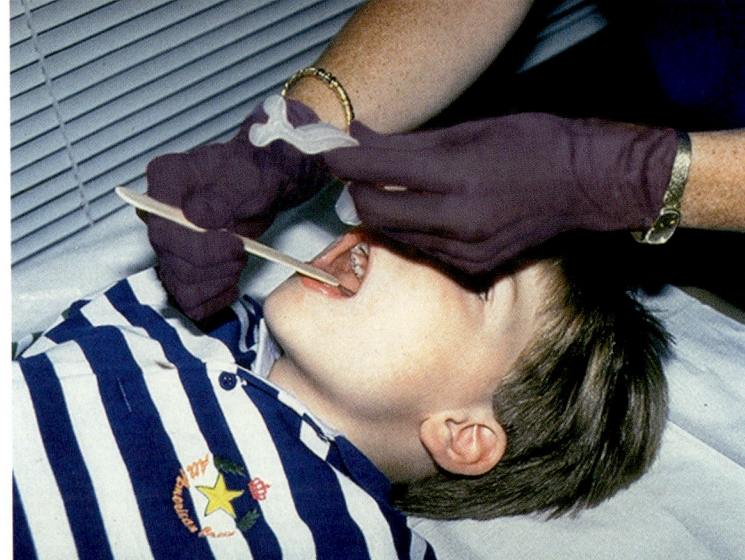

Figure 6.4 *Use a tongue depressor to depress the tongue when inserting the oropharyngeal airway.*

Bag-Valve-Mask Ventilation

Indications
Bag-valve-mask ventilation is indicated for any child with apnea, inadequate respiration, or severely altered mental status.

Contraindications
Do not use bag-valve-mask ventilation on children with an intact airway who maintain a pulse oximetry reading of greater than 95 percent. If there is upper airway obstruction or facial trauma, bag-valve-mask ventilation may complicate the process and increase the risk of pushing a foreign body into the lung.

Procedure
Carefully seal the mask from the bridge of the nose to the cleft of the chin using the E-C Clamp procedure (Fig. 6.5). An appropriately sized mask will fit across the bridge of the child's nose, not extend beyond the cleft of the chin, and should not apply pressure on the child's eyes. Hold the mask on the child's face with one hand by placing your third, fourth, and fifth digits along the bony prominence of the child's mandible, making an "E." Lifting the mandible will facilitate anterior motion, creating a manual airway. Do not apply pressure on the soft tissues under the chin as this may compromise the airway. The thumb and forefinger create a "C" on the mask; this position facilitates adjustments over the face to maintain a seal. In a two-person procedure, this position involves one person holding the mask in place while maintaining a manual airway and the other person ventilating (Fig. 6.6). Also use the Sellick maneuver (cricoid pressure) to minimize the risk of aspiration and the amount of air bagged into the stomach. In addition, ensure that the respiratory rate and tidal volume are appropriate for age to limit insufflation of air into the stomach. People tend to hyperventilate even when they do not intend to. If possible, monitor ventilation with capnography (Fig. 6.7).

Pediatric Trauma Life Support

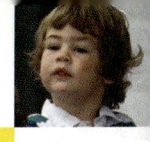

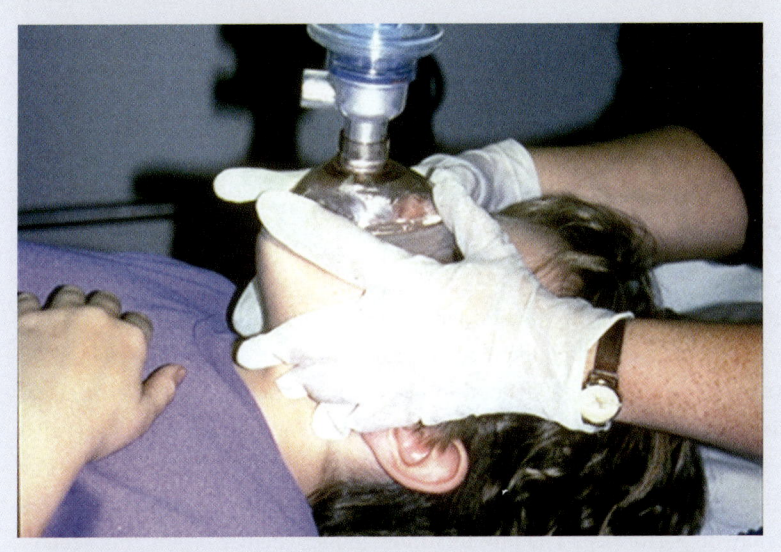

Figure 6.5 *When performing bag-valve-mask ventilation, seal the mask to the child's face using the E-C clamp method.*

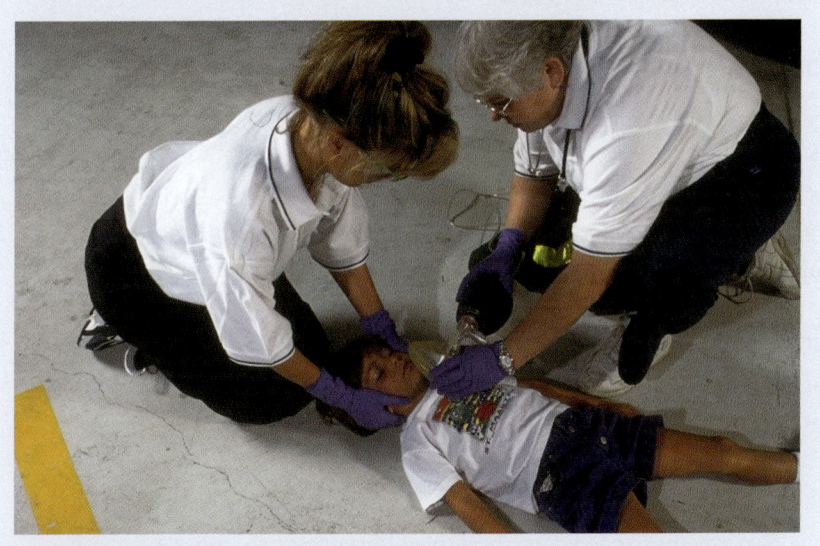

Figure 6.6 *When two rescuers perform bag-valve-mask ventilation, one rescuer ventilates when the other maintains manual restriction and holds the mask in place after it is applied.*

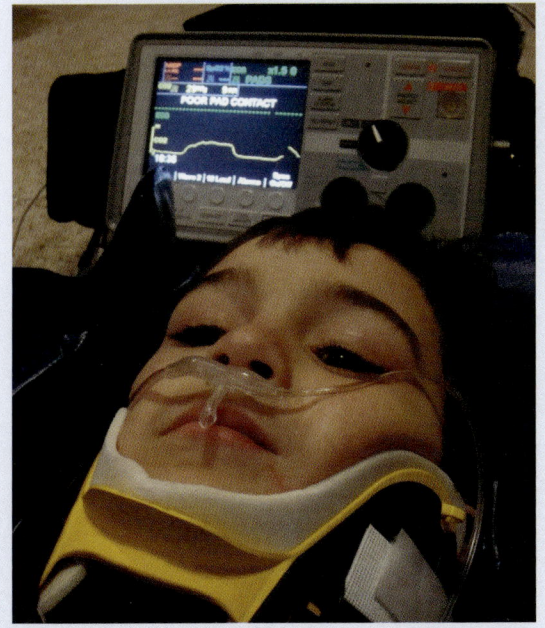

Figure 6.7 *Ventilation should be monitored with continuous wave-form capnography when available.*

Airway Management and Thoracic Trauma Skills

ADVANCED AIRWAY MANAGEMENT

Airway Assessment

When the child cannot be adequately ventilated with a bag-valve mask or is in danger of losing his airway, you may need to implement advanced airway procedures. However, this is typically a rare occurrence. Thoroughly suction the airway and begin bag-valve-mask ventilations prior to intubation. If the child can be adequately ventilated with the bag-valve mask, it is usually better not to perform endotracheal intubation. If a child is conscious but unable to manage the airway (e.g., airway burns), sedation may be needed before advanced airway maneuvers may be performed. The provider must judge whether prolonging scene or transport time to perform intubation is of greater benefit than rapid transport and airway support using noninvasive means.

Oral Intubation

Indications
Oral intubation is indicated when adequate ventilation cannot be achieved with a bag-valve mask or there is danger of losing the airway from edema (airway burns, allergic reaction, and so on) or upper airway bleeding.

Contraindications
Do not use oral intubation with a child who is maintaining his own airway or can be adequately ventilated with a bag-valve mask.

Equipment
Equipment includes correctly sized endotracheal tubes, laryngoscope, bag-valve mask, end-tidal CO_2 confirmation device, appropriate blade, and suction (Fig. 6.8).

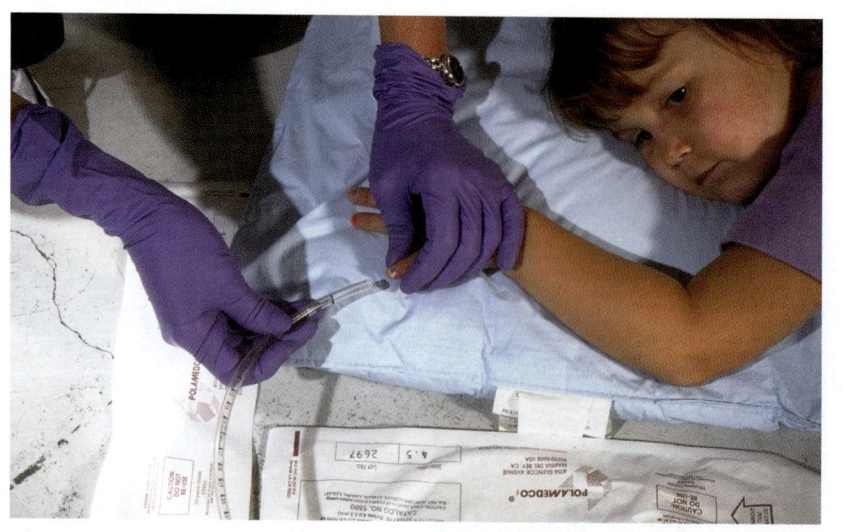

Figure 6.8 *Estimate the appropriately sized endotracheal tube by measuring it against the little finger of the pediatric patient.*

Pediatric Trauma Life Support

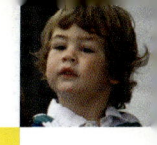

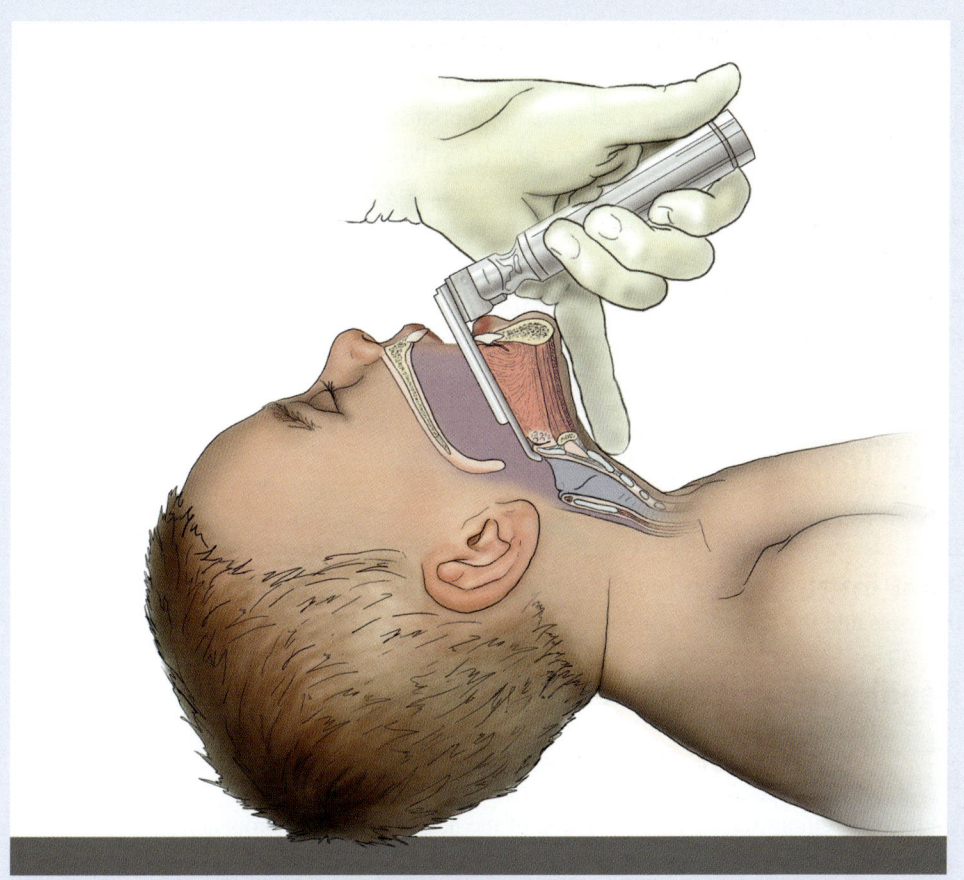

Figure 6.9 *When performing oral intubation, position the tip of the laryngoscope at the epiglottis or in the vallecula above the epiglottis.*

Procedure

The correct intubation procedure is as follows:
1. Set up equipment (suction, endotracheal tubes 0.5 mm smaller and 0.5 mm larger than the indicated size). You may select the endotracheal tube size based on the length-based tape, a card with values for age, the size of the child's little finger, or the size of the child's external nares.
2. Ventilate the patient with 100 percent oxygen before an intubation attempt.
3. A straight blade is suggested in the younger child and a curved blade in the older child.
4. Continue manual spinal motion restriction throughout the procedure.
5. Perform the Sellick maneuver during the intubation.
6. Using the left hand, position the tip of the laryngoscope blade at the epiglottis (straight blade) or in the vallecula above the epiglottis (curved blade) (Fig. 6.9).
7. Lift the tip of the blade up and away from you to directly see the glottic opening, using suction as needed to clear the pharynx.
8. Insert the tracheal tube from the right corner of the mouth, and insert the tube through the glottic opening.
9. The tube should rest with the two black lines at the vocal cords.
10. Secure the tube after confirming the correct position.

Airway Management and Thoracic Trauma Skills

Confirming Endotracheal Tube Placement

Correct endotracheal tube placement can be confirmed from the following signs:

1. The best confirmation procedures are appropriate readings with capnography, or a correct end-tidal CO_2 color reading (of yellow).
2. The child exhibits symmetrical chest movements.
3. There is a lack of breath sounds over the child's stomach.
4. There are equal breath sounds over both sides of the chest.
5. There is improvement in pulse oximetry readings.
6. Remember that condensation in the tube during exhalation, while often used as confirmation of endotracheal tube placement, is unreliable.

Blind Nasotracheal Intubation

Blind nasotracheal intubation is contraindicated in children. Inserting an endotracheal tube into the nares has a greater complication rate in children than in adults due to the size of the nares and the differences in the anatomy.

Needle Cricothyroidotomy

Indications

Under most circumstances, repositioning of the head and jaw, an oropharyngeal airway, or endotracheal intubation provides an adequate airway. Occasionally, a child with an upper airway foreign body, severe orofacial injuries, or a laryngeal fracture requires this procedure.

Contraindications

Only use this procedure in a child who has an obstructed airway for whom all other efforts to secure an airway have failed. This procedure may not be effective in children less than 12 years old because the narrowest part of the airway is the subglottic cricoid ring.

Equipment

Appropriate equipment includes an antiseptic swab, over-the-needle 14-gauge catheter, syringe, and jet insufflation device.

Procedure

Following is the correct procedure for needle cricothyroidotomy in a pediatric patient (Fig. 6.10):

1. Palpate the cricothyroid membrane anteriorly between thyroid cartilage and cricoid cartilage.
2. If time allows, prepare the area with antiseptic swabs.
3. Use a 14-gauge catheter over-the-needle device with syringe and puncture skin midline and directly over the cricothyroid membrane.
4. Direct the needle at a 45-degree angle caudally.
5. Insert the needle through the lower half of the cricothyroid membrane (Fig. 6.11). Air aspiration signifies entry into the tracheal lumen.

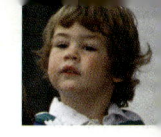

6. Withdraw stylet while advancing catheter downward.
7. Attach the catheter needle hub to a 3.0 ETT adapter and IV extension tubing and then to a jet insufflation device (ventilate at a 1:4 ratio). A second catheter may be needed to allow for exhalation. A bag-valve mask will not insufflate sufficient air to support the pediatric patient.
8. Auscultate the chest for adequate ventilation.
9. Secure the catheter.

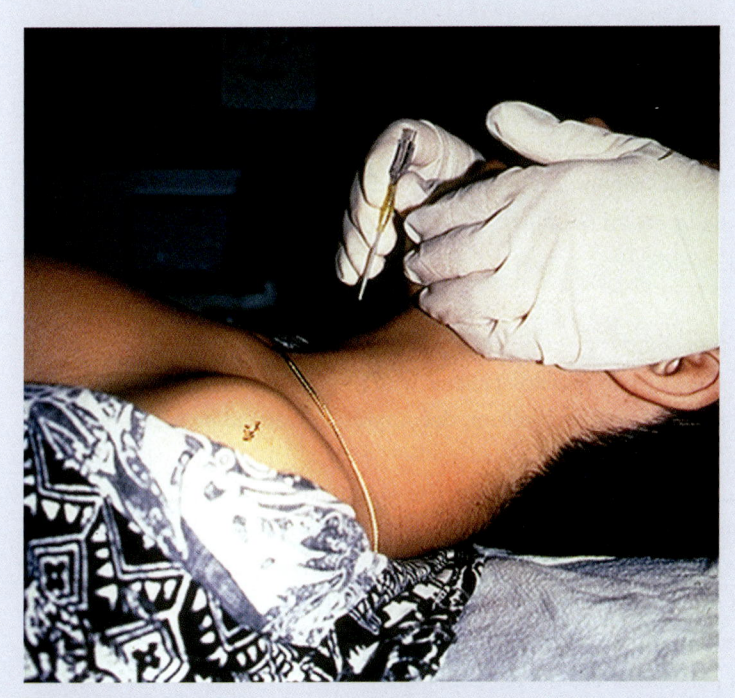

Figure 6.10 *Needle cricothyroidotomy performed on an adolescent.*

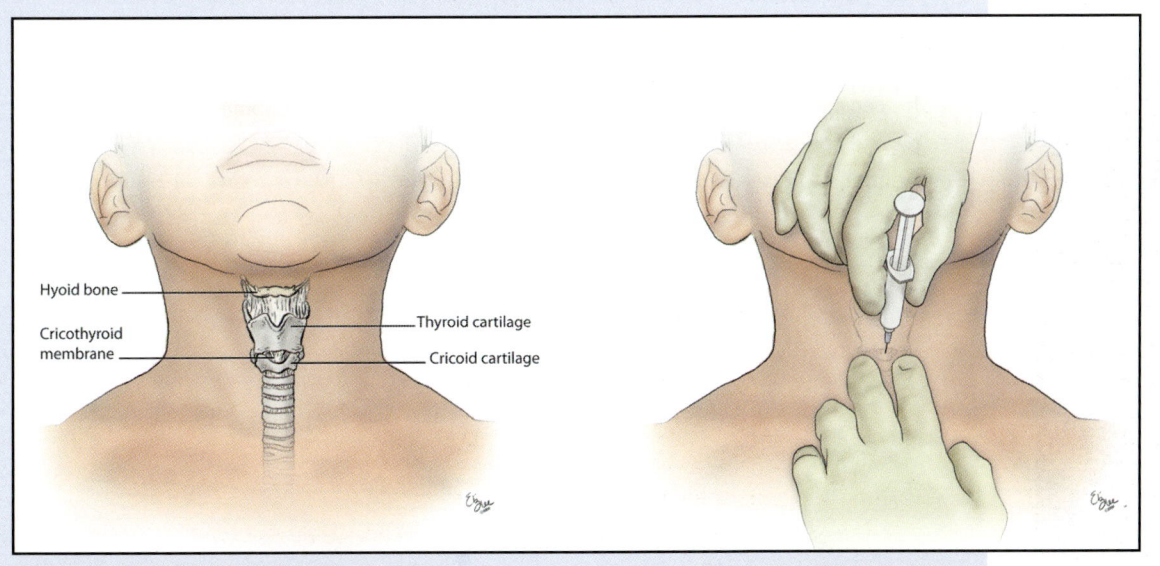

Figure 6.11 *When performing a needle cricothyroidotomy on a pediatric patient, insert the needle through the lower half of the cricothyroid membrane.*

Airway Management and Thoracic Trauma Skills

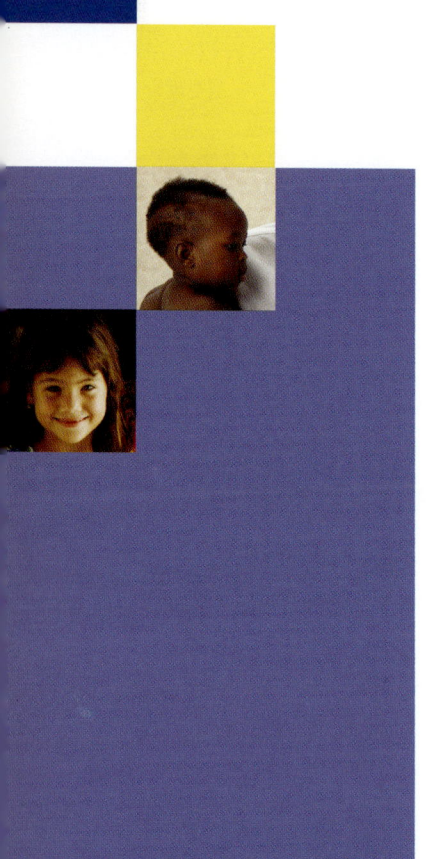

Needle Decompression of the Chest

Indications
A tension pneumothorax is diagnosed by the combination of severe respiratory distress, decreased or absent breath sounds, and signs of circulatory collapse. Distended neck veins, contralateral tracheal deviation, and ipsilateral hyperresonance to percussion are not usually present in pediatric cases.

Contraindications
Do not use needle decompression of the chest on pediatric patients with stable respiratory and circulatory status or pulse oximetry of 95 percent or greater.

Equipment
Appropriate equipment includes an antiseptic swab, 14- to 20-gauge over-the-needle catheter (see Table 5.1), and a 30 mL syringe.

Procedure
Following is the correct procedure for needle chest decompression in a pediatric patient:
1. Administer 100 percent oxygen to pediatric patients with suspected tension pneumothorax.
2. If signs of tension pneumothorax are present, decompression should be accomplished as follows (Fig. 6.12):
   a. Expose the entire chest area and clean the site vigorously with an antiseptic solution. Prepare an over-the-needle catheter (14- to 20-gauge).
   b. Insert the over-the-needle catheter in the midclavicular line on the affected side into the second or third intercostal space (Fig. 6.13). Hit the rib and then slide over it. The needle should be "walked" upward on the rib until it slides off the upper edge and penetrates into the parietal space.
   c. If the air is under tension, it will exit under pressure.
3. Remove the needle and tape the catheter in place. If available, use a one-way valve such as a Heimlich valve or an Asherman Chest Seal (Fig. 6.14). You may make a one-way valve by inserting the catheter through a rubber condom. The finger of a glove will not seal well enough to prevent air from entering the chest.
4. In teens and larger children, be sure that the catheter is long enough to enter into the pleural space.
5. Continue to reassess adequacy of ventilation.

Pediatric Trauma Life Support

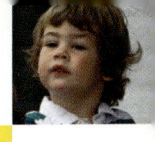

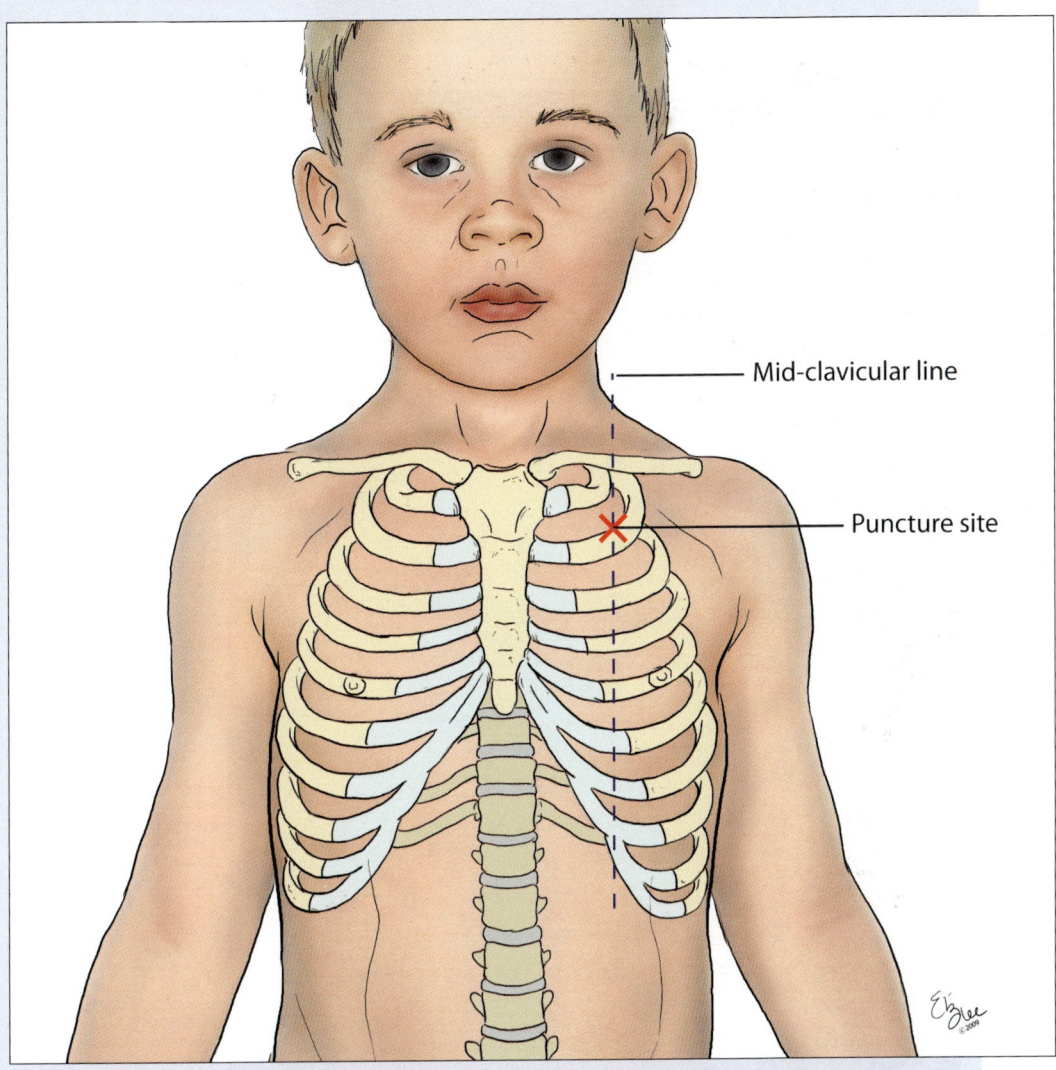

Figure 6.12 *The over-the-needle catheter should be inserted into the midclavicular line on the affected side into the second or third intercostal space when performing needle decompression on a child.*

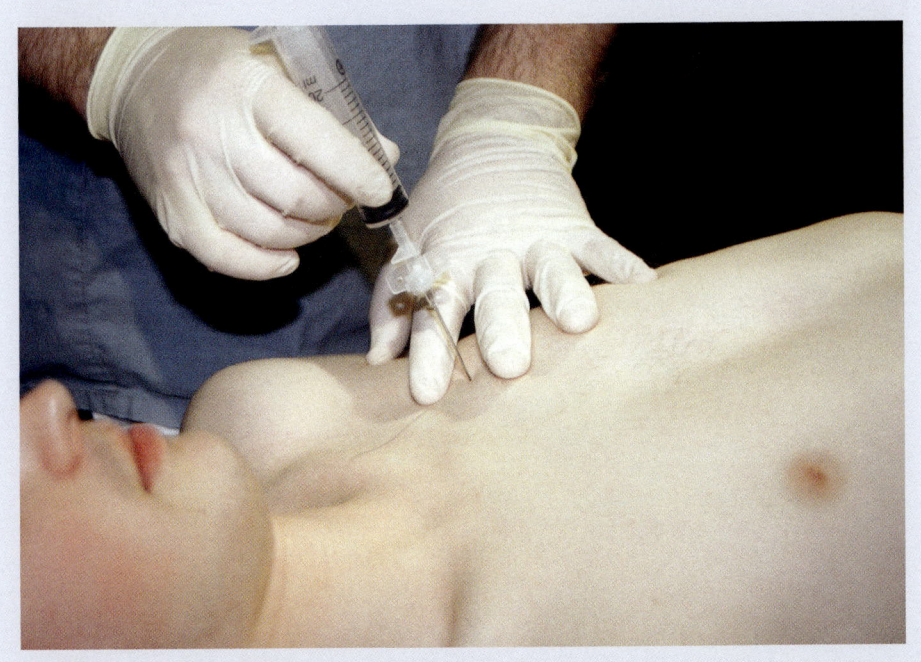

Figure 6.13 *When performing needle decompression of an older child or adolescent, be sure the catheter is long enough to enter the pleural space.*

Airway Management and Thoracic Trauma Skills

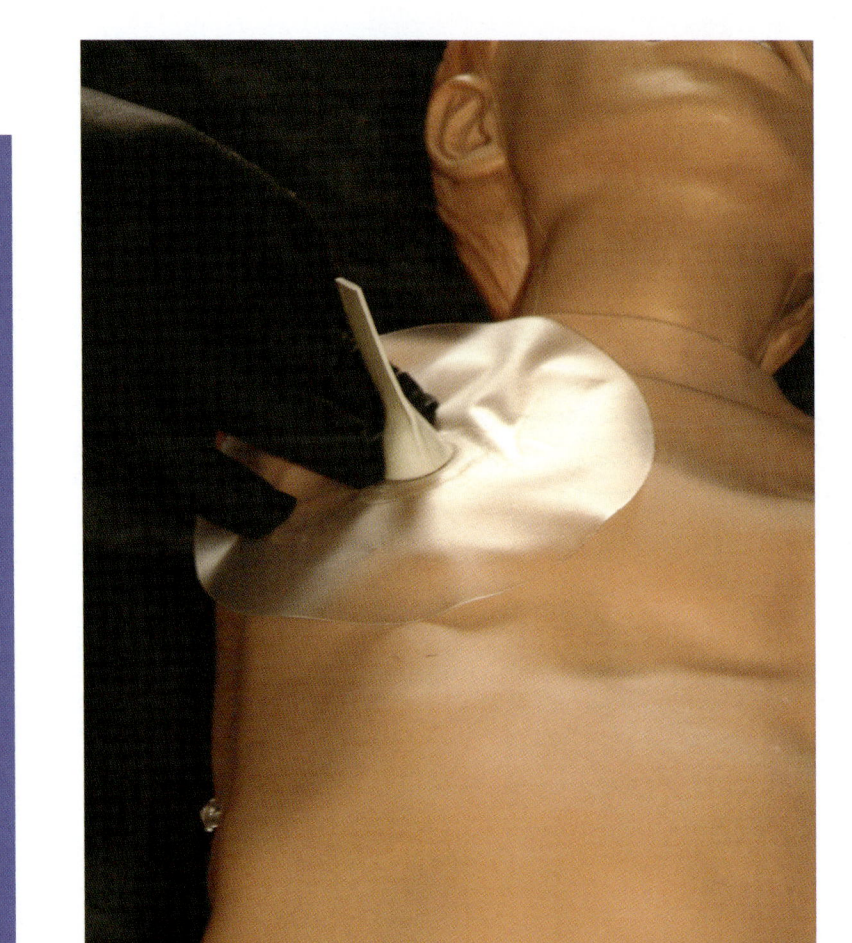

Figure 6.14 *A one-way valve like the Asherman Chest Seal should be used to tape the catheter in place if it is available.*

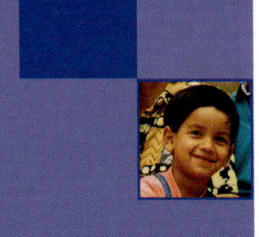

CHAPTER 7
Pediatric Shock and Fluid Resuscitation

Kathy J. Haley, RN, BSN
Linda Manley, RN, BSN
Kathryn E. Nuss, MD

Objectives
Upon completion of this chapter, you should be able to:

1. Define the term *hypovolemic shock*.

2. Recognize four early signs and/or symptoms of hypovolemic shock in the prehospital setting.

3. Describe three management strategies to treat hypovolemic shock in the prehospital setting.

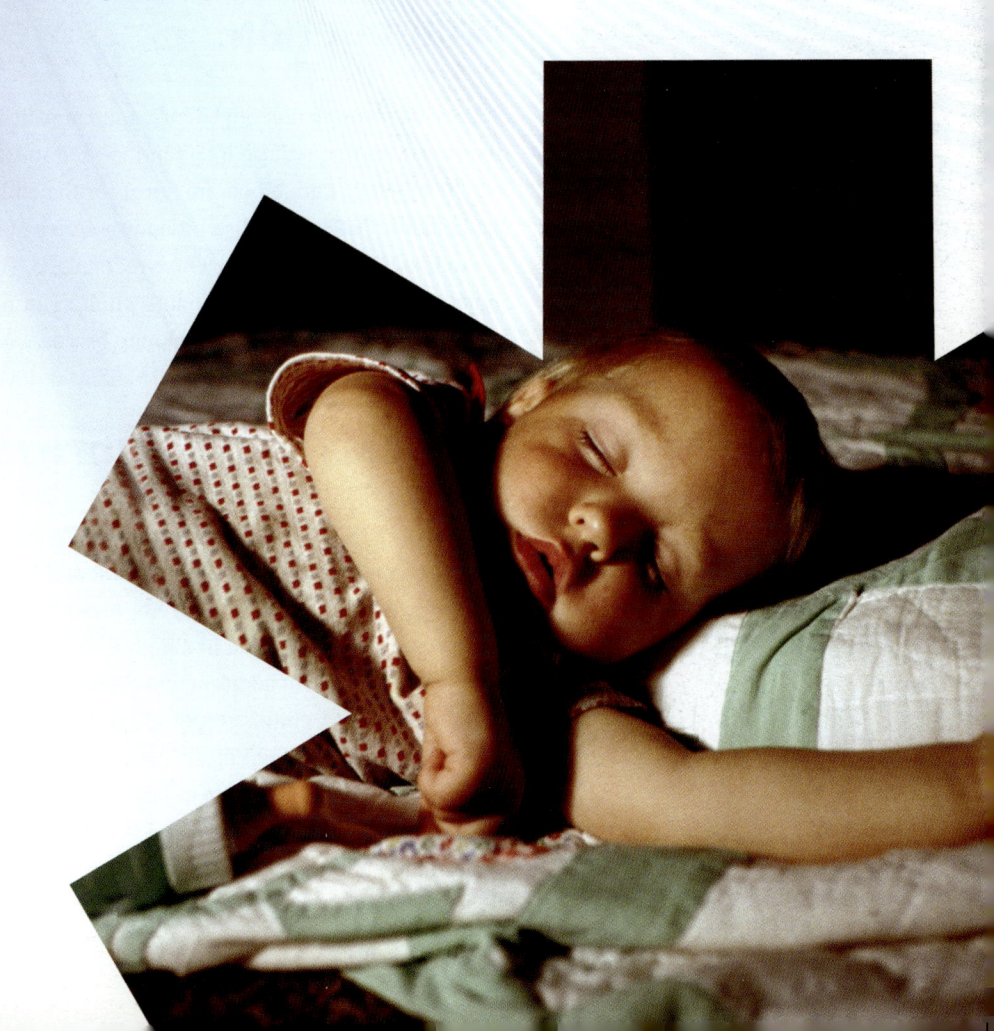

Case Study

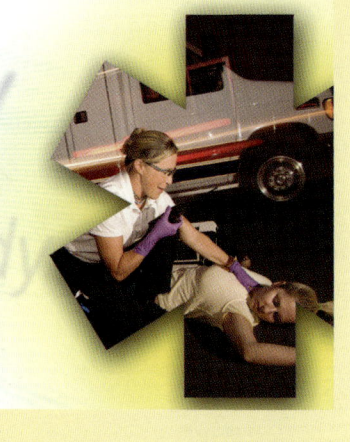

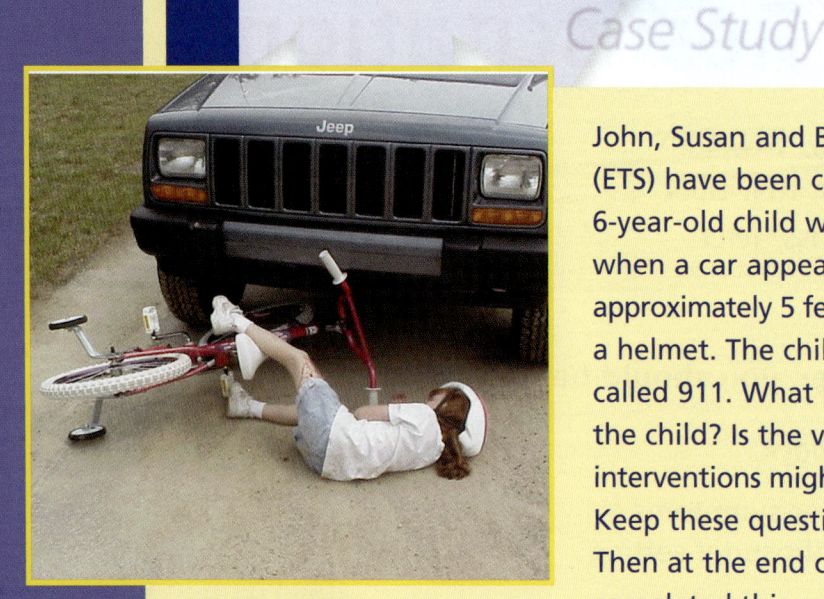

John, Susan and Bob of the Emergency Transport System (ETS) have been called to the scene of an accident. A 6-year-old child was riding her bicycle on a rural road when a car appeared and struck the child, throwing her approximately 5 feet (1.5 meters). The child was not wearing a helmet. The child's mother witnessed the event and called 911. What injuries might the team anticipate in the child? Is the victim likely to develop shock? What interventions might be required to ensure a good outcome? Keep these questions in mind as you read the chapter. Then at the end of the chapter, find out how the rescuers completed this call.

INTRODUCTION

Successful resuscitation of pediatric trauma patients begins with identifying the physiological abnormalities that require intervention. You must be familiar with normal vital signs (heart rate, respiratory rate, blood pressure) for the child. Symptoms of shock may be subtle in the pediatric patient because blood pressure can be maintained with a significant decrease in circulating blood volume. Once recognized, shock requires aggressive intervention aimed at supporting and stabilizing vital organ function. Obtaining adequate access to the vascular system is necessary and may be challenging. Optimal fluid management and blood transfusion needs are continued areas of investigation in the pediatric trauma population.

ANATOMY AND PATHOPHYSIOLOGY

The differences between children and adults make children more susceptible to certain problems, such as an airway obstruction and hypovolemic shock. Children are at higher risk for hypovolemia for a variety of reasons, including a larger extracellular fluid volume, greater insensible loss (due to a higher metabolic rate, faster respiratory rate, and greater body surface area). In addition, children have greater compensatory mechanisms for blood loss than adults. A child's response can be strong enough to mask the severity of the loss until a significant amount of the circulatory blood volume (CBV) is depleted.

Even before the assessment begins, it is important to recognize normal pediatric vital signs and be able to estimate a child's CBV. This knowledge can greatly simplify resuscitation. The CBV of a child is based on body weight and averages about 80 mL/kg.

> **PEARLS**
>
> The signs of shock in children are subtle and need to be recognized early, as aggressive treatment helps ensure a good patient outcome.

Pediatric Trauma Life Support

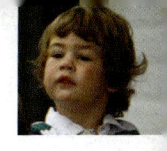

Thus, a two-year-old child weighing 12 kg has a CBV of 960 mL, or roughly one liter of fluid. If this child were to lose 25 percent of his CBV (0.25 x 960 = 240 mL), that would equal a typical 8-ounce glass of fluid. Loss of only a few hundred milliliters can be life threatening. It is important to consider not only the visible external blood loss from lacerations and abrasions, but also potential internal losses from major organ injuries, such as the liver and spleen.

In general, children can tolerate a loss of 10 percent to 15 percent of their CBV with minimal signs and symptoms. A loss of more than 15 percent of CBV, however, activates the "fight or flight" response. This response is a result of activation of the sympathetic nervous system, which secretes catecholamines, epinephrine, and norepinephrine. These catecholamines cause intense vasoconstriction and tachycardia, both of which help maintain the child's systolic blood pressure. With a significant blood loss, however, the child's compensatory responses are overwhelmed, cardiac output diminishes, and eventually cardiovascular collapse will occur if the CBV is not corrected rapidly.

PATIENT ASSESSMENT

As mentioned in Chapter 1, the mechanism of injury is important when determining the potential injuries the pediatric patient may have sustained (Fig. 7.1). It is important to remember, though, that children who are the victims of child abuse may not have a history consistent with their injuries.

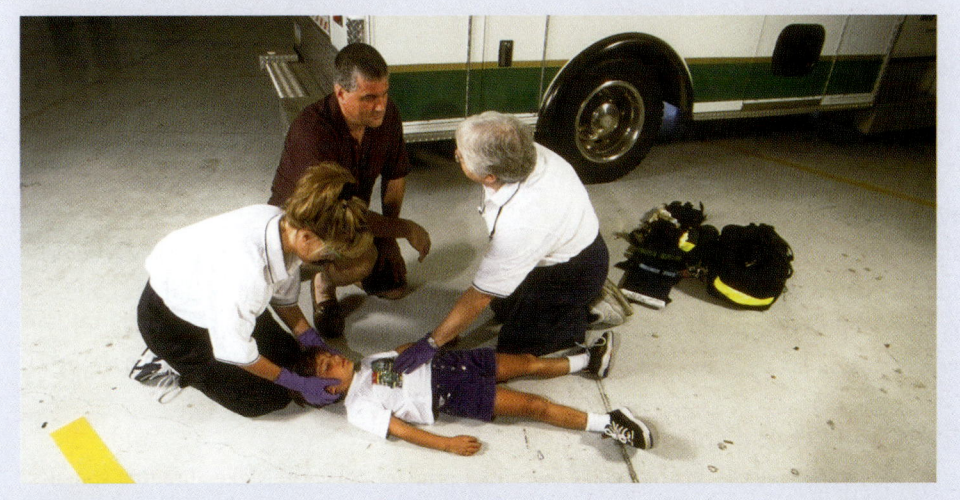

Figure 7.1 *Parents or other observers at the scene may provide details to help rescuers determine the mechanism of injury more rapidly.*

In general, all pediatric patients should be evaluated in the following manner:

1. ITLS Primary Survey
   A. Scene Size-Up
   B. Initial Assessment
   C. Rapid Trauma Survey or Focused Exam
   D. Critical Interventions and Transport Decisions
   E. Contact medical direction as needed.
2. ITLS Secondary Survey and/or Ongoing Exam

> **PEARLS**
>
> A loss of only a few hundred milliliters can be life-threatening in a child; consider visible blood loss from lacerations and abrasions, as well as potential internal losses from major organ injuries, such as the liver and spleen.

Pediatric Shock and Fluid Resuscitation

ITLS Primary Survey

Scene Size-Up
The mechanism of injury may be helpful for identifying the source of blood loss when a child is in shock (Fig. 7.2). A low-energy injury indicates a more focused site for blood loss, whereas a high-energy injury suggests a child at risk for multisystem injury.

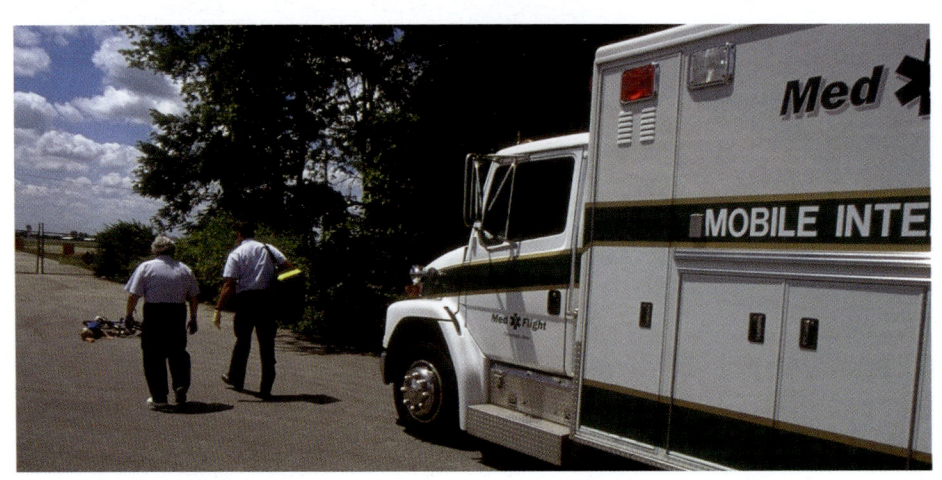

Figure 7.2 *Consider the mechanism of injury during the Scene Size-Up.*

Initial Assessment
General Impression
The general impression is particularly important in children. Does the child see you coming? What is his position, both in relation to his surroundings and in terms of posture? Is he struggling to breathe? Is his color markedly changed? Is he bleeding?

Level of Consciousness
Often, children with signs and symptoms of shock may appear agitated and restless due to poor circulation to their brain. Conduct a brief neurological assessment, and if the child has an altered mental status, prepare for a rapid transport. *Remember, hypoxia can also cause mental status changes.* Maintain a patent airway and administer supplemental oxygen.

Airway and Cervical Spine
As stressed in Chapter 4, this is always the initial primary concern. Make sure that spinal motion restriction is maintained throughout the entire assessment and management of the child. If the child has a compromised airway, it must be treated *immediately*.

Breathing
All children with significant trauma should receive supplemental oxygen and have their respiratory status carefully monitored (Fig. 7.3). If their rate or tidal volume is inadequate, you must assist their breathing. Children in shock may also exhibit tachypnea (increased respiratory rate), even without airway or breathing problems, as the body tries to maximize oxygen intake. As mentioned, shock is defined simply as inadequate tissue oxygenation; thus, the mainstay of therapy is to improve oxygenation. The importance of administering oxygen cannot be overemphasized. Children are not harmed by the administration of oxygen in the field.

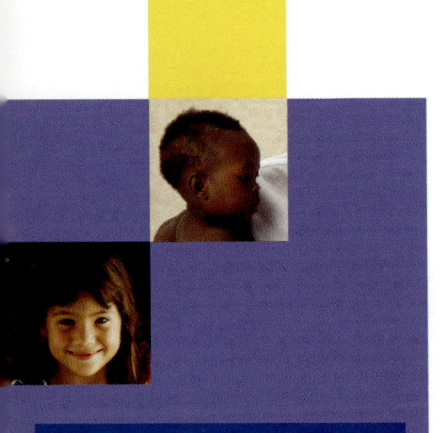

PEARLS

A change in mental status such as agitation or restlessness may mean early signs of shock; consider rapid "load-and-go" transport.

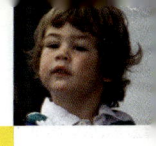

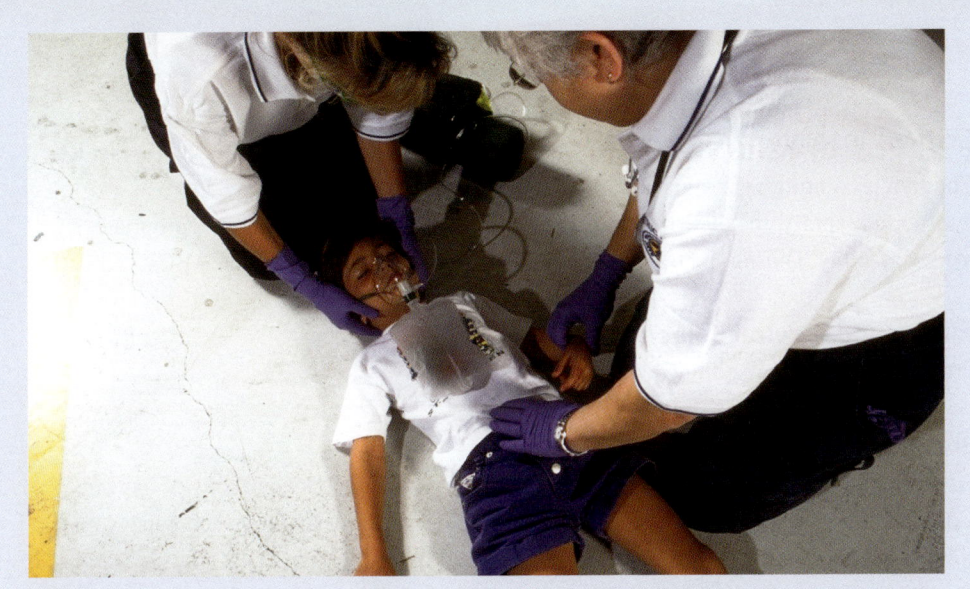

Figure 7.3 *The importance of administering oxygen to a child in shock cannot be overemphasized.*

Circulation

As mentioned in Chapter 2, early signs and symptoms of hypovolemic shock in children are subtle. Initial assessment includes observing for signs of central and peripheral perfusion. In general, these signs are the result of the body's catecholamine (fight-or-flight) response, and include tachycardia (remember age-dependent heart rates), weak or thready peripheral pulses, and pale or mottled skin with slow capillary refill. Normal capillary refill is less than 2 seconds. A blood pressure reading on a child can be very difficult to obtain in the field and should be obtained en route to the hospital (remember age-dependent pressures). In early stages of hypovolemic shock, catecholamines cause increased vascular resistance and an increase in the diastolic pressure without changing the systolic pressure. This results in a narrowing of the pulse pressure (the difference between systolic and diastolic pressures), which is often not recognized. Children can maintain a "normal" systolic pressure despite a 25 percent CBV loss, misleading pre-hospital providers to believe the child is stable. In general, *shock is best recognized in a child by tachycardia and poor perfusion*.

During circulatory assessment, *note any evidence of external bleeding and carefully control with direct pressure*. It is surprising how much blood loss can occur from a simple scalp laceration, especially in a child. Some scalp lacerations are severe enough to cause hypovolemic shock. Direct manual pressure to the laceration is usually effective in minimizing blood loss.

Rapid Trauma Survey

The Rapid Trauma Survey should reveal the possible source of acute blood loss and help differentiate hemorrhagic shock from other causes of shock, including tension pneumothorax and pericardial tamponade. Remember that in the presence of a spinal cord injury, there may be no catecholamine response. Children with a spinal cord injury will have hypotension and bradycardia. If possible, obtain a blood pressure en route to the hospital. Compare it with the normal range of blood pressures for the child's age (at a minimum, 70 + 2 x age for systolic blood pressure). *Remember that hypotension is a late and ominous sign of shock in children.* It takes a loss of 30 percent to 35 percent of the CBV before hypotension occurs.

Pediatric Shock and Fluid Resuscitation

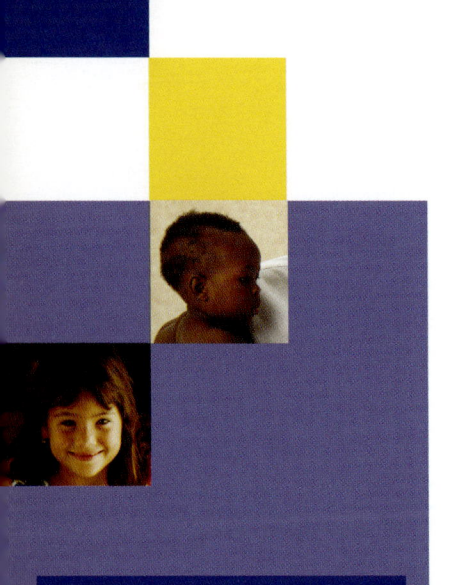

Critical Interventions and Transport Decisions

Children presenting with signs and symptoms of hypovolemic shock need to be transported rapidly, ideally to a Level I Pediatric Trauma Center or other appropriate medical facility. During the transport, continually assess and reassess the ABCs.

Airway and Cervical Spine
Provide care as discussed in Chapter 4.

Breathing
Assist ventilations as needed and maintain the child on high concentrations of oxygen. Continually reassess the patient for signs of respiratory failure that may accompany shock. If respiratory failure develops, manage as discussed in Chapter 4.

Circulation
The treatment of shock consists of ensuring a patent airway and adequate ventilation, providing supplemental oxygen, controlling external bleeding, positioning and immobilization, thermal regulation, and restoring CBV. Restoring the CBV depends on (1) preventing further blood loss, (2) establishing vascular access, and (3) replacing intravascular fluids and later stopping the primary source of bleeding. It is also important to keep the child warm.

Prevent Further Blood Loss. To prevent further blood loss, apply direct pressure to external wounds and elevate the part if possible. If you cannot stop severe bleeding with pressure nor can you use a tourniquet (groin, axilla, neck, face, scalp), you may use one of the hemostatic agents (Celox, QuikClot 1st Response, and so on). Skeletal fractures will bleed until immobilized; thus, splinting is important.

Establish Vascular Access. Intravenous access can be established en route to the receiving facility. This intervention can be difficult and time-consuming in a healthy child, let alone one who is hypovolemic. If IV access is indicated, over-the-needle cannulas can be started in the hand, forearm, or antecubital fossa. It is best to use the largest cannula diameter with the shortest length. Prehospital care providers are often successful using a catheter one size larger than originally anticipated.

The truly hypovolemic child will most likely present with mottled, cold extremities and unstable vital signs. In this case, vascular access may be possible only by an alternate route: intraosseous (IO) infusion. IO infusion is the infusion of fluids, blood, and/or drugs directly into the bone marrow cavity. In the field and emergency department settings, it is an established popular route for venous access if the child is *unstable*. If IV access is not readily available, an IO infusion should be placed in a child who is unconscious, in arrest, or rapidly deteriorating.

It is important to understand the basic principles of IO infusion. Fluids enter directly into the bone marrow cavity and are absorbed into the central circulation by a network of venous sinusoids. In children less than 4 years old, the bone marrow cavity is responsible for the production of red blood cells. After this age, some fat cells occupy the marrow cavity of the long bones, gradually filling them with yellow "fatty" marrow. Serious complications are rare with this procedure if done correctly.

PEARLS
Treatment of shock in children is the same as with adults and includes preventing further blood loss, establishing vascular access, and replacing intravascular fluids.

PEARLS
Consider placement of an IO line in a child who is unconscious, in arrest, or who is rapidly deteriorating. Estimate the child's weight with a length-based tape and administer fluids via the IO the same as any IV line at 20 mL/kg.

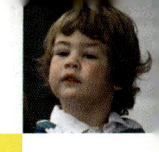

The sites of choice for an IO infusion in a pediatric patient are the long bones of the lower extremity. The most frequent site for insertion is the anterior proximal medial aspect of the tibia, 1 cm below the tibial tuberosity, as there are no vital structures in that area that could be injured. Absolute contraindications to inserting an IO line include a fracture of the bone or previous attempts in the same bone. An alternative site is the distal third of the anterior femur, although there is greater muscle mass at this site.

Once the IV or IO line is established, tape it securely and immobilize it properly so that it does not become dislodged. All medications, fluids, and even blood can be administered safely through the IO route. This technique is addressed further in Chapter 8.

Replace Intravascular Fluids. Rapid administration of fluids is essential in the treatment of hypovolemic shock. IV or IO access should be attempted en route to the hospital, as it is important to begin early, aggressive fluid resuscitation; at the scene for patients awaiting helicopter transfer; or if there is a prolonged extrication (Fig. 7.4). Normal saline or other medically approved crystalloids are the fluids of choice. Intravascular fluid replacement must be managed in a controlled manner. Fluids are administered to children by a fluid bolus of 20 mL/kg.

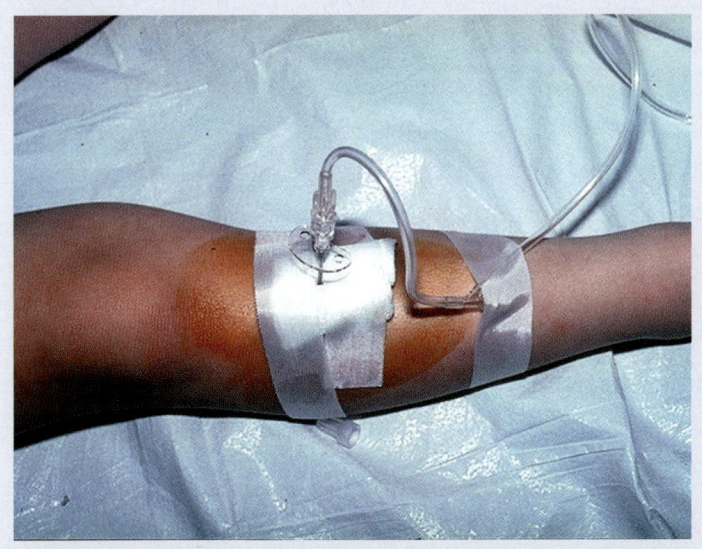

Figure 7.4 *Intraosseous infusion in a pediatric patient is best performed on the long bones of the lower extremities.*

A fluid bolus is given as a rapid way to correct hypovolemia. The child's response to the bolus can be an early, reliable indicator of continued blood loss. Most children who receive a fluid bolus show marked improvement. If that does not happen, consider ongoing blood loss. If there is continued evidence of shock (tachycardia and delayed capillary refill), a second 20 mL/kg may be administered. Additional boluses may be repeated if indicated by medical direction. On arrival at the hospital, report the total volume of fluids that have been administered. Fluids should never be restricted in a child with a head injury, pulmonary contusion, or shock; inadequate perfusion will result in a worse outcome for a child with a severe head injury.

Keep the Child Warm. Children are prone to hypothermia because of their greater body surface area and lack of subcutaneous tissue. Administer warm fluids whenever possible, and keep the child wrapped (including the head) between assessments and during transport.

ITLS Secondary Survey

Complete an ITLS Secondary Survey, looking carefully for sources of blood loss. An abdominal or pelvic injury may result in shock in a pediatric patient. These injuries cannot be corrected in the field and require close management at a pediatric trauma center.

Case Study continued

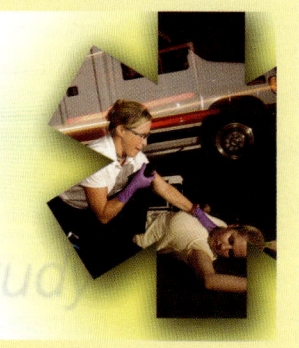

John, Susan and Bob of the Emergency Transport System (ETS) have been called to the scene of an accident. A 6-year-old child was riding her bicycle on a rural road when a car appeared and struck the child, throwing her approximately 5 feet (1.5 meters.) The child was not wearing a helmet and is now lying on the side of the road.

On arrival, Bob gets the trauma box and cervical collars and begins the Scene Size-up. John gets the oxygen and airway equipment, and Susan gets the pediatric long-board. The police are on-scene and signal that the scene is safe. There is no other patient.

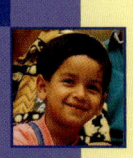

Bob starts the Initial Assessment. The general impression is poor. The child is not responsive and is breathing noisily. John stabilizes the head and neck and opens the airway with a modified jaw thrust, and Bob clears the airway using gentle suction. The respiratory rate and effort is now adequate and a nonrebreather mask is applied with an oxygen flow rate of 12 liters per minute. The child's color immediately improves. After attending to the child's airway and breathing/ventilation, circulation is assessed by checking the pulse and capillary refill. Bob records a thready, rapid radial pulse with cool extremities and delayed capillary return. Team leader Bob recognizes the signs of shock in this child and makes the decision to load and go. Bob performs a Rapid Trauma Survey that reveals bleeding from the right ear, a contusion/abrasion over the right anterior costal margin, and a deformed, swollen right thigh. While dispatching a helicopter to the scene, the child is log-rolled onto a backboard, checking the back in the process. The neurologic survey shows pupils that are equal and reactive and the Glasgow Coma Score is 10 (E2, V3, M5). The decision is made to carefully monitor airway and breathing adequacy and establish intravenous (IV) access. After a 20 mL/kg bolus of normal saline is given, the heart rate decreases and the peripheral pulses are stronger. The child is transferred directly to a Pediatric Level I Trauma Center with neurosurgical capability; en route, vital signs including pulse oximetry were monitored and the ITLS Ongoing Exam was performed. The trauma team was waiting on their arrival.

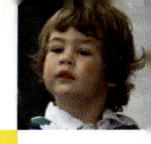

Further in-hospital assessment and investigations revealed that the child had sustained cerebral contusion, basal skull fracture, and a closed fracture of the right femur. After a period on the neurosurgical intensive care unit, she was cared for on an orthopedic ward. Several weeks post-injury, the child was discharged home with an excellent prognosis and a bike helmet!

Case Study wrap-up

Bicycle injuries are a significant cause of death and disability for children in our communities. Children may sustain a variety of injuries from this mechanism, ranging from minor to major trauma. Head and spinal trauma, facial wounds, thoracic and abdominal trauma, and fractures are commonly associated with this mechanism.

This is a child with significant primary head injury with airway compromise and hemorrhagic shock from a closed right femoral fracture. Using the ITLS patient assessment skills and critical interventions, secondary brain injury was prevented. Early recognition of shock and the prompt load-and-go decision ensured early transport of the injured child to a dedicated Pediatric Level I Trauma Center for definitive care. Hypovolemic shock remains a significant contributor to poor outcome in pediatric trauma. Early recognition and fluid resuscitation followed by definitive care in hospital usually optimizes outcome. Some injuries are preventable and injury prevention programs should be a strategy that should not be overlooked.

Pediatric Shock and Fluid Resuscitation

SUMMARY

1. Shock is defined as inadequate tissue oxygenation. Hypovolemic shock is the most common type of shock in children.
2. Subtle, early signs of hypovolemic shock include tachycardia, weakness of the peripheral pulses, poor peripheral perfusion (capillary refill of more than 2 seconds, pallor, or mottled skin), tachypnea, and agitation or restlessness. Hypotension is a late and ominous sign of shock.
3. Control external blood loss with direct pressure. Hemostatic agents may be needed on rare occasions.
4. IV or IO access can be life-saving. IO infusion can be used to administer fluids, blood, and/or drugs directly into the bone marrow cavity and is most often performed on the young child in whom you cannot rapidly obtain vascular access.
5. Once vascular access is established, administer an isotonic solution by a fluid bolus (20 mL/kg), and carefully reevaluate the child. If there is no improvement, administer a second bolus (same amount). Notify the receiving hospital of the total amount of fluid administered and the child's response.
6. It is important to reassess ABCs frequently and ensure that the child does not become hypothermic.
7. Rapid transport to a pediatric trauma center is indicated for children with signs and symptoms of hypovolemic shock, especially those who do not respond to one fluid bolus.

Recommended Reading

American College of Surgeons. "Shock." In *Advanced Trauma Life Support Program for Doctors*, 8th ed. Chicago: Author, 2008.

Brain Trauma Foundation. *Guidelines for the Prehospital Management of Severe Traumatic Brain Injury*, 2nd ed. New York: Author, 2007.

Campbell, John Emory, ed. "Shock Evaluation and Management." In *International Trauma Life Support for Prehospital Care Providers*, 6th ed., 118–35. Upper Saddle River, N.J.: Pearson/Prentice Hall, 2008.

Gwinnutt, Carl L., and Peter A. Driscoll, eds. "Shock" In *Trauma Resuscitation: The Team Approach*, 2nd ed., 78–106. Oxford, U.K.: BIOS Scientific Publishers Limited, 2003.

National Center for Statistics and Analysis. *Traffic Safety Facts 2004: Pedal Cyclists*. Washington, D.C.: National Highway Traffic Safety Administration, 2006.

Ralston, Mark, Mary Fran Hazinski, Arno L. Zaritsky, Stephen M. Schexnayder, and Monica E. Kleinman, eds. *Pediatric Advanced Life Support Provider Manual*. Dallas: American Heart Association, 2007.

Turnage, Bryce and Kimball I. Maull. "Scalp Laceration: An Obvious 'Occult' Cause of Shock." *Southern Medical Journal* 93 (2000): 265–66.

CHAPTER 8
Fluid Resuscitation Skills

Kathy J. Haley, RN, BSN
Linda Manley, RN, BSN

Objectives

On completion of this skill station, you should be able to:

1. Identify two sites for peripheral venous cannulation.
2. Describe the indications for intraosseous cannulation.
3. Demonstrate the technique of intraosseous and peripheral venous cannulation.
4. Demonstrate how to administer a fluid bolus to a child.

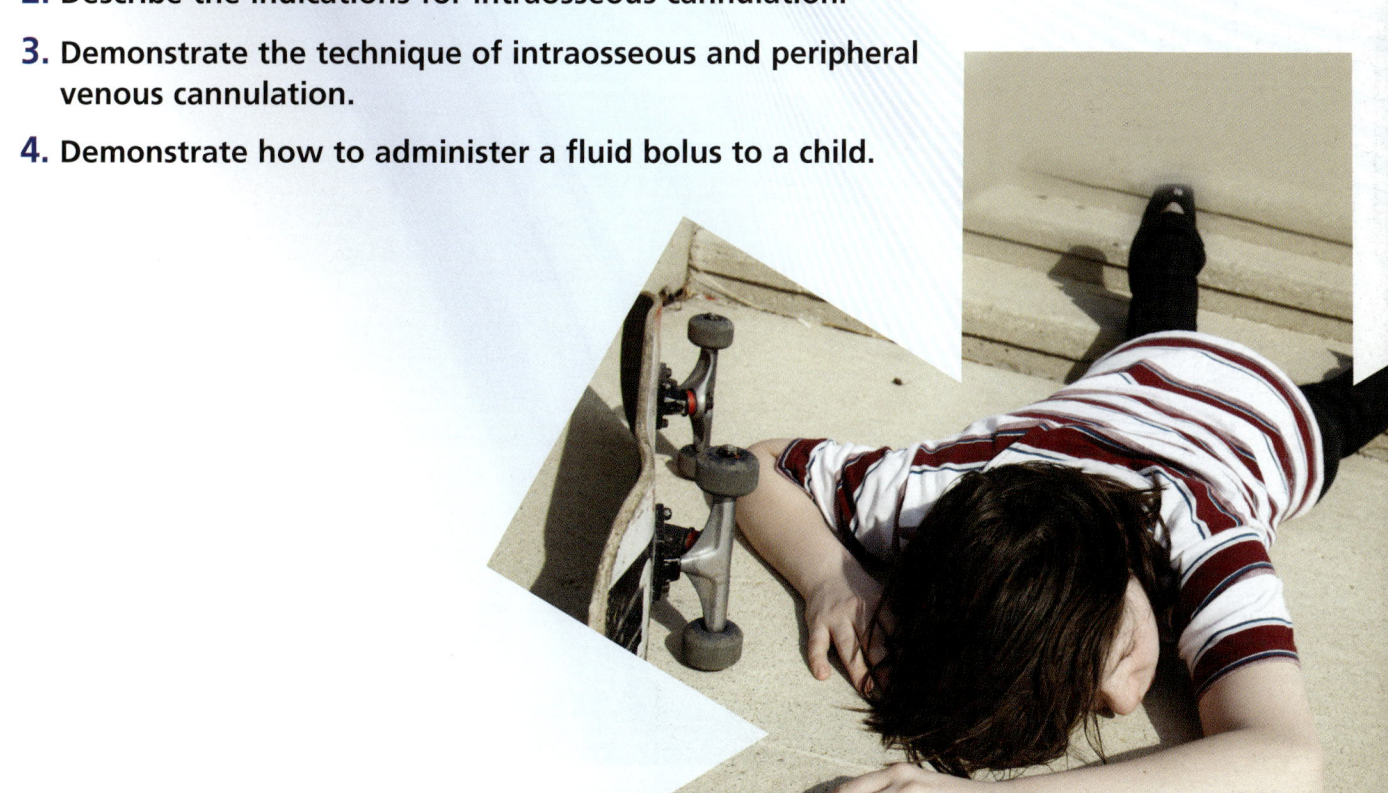

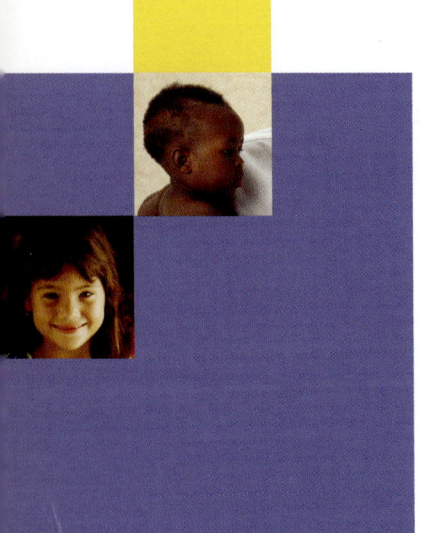

INTRAVENOUS ACCESS VIA PERIPHERAL CANNULATION

Determine the need for the procedure and follow written protocol or obtain permission from medical direction.

Indications

Peripheral IV access is indicated if there is a need or anticipated need for IV fluid resuscitation or administration of IV medications.

Contraindications

Peripheral IV access may be contraindicated if the patient is at risk for fluid extravasation or inadequate flow. Examples include extremities that have massive edema or burns. Extremities with other injuries or a dysfunctional or impaired arm dialysis shunt should also be avoided. In all of these cases, assess alternative sites.

Equipment

Equipment includes an over-the-needle cannula, skin cleansing solution, gloves, tape, extremity immobilization board, and IV setup.

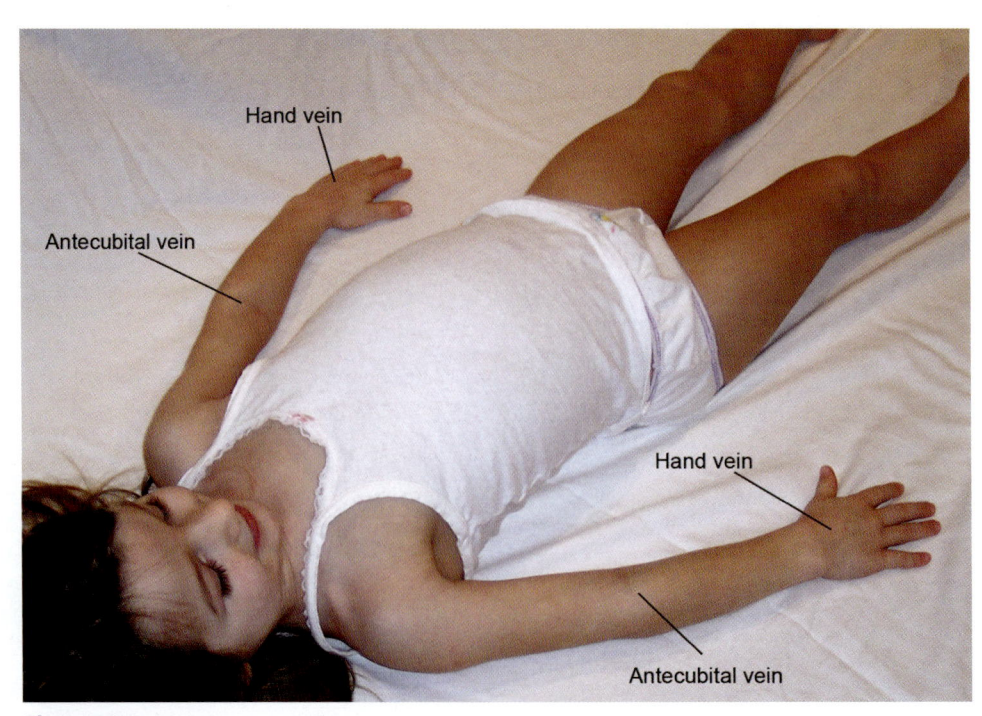

Figure 8.1 *Hand or antecubital veins are preferred for inserting an intravenous line.*

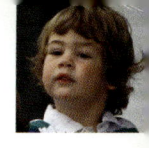

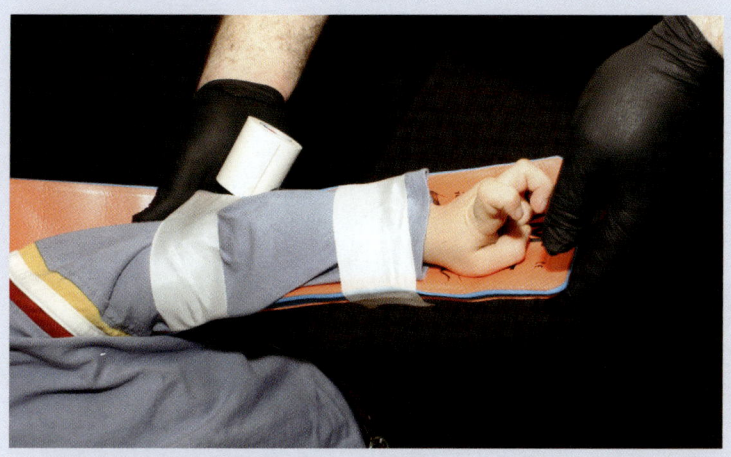

Figure 8.2 *The arm or hand should be immobilized and taped into position. If the antecubital vein will be used, the child's sleeve should be pulled up or shirt removed.*

Procedure

Select a site (Fig. 8.1). Usually, the hand or antecubital veins are preferred. (Scalp veins are not typically recommended because the area around the child's head is usually congested with persons facilitating airway management and the use of scalp veins in a child with head trauma is controversial.)

1. Immobilize the hand or arm with an arm board and tape in a position of function (Fig. 8.2). A venous tourniquet may be used.
2. Cleanse the site with a cleansing wipe.
3. Insert the over-the-needle catheter device (usually a 22-gauge or larger if possible) in the skin and into the vein.
4. Secure with tape, attach standard IV tubing, and infuse fluid and/or medication. A three-way valve and a 60 mL syringe may be used in order to carefully control the amount of each fluid bolus.

INTRAOSSEOUS INFUSION

Indications

Intraosseous (IO) access is indicated when immediate vascular access is needed for the critically ill or injured pediatric patient who requires fluid, blood, or medications, or the patient for whom you cannot quickly obtain peripheral venous access.

Contraindications

Do not perform IO infusion on children with a history of "brittle-bone" disorder (i.e., osteogenesis imperfecta).

An IO needle should not be inserted in an extremity with a recent or new fracture. If a bone has been stuck once, avoid a second attempt in the same extremity. Fluid, blood, and medications will seep out of the second hole, lessening the infusion of agents to their site of action.

Fluid Resuscitation Skills

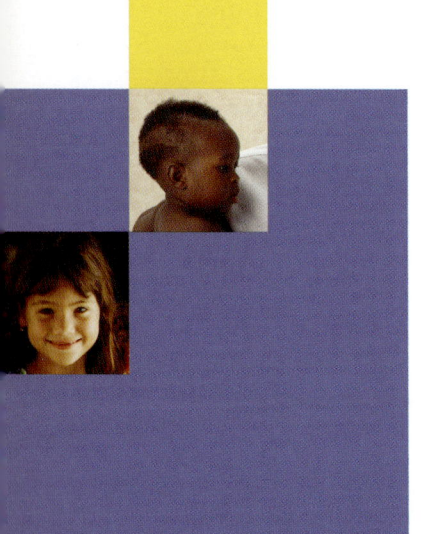

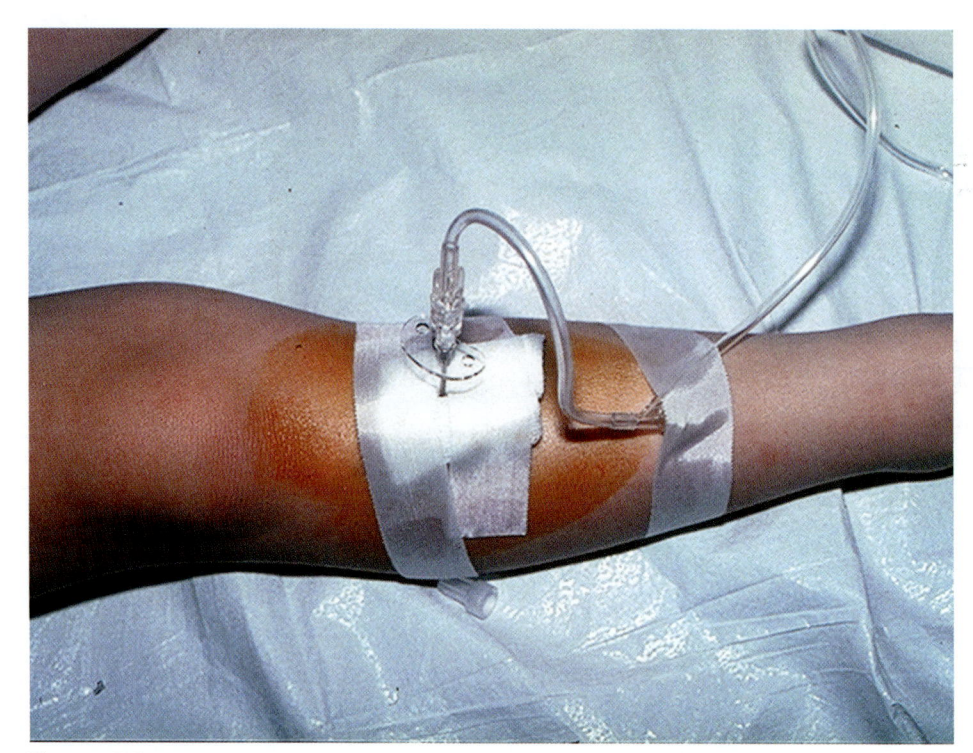

Figure 8.3 *The best site for intraosseous access is the proximal tibia.*

Equipment

Equipment includes a disposable 15- or 16-gauge intraosseous cannula/needle (an 18-gauge may be used in small infants), a syringe for bone marrow aspiration, skin cleansing solution, and a syringe with infusion fluid. There is also an option to use a commercially available IO drill using their recommended technique for manual IO infusion.

Procedure

Select the site for insertion (Fig. 8.3). The best site is usually the proximal tibia, one finger width or 1 cm below the tibial tuberosity over the medial flat surface of the tibia.

1. Clean the site with a cleaning solution.
2. Place the needle perpendicular to the bone and point it away from the nearest joint (to avoid the growth plate). Insert the needle with a screwing, to-and-fro motion. Often, a "pop" will be felt as the needle penetrates the bone cortex.
3. At this point, remove the inner stylet and apply a sterile syringe. Aspiration of red marrow fluid may help confirm placement, but may be absent even with proper placement.
4. If you obtain bone marrow, save it so it can be sent to the laboratory for testing. In the field, you can obtain serum blood glucose, an important test in the pediatric patient.

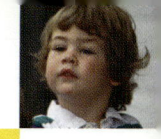

5. Attach a pressure infusion device (e.g., blood pressure cuff) to the bag of fluid to ensure continuous fluid administration or a three-way valve and syringe to accurately infuse the volume calculated for resuscitation.
6. Examine the site frequently for extravasation of fluid and swelling. If you observe these, the needle has been dislodged and requires removal. Secure the needle with tape.

FLUID BOLUS ADMINISTRATION

Indications

A fluid bolus is indicated in the child showing symptoms of hypovolemic shock a discussed in Chapter 7.

Contraindications

Do not administer a fluid bolus to any child who is hemodynamically stable or has pulmonary edema/congestive heart failure.

Equipment

Equipment includes maxi-drip tubing, a 60 mL syringe, and extension tubing (Fig. 8.4).

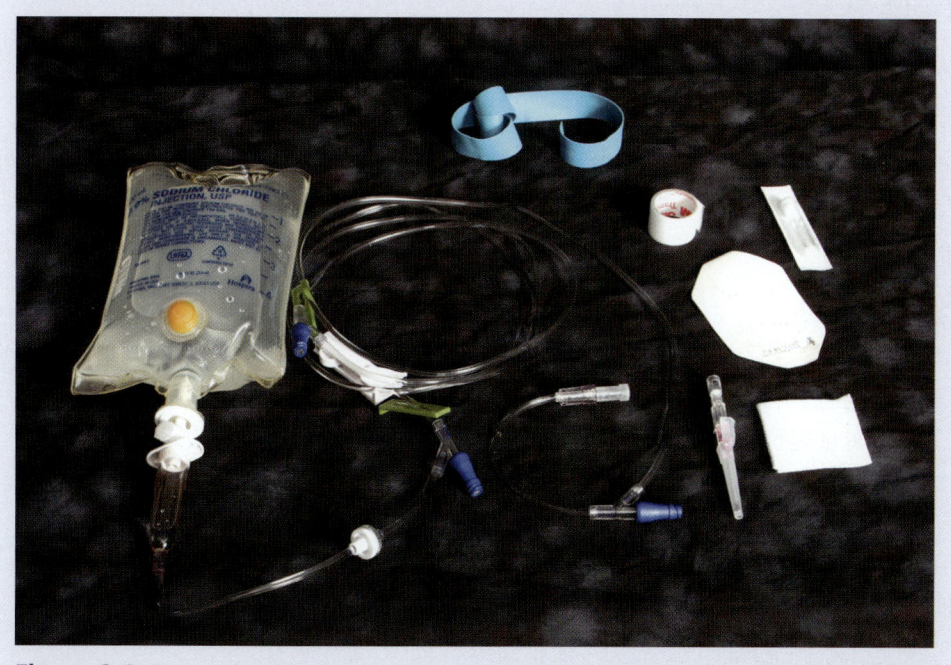

Figure 8.4 *Setup for administering a fluid bolus includes a syringe, tubing, and fluid bag.*

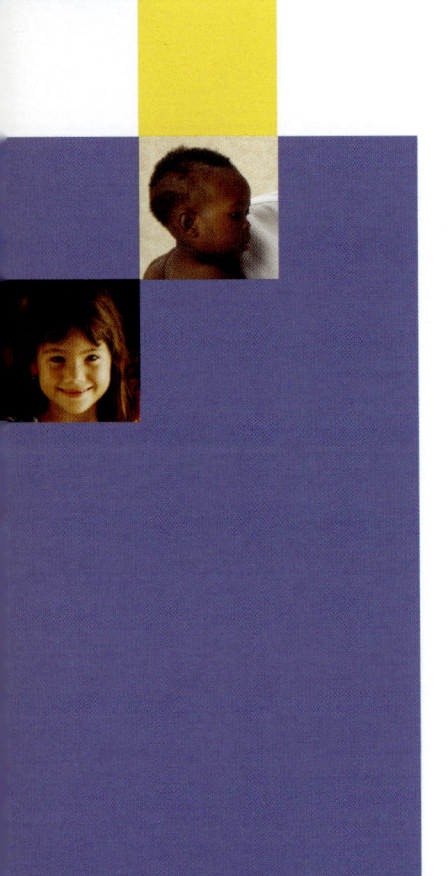

Procedure

1. Determine the fluid amount (20 mL/kg) and draw the fluid from the bag into the syringe.
2. Administer the fluid from the syringe to the child through the peripheral IV or IO line.
3. After administering the predetermined amount, maintain the line at a keep-open rate and reassess the child.
4. Most often, you will notice a dramatic improvement in the child's circulatory status, the pulse will decrease, and the capillary refill will improve. If this does not happen, the child may need a second, and possibly third, fluid bolus.
5. It is imperative that the receiving hospital be aware of the child's response to the fluid bolus and total fluid administered, as the child may require blood products.

CHAPTER 9
Pediatric Abdominal Trauma

Sharon Deppe, BSN, RN
Kathy J. Haley, RN, BSN
Kathryn E. Nuss, MD

Objectives
Upon completion of this chapter, you should be able to:

1. Describe how undetected abdominal trauma can lead to shock and death.
2. Discuss why abdominal trauma in children usually is associated with other injuries.
3. Describe the assessment and management of a child with abdominal trauma.

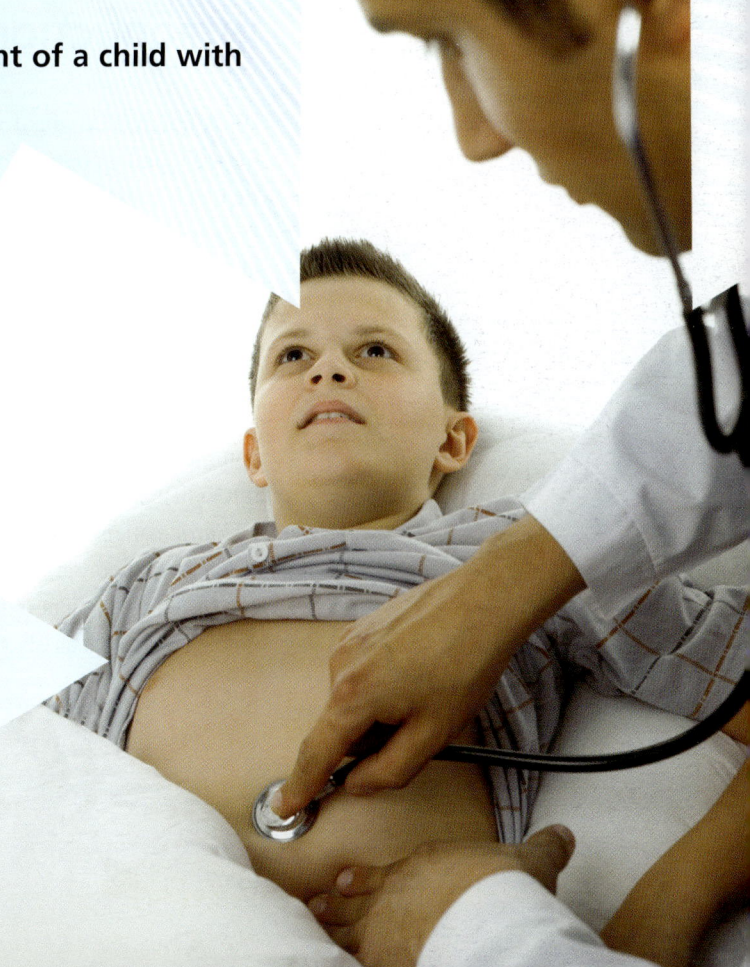

Case Study

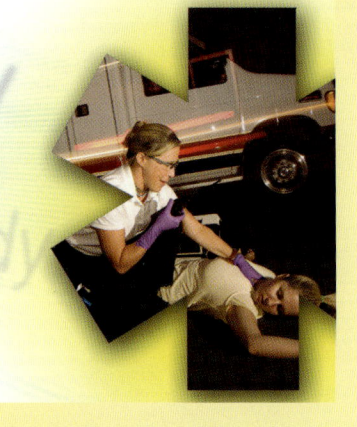

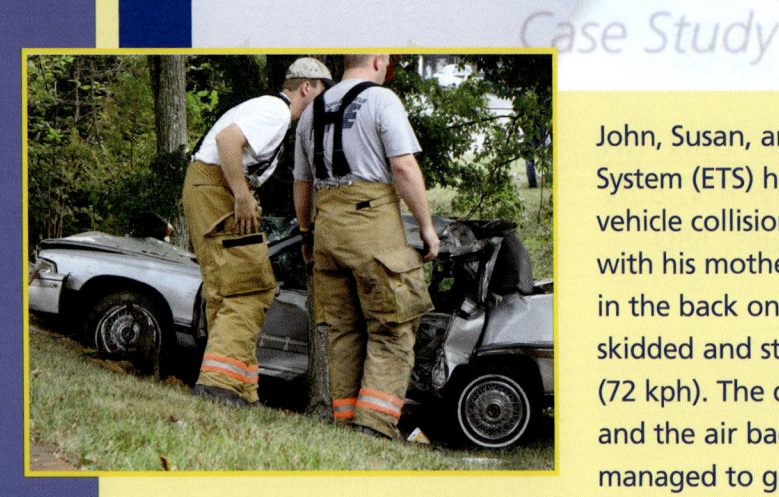

John, Susan, and Bob of the Emergency Transport System (ETS) have been called to the scene of a motor vehicle collision. A 4-year-old child was riding in a car with his mother on a wet day. The child was restrained in the back only loosely with a lap belt. The vehicle skidded and struck a tree at approximately 45 mph (72 kph). The driver was wearing a cross-chest lap belt and the air bag was deployed on impact. The mother managed to get out of the car. Concerned that her son may have been hurt, she calls for assistance. What injury should the team expect in the child with this mechanism of injury? What should be their assessment and treatment plan? How is it different from an adult? Keep these questions in mind as you read the chapter. Then, at the end of the chapter, find out how the rescuers completed this call.

INTRODUCTION

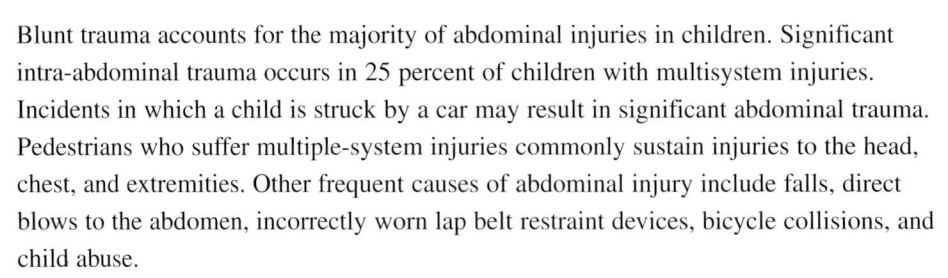

Blunt trauma accounts for the majority of abdominal injuries in children. Significant intra-abdominal trauma occurs in 25 percent of children with multisystem injuries. Incidents in which a child is struck by a car may result in significant abdominal trauma. Pedestrians who suffer multiple-system injuries commonly sustain injuries to the head, chest, and extremities. Other frequent causes of abdominal injury include falls, direct blows to the abdomen, incorrectly worn lap belt restraint devices, bicycle collisions, and child abuse.

It is often difficult to recognize when a child has sustained an abdominal injury. Patient anxiety, difficulty with the abdominal exam, your comfort level, and the child's limited communication skills may affect the ability to discover subtle changes that warrant immediate intervention and further evaluation. Undetected abdominal trauma in the pediatric patient can lead to shock and death. With a brief and accurate systematic assessment, appropriate intervention, and rapid transport, the child with abdominal trauma can have an excellent outcome. Children with penetrating injuries to the abdomen, while not as common, can also have a positive outcome if managed appropriately.

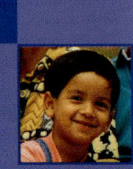

Pediatric Trauma Life Support

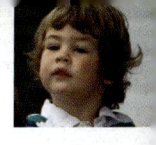

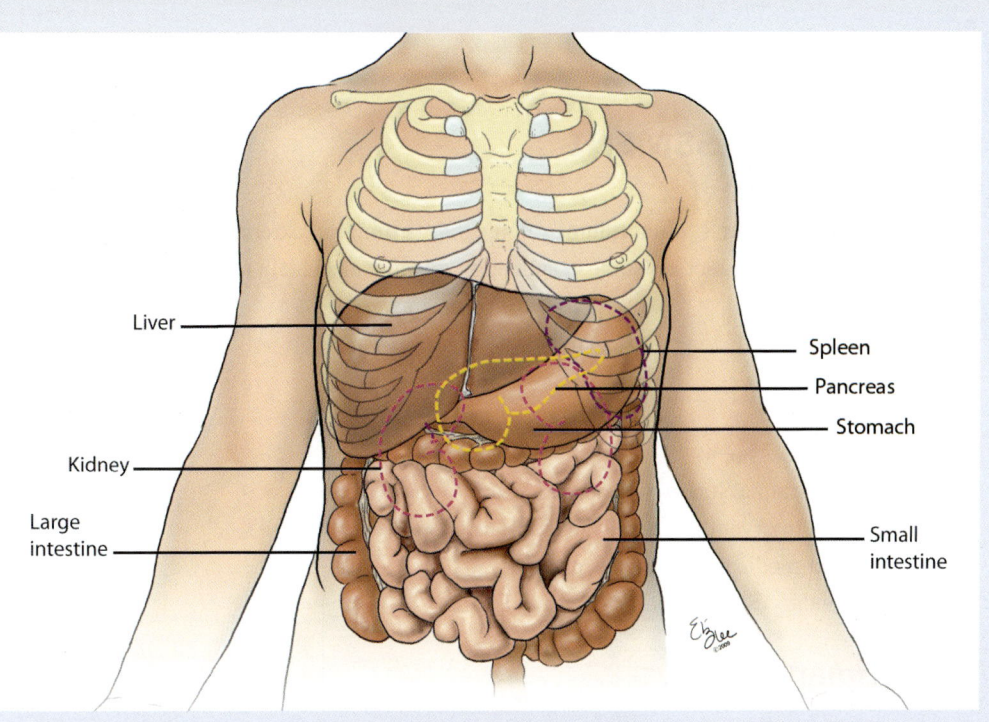

Figure 9.1 *The anatomy of the abdominal cavity of a child.*

ANATOMY AND PATHOPHYSIOLOGY

The child's abdomen can be divided into four quadrants: right upper quadrant, left upper quadrant, and right and left lower quadrants. The abdominal cavity is located below the diaphragm and contains both solid and hollow organs (Fig. 9.1). Blunt trauma to any of the quadrants can cause a rupture or tear of an organ.

The spleen is a blood-filled organ located in the left upper quadrant and is partially protected by the lower ribs. Despite this protection, it is the most commonly injured organ. Blunt force can cause the spleen to rupture but the spleen also could be lacerated by a fractured rib (although this is less common).

The liver is a solid, vascular organ in the right upper quadrant located under the right lower rib cage. While less commonly injured than the spleen, liver rupture or laceration can cause severe hemorrhage. *Liver injury is the most common fatal abdominal injury.*

The true abdomen (right and left lower quadrants) contains the large and small intestines and the bladder. Damage to these organs can result in infection and shock.

Behind the true abdomen lies the retroperitoneal space that contains the kidneys, ureters, pancreas, duodenum, abdominal aorta, and inferior vena cava. A child's kidneys are more vulnerable to blunt injury than an adult's because it is proportionately larger and less protected by bone, fat, and muscle. Because the pancreas and duodenum are relatively protected in the retroperitoneal space, they are injured less often than other organs. However, when these organs are involved, severe consequences often result.

Pediatric abdominal muscles are less developed than those of adults and, therefore, are less defined. This accounts for the "pot-bellied" appearance that infants and toddlers exhibit when laying or standing. A thinner muscle wall should make the pediatric abdomen easier to assess than that of the adult. However, anxiety and pain can cause a child to cry, which then causes muscles to tighten and makes abdominal assessment more difficult. Air swallowed while the child cries can also distort the abdomen, making it appear more distended. This causes increased discomfort and may impair respiratory effort by displacing the diaphragm into the thorax. Positive-pressure ventilation may also result in abdominal distention.

PATIENT ASSESSMENT

As discussed in Chapter 1, blunt trauma often exhibits minimal external signs, and the infant or young child cannot assist the examiner by relating adequately to describe the pain.

In general, use the following approach:
1. ITLS Primary Survey
   A. Scene Size-Up
   B. Initial Assessment
   C. Rapid Trauma Survey or Focused Exam
   D. Critical Interventions and Transport Decisions
   E. Contact medical direction as needed.
2. ITLS Secondary Survey and/or Ongoing Exam

ITLS Primary Survey

Scene Size-Up

At the scene, it is important to note the circumstances surrounding the traumatic event. If the child is involved in a motor vehicle collision, observations related to speed of vehicle, extent of damage, extrication procedures, distance thrown or ejected, surface or object of contact, and use of shoulder or lap belt help determine the degree of suspicion for multisystem injury with potential abdominal involvement. If the incident is a pedestrian- or bicycle-related accident or other blunt trauma, inquire about any trauma to the abdomen, including handlebars or bumpers (Fig. 9.2).

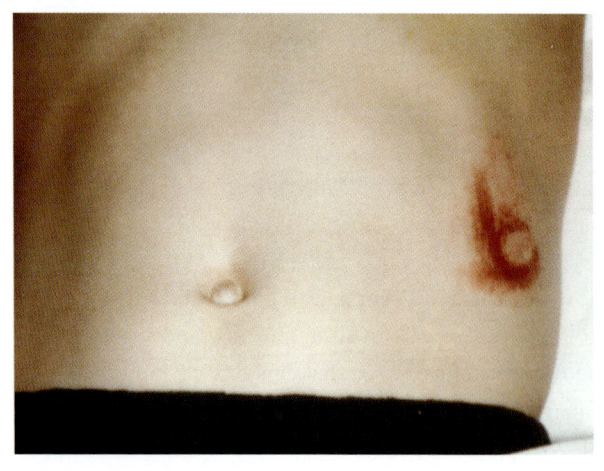

Figure 9.2 *Injury to the abdomen caused by the handlebar of a bicycle.*

Initial Assessment

General Impression and Level of Consciousness

Form a general impression of the child on approach and evaluate the initial level of consciousness.

PEARLS

Blunt trauma to the abdomen often exhibits minimal external signs, and children may not be able to describe pain. Carefully assess the mechanism of injury and have a high index of suspicion for abdominal trauma.

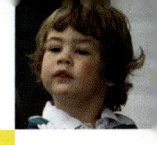

Airway and Cervical Spine
Because abdominal trauma is usually associated with injury to other systems, the ITLS Primary Survey begins with the ABCs. Provide spinal motion restriction and manage the airway as discussed in Chapter 4. Any patient suspected of having an abdominal injury should be placed on 100 percent oxygen.

Breathing
Assess the child's breathing next. Use the assessment skills outlined in Chapters 4 and 5 to recognize and manage any respiratory distress or failure. When internal bleeding is present, the normally soft, round pediatric abdomen becomes rigid, distended, and guarded. The child's respiratory effort is marked by expiratory grunting in an attempt to splint pain and to increase force on the diaphragm for improved exhalation. Large amounts of blood in the abdomen can impair ventilation as the accumulation of fluid begins to restrict diaphragmatic movement. Blood and bile are irritants to the diaphragm, and the presence of either can exhibit as referred pain. Injury to the spleen or liver can produce referred pain to the left or right shoulder through diaphragmatic irritation.

Circulation
Many children with intra-abdominal injuries will show signs and symptoms suggestive of shock. As indicated previously, tachycardia can be an early sign of intra-abdominal bleeding. The heart rate increases in an attempt to circulate blood and maintain blood pressure. Tachycardia continues until the cardiac reserve is depleted and blood pressure drops. Hypotension is a late and ominous sign of hypovolemic shock. During the ITLS Primary Survey, control all external bleeding with pressure dressings.

Rapid Trauma Survey
The Rapid Trauma Survey will identify other injuries as well as provide more information related to the abdomen. Do not overlook other injuries, as abdominal injures are often associated with other injuries such as head and extremity trauma. Isolated abdominal injuries may also be very significant, yet subtle; therefore, it is important to take children with potential abdominal injuries seriously.

Brief Neurological Assessment
A brief neurological assessment should be performed if there is altered mental status. As with adults, it is not easy to assess abdominal pain in the child with a decreased level of consciousness.

Critical Interventions and Transport Decisions
Many pediatric patients with a significant abdominal injury will show signs of shock. As with a child who has an unstable airway, respiratory insufficiency, or altered mental status, immediately package and transport any pediatric patient who exhibits signs of shock. As discussed in previous chapters, place the child on 100 percent oxygen. It is important to keep a child with an abdominal injury well oxygenated. Remove the child with potential abdominal injury from the car seat and secure him to a spinal motion restriction device. Because the extent of internal injuries is unknown, spinal motion restriction can help limit further injury and internal hemorrhage. When possible, procedures should be performed en route to the hospital. If a child is in shock, venous access may be attempted at the scene while waiting for air transport

> **PEARLS**
>
> **Do not to overlook other injuries; abdominal injuries are often associated with other injuries such as head and extremity trauma.**

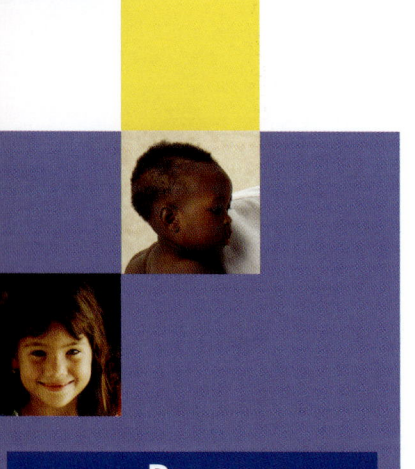

or during a prolonged extrication. Administer fluid boluses of normal saline or other medically approved crystalloid to increase circulating volume (see Chapter 7). An initial bolus of 20 mL/kg is appropriate. The child who continues to be hemodynamically unstable and has failed to respond to aggressive fluid resuscitation may require emergency surgery; transport this child rapidly to a pediatric trauma facility.

ITLS Secondary Survey

Abdominal Examination

With the child's clothing removed, conduct a rapid assessment of the abdomen. Inspect the skin for ecchymosis, abrasions, and marks. Bruising to the umbilicus, flank, scrotum, or labia indicates potential internal bleeding. Pain and linear markings over the chest and abdomen, along with lower back pain, can be an indication of a shoulder lap belt injury. Rib fractures, intestinal perforations, and lumbar compression fracture have been associated with "seat belt syndrome." For children that have sustained blunt abdominal trauma, examine the abdomen carefully for any marks or bruises. Handlebar marks from a bicycle injury represent concentrated focal trauma to an area and may indicate a liver injury (right upper quadrant) or spleen injury (left upper quadrant). Recent pediatric literature shows that most blunt abdominal injuries in children can be managed conservatively with fluid therapy and close observation

Operative intervention is used if the volume deficit cannot be corrected or there is evidence of persistent bleeding. This conservative approach has led to a drastic reduction in unnecessary surgery and a lower complication rate.

In the emergency department, children with blunt abdominal injury receive either a Focused Assessment with Sonography for Trauma Examination (FAST exam) ultrasound or a CT scan of their abdomen to delineate internal injuries. These investigations assist in the management of blunt abdominal trauma by giving insight into the nature of the internal injury.

Penetrating Trauma

If there is evidence of penetrating injury upon physical examination, treatment for the pediatric patient is the same as for an adult (Fig. 9.3). Do not remove objects protruding from the abdomen. Stabilizing the object to the body with a bulky dressing can help prevent further damage. If entrance and exit wounds are visible, a penetrating traumatic injury is obviously present. Occasionally, only an entrance wound may be seen. The extent of injury cannot be determined by the location of the entrance wound. For example, a bullet may pass erratically through many organs in an irregular course. If penetrating trauma occurs to the lower chest area (below the level of the nipple), also assess the abdomen for involvement. Penetrating injury to the abdominal wall can cause internal contents to protrude to the outside. Cover evisceration injuries with a moist, sterile saline dressing. Do not attempt to return the visible organ into the abdominal cavity.

> **PEARLS**
>
> A child with abdominal injury may show signs of shock. As with any unstable patient, immediately package and transport the pediatric patient with abdominal trauma.

> **PEARLS**
>
> A child with penetrating trauma should be treated the same as you would an adult: immobilize any impaled objects, control bleeding, and cover any visible organs.

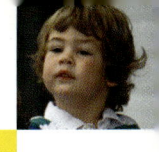

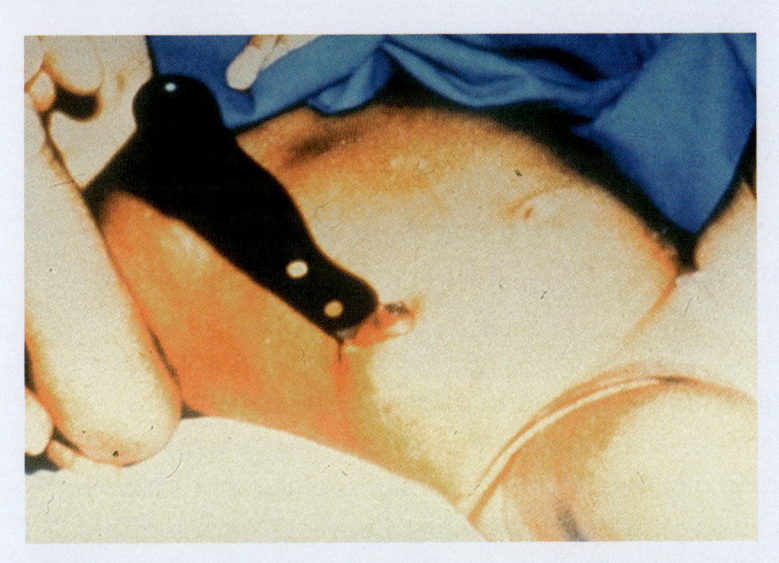

Figure 9.3 *A knife wound to the abdomen is an example of penetrating trauma.*

Case Study continued

John, Susan and Bob have been called to the scene of an accident involving a car and a tree. As they respond, they decide that Susan will act as team leader and prepare for a 4-year-old patient with injuries to the chest, abdomen, extremity and spine.

Upon their arrival, they find the police already on scene. The scene is safe. The mother of the child is unhurt but concerned about her son. He is still in the car, conscious and crying for his mother.

Susan and John approach the patient while Bob quickly checks the patient's mother to ensure she has no injuries. Bob and the patient's mother then join Susan and John.

Initial assessment reveals a conscious child with a clear airway and grunting respiration at a rate of 40 per minute. His radial pulse is 140 bpm and weak. Capillary refill is delayed and his hands are moist and cool.

The cervical spine is protected and a nonrebreather oxygen mask of appropriate size is applied. The team uses a pediatric long board to extricate him, noting there are no obvious injuries to the back.

Susan identifies him as a load-and-go patient because of the mechanism and signs of shock. She performs a Rapid Trauma Survey and confirms pain and tenderness with guarding in the left upper quadrant of his abdomen.

En route to hospital, IV access is established and a normal saline fluid

Pediatric Abdominal Trauma

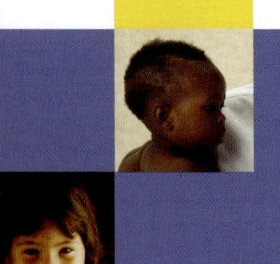

bolus of 20 mL/kg of body weight is given. His vital signs improve with fluid replacement.

Susan reports to medical direction, stating that she is bringing in a 4-year-old boy with a possible splenic injury. The patient is taken to a pediatric trauma center.

Further assessment and CT imaging confirmed the presence of a splenic hematoma with little intraperitoneal collection of blood. The patient was admitted to the hospital and observed closely. Immediate surgery was not indicated and he was managed conservatively. Vital signs remained stable, and the abdominal symptoms and signs settled gradually. Repeat CT imaging of the spleen excluded any further bleeding. The patient was discharged home in a week with a diagnosis of a splenic hematoma.

Case Study wrap-up

Proper restraints are not always used on children riding in motor vehicles, and when used, they are frequently applied incorrectly. In this case, the child did not have a shoulder restraint in place, putting all of the force from the collision onto the lap belt and the child's abdomen.

You should approach the scene not only looking for mechanism of injury, but also for placement of the child in the vehicle and the type of restraint devices in use. When a lap belt is used alone, the child is more likely to suffer abdominal trauma from the belt sliding up from the pelvis to the more compressible portion of the abdomen during a collision. This typically causes small bowel and lumbar flexion injuries ("seat belt syndrome"). In this scenario, the seat belt has compressed high on the abdominal wall, causing injury to the spleen. The findings of the ITLS Primary Survey, which are increased respiratory rate and signs of shock, confirm that the child is a load-and-go patient. Perform a Rapid Trauma Survey, extricate the child to a child-sized spinal motion restriction device, and transport the child to an appropriate medical facility.

SUMMARY

1. Because most pediatric abdominal injuries are subtle, maintain a high degree of suspicion.
2. Perform a rapid, systematic assessment.
3. Patients exhibiting signs of shock need rapid package and transport. Perform procedures en route to hospital.

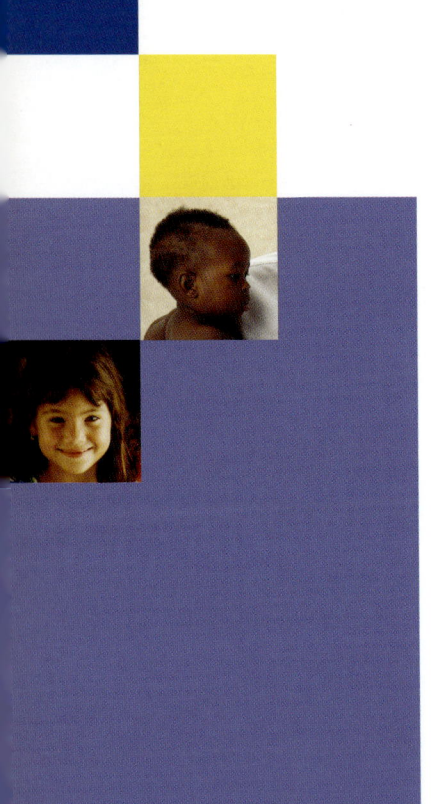

Recommended Reading

American College of Surgeons. "Pediatric Trauma." In *Advanced Trauma Life Support for Doctors*, 8th ed. Chicago: Author, 2008.

Alpar, E. K., and Robert Owen. "Abdominal Injuries." In *Paediatric Trauma*. Oxford, U.K.: Oxford University Press, 1988.

Campbell, John Emory, ed. "Abdominal Trauma." In *International Trauma Life Support for Prehospital Care Providers*, 6th ed., 203–10. Upper Saddle River, N.J.: Pearson/Prentice Hall, 2008.

Davies, Kimberly. "Buckled-up Children. Understanding the Mechanism, Injuries, Management, and Prevention of Seat-belt Related Injuries." *Journal of Trauma Nursing* 11 (Jan-Mar 2004): 16–24.

Foltin, George and Arthur Cooper. "Abdominal Trauma." In *Pediatric Emergency Medicine: Concepts and Clinical Practice*, 2nd ed., edited by Roger M. Barkin, et al., 335–54. St. Louis: Mosby; 1997.

Holmes, James F., Aaron Gladman, and Cindy Chang. "Performance of Abdominal Ultrasonography in Pediatric Blunt Trauma Patients: A Meta-analysis." *Journal of Pediatric Surgery* 49 (September 2007): 1588–94.

Jordan, B. "Lapbelt Complex. Recognition and Assessment of Seatbelt Injuries. Pediatric Trauma Patients." *Journal of Emergency Medical Services* 26 (May 2001): 36–43.

Ralston, Mark, Mary Fran Hazinski, Arno L. Zaritsky, Stephen M. Schexnayder, and Monica E. Kleinman, eds. *Pediatric Advanced Life Support Provider Manual*. Dallas: American Heart Association, 2007.

Tepas III, Joseph J., Mary E. Fallat, and Thomas M. Moriaty. "Trauma" In *APLS: The Pediatric Emergency Resource*, 4th ed., edited by Susan Fuchs, Marianne Gausche-Hill, Loren Yamamoto, et al., 269-23. Sudbury, M.A.: Jones and Bartlett, 2007.

Tuggle, David W. and Jennifer Garza. "Pediatric Trauma." In *Trauma*, 6th ed., edited by Ernest Moore, David Feliciano, and Kenneth Mattox, 988-1001. New York: McGraw-Hill, 2008.

CHAPTER 10
Pediatric Head Trauma

Lori Dandrea, MD
Jeffrey Kempf, DO
Laurie Weaver, RN, BSN, EMT-P

Objectives
Upon completion of this chapter, you should be able to:

1. Describe the anatomy of the pediatric head and brain.
2. Describe the pathophysiology of pediatric traumatic brain injury.
3. Discuss primary versus secondary brain injury.
4. Describe the development of secondary brain injury.
5. Describe the assessment and management of the pediatric patient with traumatic brain injury.

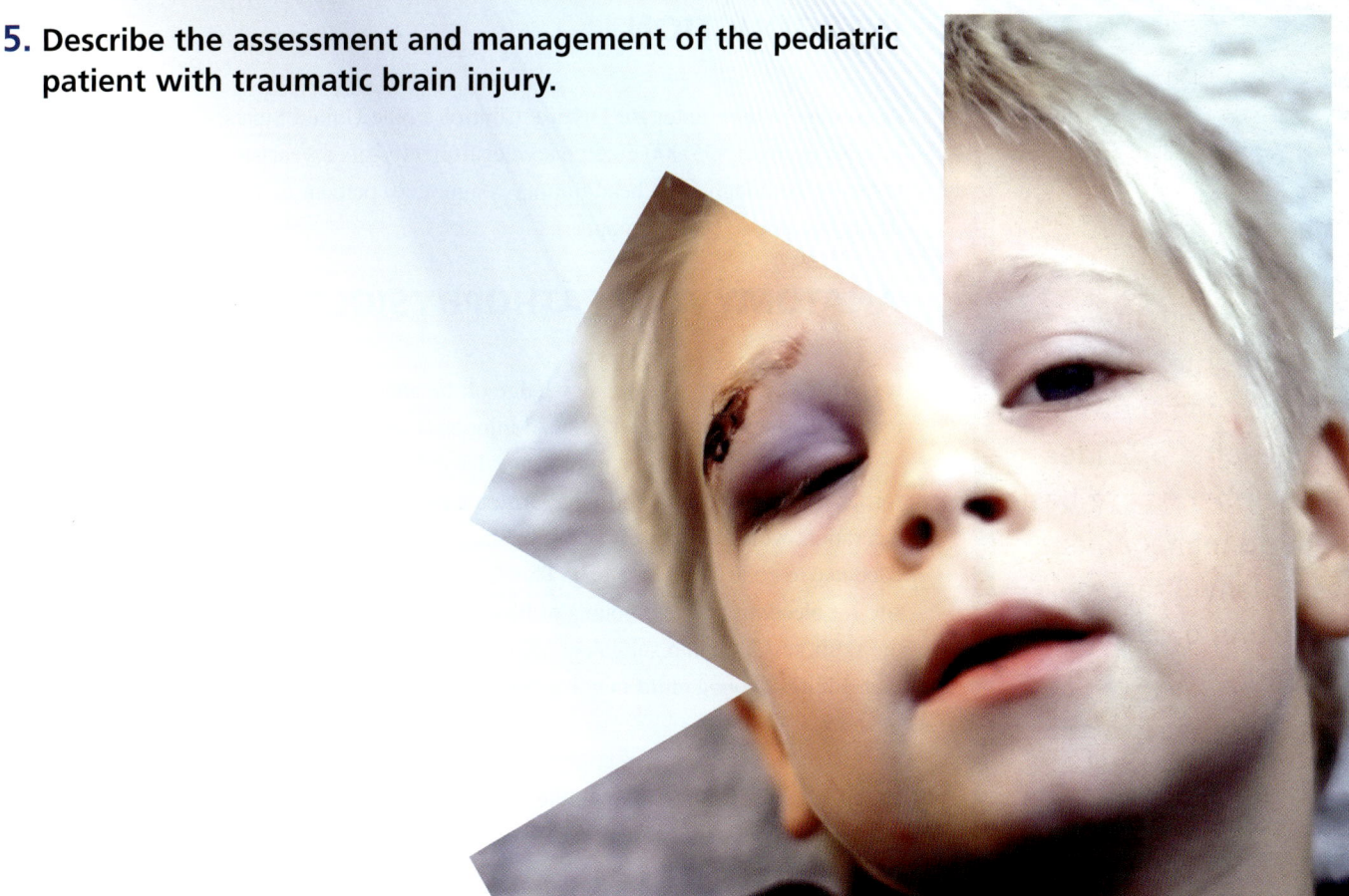

Case Study

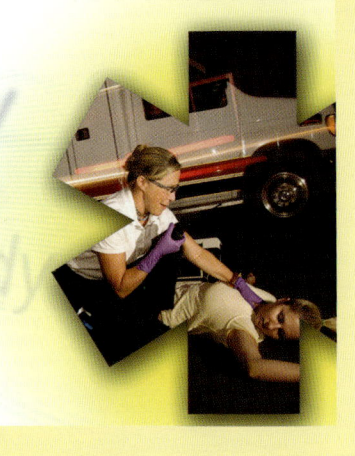

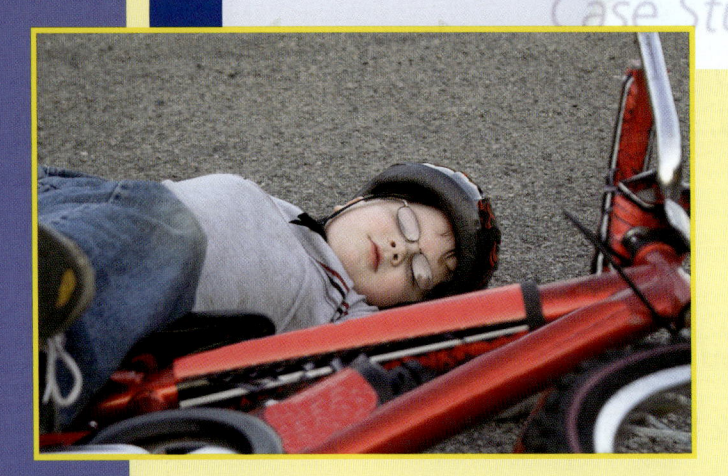

Susan, John, and Bob of the Emergency Transport System (ETS) have been dispatched to the scene where an 8-year-old boy was involved in a bicycle accident. While jumping his bicycle over a bale of hay, the child flew approximately 5 feet (1.5 meters) and lost control, landing on a gravel road. The child was not wearing a helmet. When they arrive, the child is motionless. How should the team approach this patient? What injuries should they suspect from this mechanism of injury? How should they care for this patient? Keep these questions in mind as you read the chapter. Then, at the end of the chapter, find out how the rescuers completed the call.

INTRODUCTION

According to the Center for Disease Control, in the United States, children with head injuries result in 435,000 emergency department visits a year and more than 2,600 deaths annually. Although most head trauma is minor, 80 percent to 90 percent of pediatric trauma deaths are due to head trauma.

ANATOMY AND PATHOPHYSIOLOGY

It is important to have basic knowledge of the anatomy of the skull and its contents to understand the various types of head injuries (Fig. 10.1).

The scalp in children is highly vascularized, as it is in adults, and it is a common site for lacerations. A young child may lose a significant amount of blood from even a simple laceration, which may rarely result in shock. Fortunately, direct pressure is usually adequate to control the bleeding. The deeper layer of the scalp, the galea, is also a potential site for bleeding. Large amounts of blood may collect in the space between the galea and the skull, resulting in a subgaleal hematoma. Because infants have a smaller blood volume than adults, a young child may lose enough blood into a subgaleal hematoma to result in shock.

Mechanical factors also contribute to the severity and pattern of head injuries seen in pediatric patients. In childhood, the head comprises the largest part of the body mass, and may be more than 25 percent in early infancy. Weak upper extremity and neck muscles

PEARLS

Bleeding may be significant from a scalp wound and frighten the child, parents and the prehospital provider. Remember to use basic wound management, especially direct pressure, on the wound.

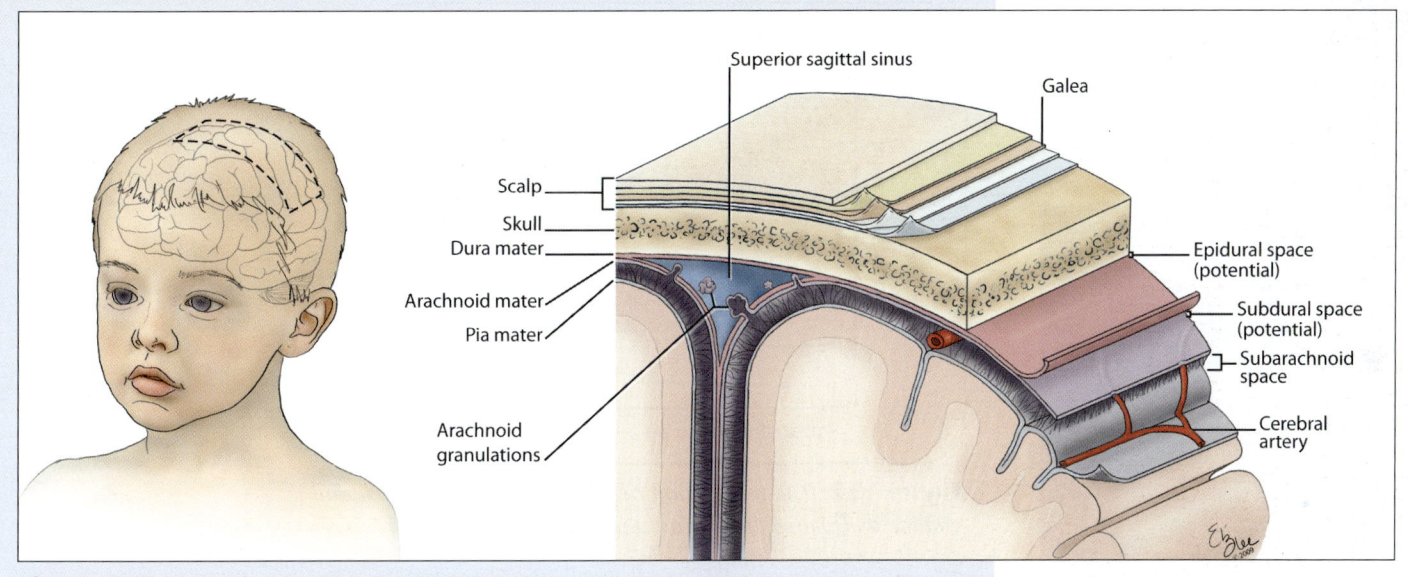

Figure 10.1 *The anatomy of the brain of a child.*

make it very difficult for a child to protect himself from head injury. In addition, the skull of the infant is very soft; thus, a direct blow will easily deform the skull and may cause underlying cerebral injury. Fortunately, children have suture lines, which allow the skull to expand without causing compression of the brain. This enables the infant to suffer fewer effects of increased intracranial pressure applied over a short time.

Brain Injuries

The brain, as a result of trauma, can sustain both primary and secondary injury. Primary injury occurs as a direct result of the trauma (i.e., skull fractures, contusions, lacerations, and concussions). Once incurred, this damage is seldom influenced by therapeutic interventions. Secondary injury occurs as a result of the brain's response to the primary injury. It may be from bleeding, swelling or infection. Complications from other injuries, such as hypoxia (lack of oxygen), hypercapnia (lack of ventilation), or shock (lack of adequate tissue perfusion) all further aggravate the overall severity of the brain injury.

Treatment of the head-injured child is aimed at preventing the secondary injury and, thus, improving outcome. Although many factors interact to determine the degree of secondary injury, the most crucial of such factors is increased intracranial pressure. Understanding what factors influence intracranial pressure will aid in the treatment of severe head trauma.

Cerebrospinal fluid, blood, and brain parenchyma are enclosed by the cranium. Always changing, these three components attempt to maintain a relatively constant intracranial pressure. When one component increases in volume, the other two will decrease to maintain a constantly normal intracranial pressure—usually less than 15 mmHg (Fig. 10.2). Pulse, respiration, position changes, and valsalva maneuvers also may cause some fluctuation in the intracranial pressure. When the brain is injured, the other intracranial components, cerebrospinal fluid and cerebral blood flow, attempt to buffer the system through compensation.

Cerebrospinal fluid contributes 10 percent of the total intracranial volume and is the first area affected when volume must be regulated. With an increase in intracranial volume, cerebrospinal fluid can be displaced easily into either the spinal subarachnoid space or the ventricular system to diminish cerebrospinal fluid volume. Both are

> **PEARLS**
>
> **A child's head is the largest part of his body, especially in infancy, when it is 25 percent of their total body. Suspect head injury in any child with a significant mechanism of injury.**

> **PEARLS**
>
> **It is the prehospital provider's job to prevent secondary injury to the brain by providing adequate oxygenation, ventilation and perfusion. Careful attention to ABCs can help to identify the need for the correct intervention.**

Pediatric Head Trauma

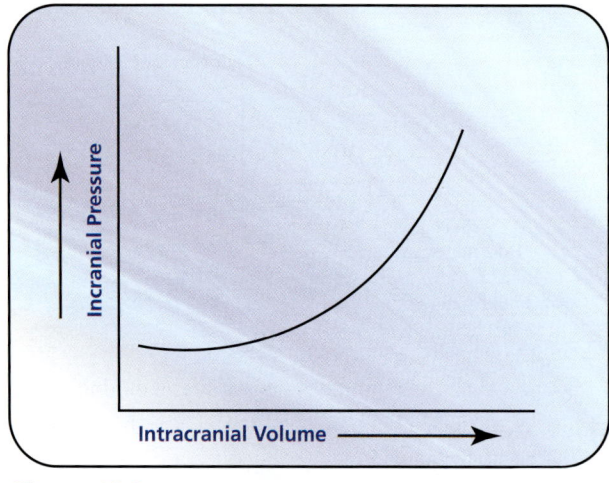

Figure 10.2 *The correlation between increasing intracranial volume and increasing intracranial pressure.*

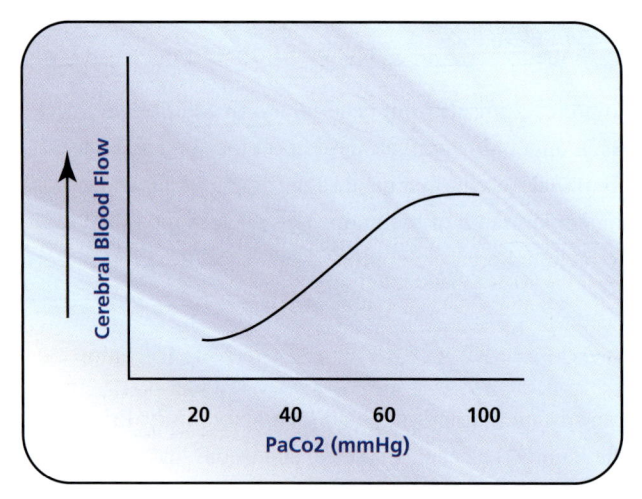

Figure 10.3 *Association between increasing carbon dioxide levels and increasing cerebral flow.*

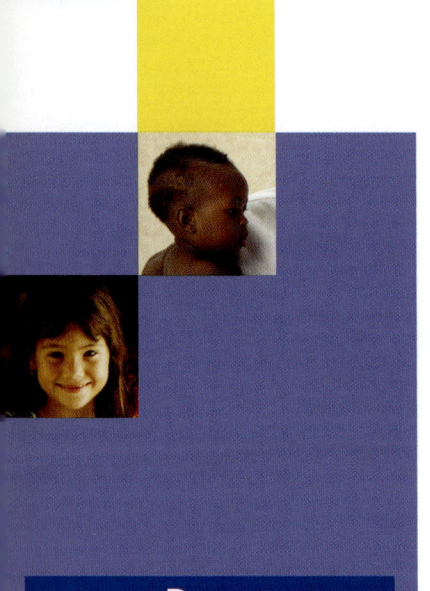

PEARLS

Avoid hyperventilation; provide adequate ventilation with 100 percent oxygen to the head-injured child. Contact medical direction for instruction in the event of rapid deterioration of the child.

attempts to maintain a constantly normal intracranial pressure. Marked changes in the intracranial pressure can occur with very small volume changes. When the cerebrospinal fluid shifts can no longer lessen the intracranial pressure, cerebral blood flow attempts to lower pressure by altering flow. Cerebral blood flow comprises only 8 percent of the intracranial volume, and changes in its volume can occur via several physiological relationships. Thin-walled veins contain most of the cerebral blood volume, and with extrinsic tissue pressure, as occurs in cerebral edema, the cerebral veins compensate by decreasing their volume of cerebral blood.

Cerebral blood flow is also responsive to changes in carbon dioxide levels. Cerebral blood volume and, thus, intracranial pressure, will decrease due to cerebral vasoconstriction, which is caused by rapidly lowering levels of carbon dioxide (Fig. 10.3). Thus, hyperventilation to prevent the accumulation of carbon dioxide will lower intracranial pressure. However, hyperventilation will also lower intracranial perfusion (to an even greater degree) and studies have shown that the routine use of hyperventilation in patients with severe head trauma decreases their survival rate. Hyperventilation is recommended only for the head-injured child with signs of impending herniation. This is because desperate measures are needed to buy precious time to try to get the child to a trauma center that may be able to surgically relieve the pressure. Adequate oxygenation is also essential, as hypoxia may lead to increased cerebral blood flow and, thus, increased intracranial pressure.

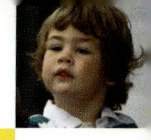

Brain matter/tissue comprises the last 80 percent of the intracranial volume. Obviously, with acute trauma there is little this fixed mass can do to maintain normal intracranial pressure.

Head Injuries

Most pediatric head trauma involves extracranial injuries, such as lacerations and hematomas. Intracranial injuries are injuries to the brain that can cause serious morbidity and mortality. Other trauma that can occur to the skull, such as fractures, may be accompanied by intracranial injuries or, as is more common, occur as isolated injuries.

Extracranial Injuries

Lacerations and hematomas of the head are extremely common in children. Apply a sterile dressing to every scalp laceration, and stop all active bleeding. Note the location of all lacerations and hematomas because there may be more serious injuries underneath, such as fracture or intracranial bleeding.

Skull Fractures

Skull fractures are distinguished as either open or closed fractures. There are three basic types of closed skull fractures: linear, depressed, and basilar.

Open. A depressed fracture (or avulsed portion of skull) with an overlying laceration poses the added danger of infection of the brain or brain coverings. Carefully cover this type of fracture with a sterile dressing without applying any pressure to the underlying brain tissue.

Linear. Most linear skull fractures occur in young children and are fairly benign, unless accompanied by cerebral injury.

Depressed. A depressed skull fracture may be associated with blunt trauma, a penetrating object, or an overlying laceration, creating an open fracture. If a step-off or irregularity of the skull is palpable, avoid placing pressure on that area. If an impaled object is present in the skull, stabilize it and do not attempt to remove it in the field. This type of fracture usually requires an operation to place the piece of bone into the correct location. Monitor these children closely because the brain may bleed where the skull pushes in on it.

Basilar. A basilar skull fracture is diagnosed clinically. Signs associated with basilar skull fractures are cerebral spinal fluid leakage from the ears or the nose, postauricular or mastoid ecchymosis (Battle's sign), and raccoon or panda eyes (bruising or discoloration of the periorbital areas). These fractures may involve the frontal, ethmoid, sphenoid, temporal bones, or occipital bones and may be accompanied by cerebral injury. A risk from these fractures is infection. With the cerebrospinal fluid communicating with the outside environment, bacteria can migrate into the fluid and cause infections such as meningitis.

Intracranial Injuries

It is critical to identify an intracranial injury early. The different types cannot be differentiated by the clinical exam and will require further in-hospital imaging. Children with these injuries need aggressive medical and surgical management to give them the best chance for a positive outcome.

Epidural Hematomas

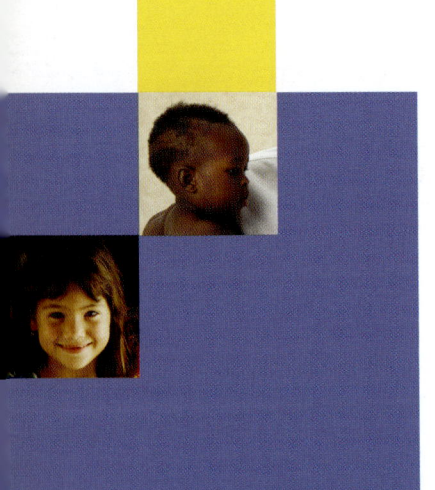

The epidural space lies just beneath the skull. This area is important because the meningeal arteries run through it and, if they are damaged, severe hemorrhage can occur here (Fig. 10.4). Fortunately, epidural hematomas are less common in children than adults. The most frequent cause of epidural hematoma is a temporal bone fracture that crosses the middle meningeal artery.

The usual presentation of an epidural hematoma is a rapid deterioration of neurologic function with associated symptoms of increased intracranial pressure. These patients may have a subacute presentation or may be fine (lucid) following the injury, and then become progressively lethargic. That is why it is so important to reassess and monitor children with head trauma. Surgical removal of the hematoma prior to developing an impaired level of consciousness and neurologic deficits usually results in a complete recovery.

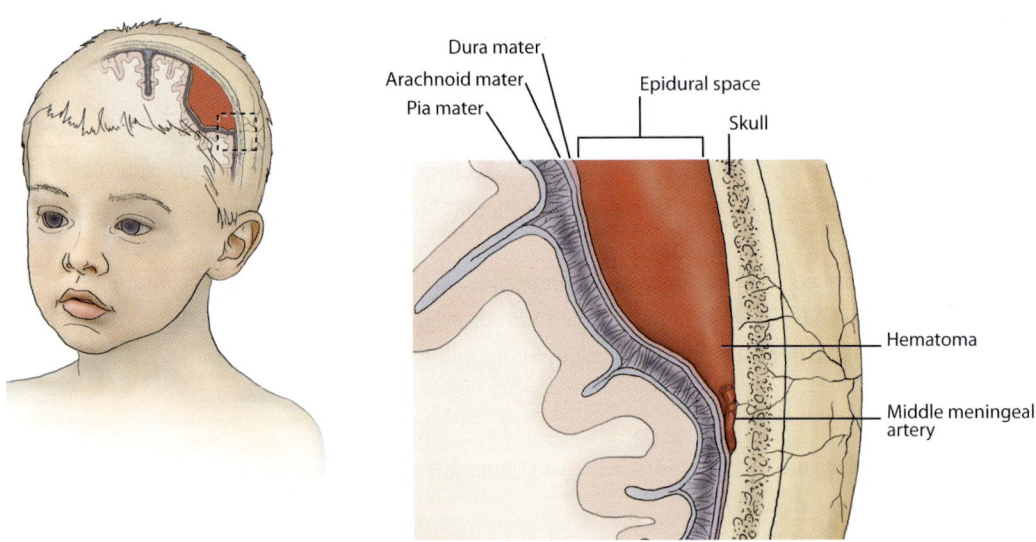

Figure 10.4 *An epidural hematoma occurs when the meningeal arteries are damaged and blood fills the epidural space just beneath the skull.*

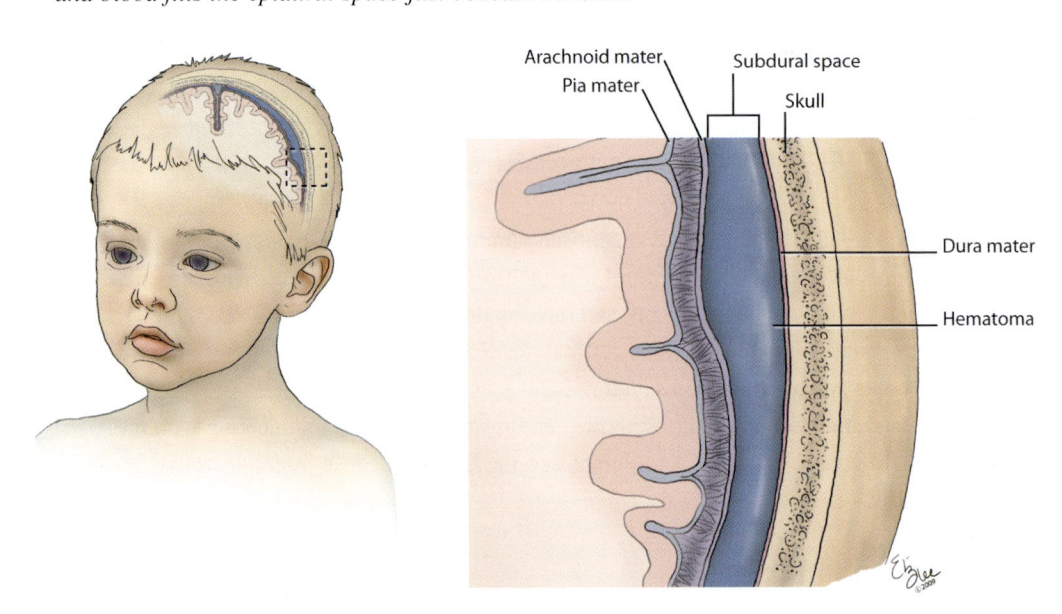

Figure 10.5 *A subdural hematoma results from blood between the dura mater and the arachnoid membrane.*

Pediatric Trauma Life Support

Subdural Hematomas

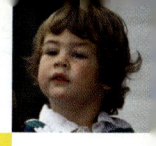

The dura mater, a fibrous layer that covers the brain, sits beneath the epidural space. Immediately below is another layer, the arachnoid membrane. Subdural hematoma is the result of bleeding between the dura and the arachnoid and is associated with injury to the underlying brain tissue (Fig. 10.5). Subdural hematomas are more common in children than are epidural hematomas. Because the bleeding is from veins instead of arteries, intracranial pressure increases more slowly, and the onset of symptoms may take hours to days after the injury to develop. There is impaired level of consciousness associated with lethargy and irritability. Focal or generalized seizures can also occur. Infants also may have a bulging fontanel (a sign of increased intracranial pressure). It is important to bear in mind that subdural hemorrhages are often associated with shaken baby syndrome. This syndrome is a form of child abuse in which the infant is held and shaken; there usually are minimal signs of external injury, but the shaking results in serious brain injury.

Diffuse Axonal Injury

This is the most common type of injury associated with severe head trauma. The brain is injured so diffusely that there is diffuse subarachnoid blood and edema. The subarachnoid blood causes diffuse irritation that results in increased pressure and "leaking" of fluid into the brain. Patients with this injury also may have seizure activity and vomiting from the irritation.

Cerebral Edema

Cerebral edema, or diffuse brain swelling, is the most difficult type of injury to manage. This swelling increases the intracranial pressure and may even lead to herniation, the movement of brain tissue through the fibrous layers that surround the brain. Cushing's triad (irregular respirations, bradycardia, and hypertension) is a sign of impending herniation, which is usually a terminal event for the brain. Herniation also may cause dilated, unreactive pupils, impairment of lateral or upward gaze, decreased level of consciousness, increased muscle tone with decorticate or decerebrate posturing, and cardiopulmonary arrest. The management of a head-injured child with signs of impending herniation (unequal pupils, extensor posturing, progressive neurologic deterioration) is directed at keeping the intracranial pressure low by elevating the head of the backboard and in decreasing the intracranial pressure through hyperventilation (this is the only indication for hyperventilation), in order to maintain blood flow to the brain. It is also important to keep the patient well oxygenated. Ventilate the child at 15 to 20 breaths per minute (bpm) and hyperventilate at 30 bpm. Ventilate infants at 25 bpm and hyperventilate at 35 bpm. If you are able to monitor end-tidal CO_2, ventilate at a rate to maintain an end-tidal CO_2 between 35-40 mmHg and hyperventilate to maintain an end-tidal CO_2 of 30 mmHg.

Other Injuries

Another injury is cerebral hematoma. This is a collection of blood within the brain tissue. It is usually quite serious and the result of severe head trauma. Other less severe forms of cerebral damage include contusions and concussions. Brain contusions are focal areas of swelling and bruising within the brain tissue. The neurological findings are variable and depend on the location and extent of the bruising. Concussions represent a transient neurological deficit secondary to trauma. This may include an altered level of consciousness, abnormal behavior, vomiting, headache, or amnesia that improves over time. Early in their course, concussions cannot be differentiated from intracranial injury; all children with the preceding symptoms need complete medical evaluations and continuous monitoring.

PATIENT ASSESSMENT

The assessment of the pediatric trauma patient follows the standard ITLS procedure:

1. ITLS Primary Survey
   A. Scene Size-Up
   B. Initial Assessment
   C. Rapid Trauma Survey or Focused Exam
   D. Critical Interventions and Transport Decisions
   E. Contact medical direction as needed.
2. ITLS Secondary Survey and/or Ongoing Exam

ITLS Primary Survey

Scene Size-Up

The mechanism of injury is particularly important to ascertain. In pediatric patients, it is also useful to note any clues of possible child abuse, such as a chaotic home environment, discrepancies in caretakers' stories, or a reported mechanism of injury that does not fit with either the child's injuries or his developmental age. Necessary historical information to obtain following a head injury includes loss of consciousness, amnesia for the event, severe headache, vomiting, or any change in behavior. A short seizure immediately following a head injury is often benign but requires a complete medical assessment. A child who has a head injury followed by a seizure should be stabilized in the manner described in the following section and transported. Assume that any child with an altered mental status has a possible head injury and stabilize the child as described.

Initial Assessment

General Appearance of the Child

As you approach, note the child's approximate age, sex, weight, and general appearance. Observe the position of the child, both body position and position in relation to the surroundings. Note the child's activity. Is the child aware of surroundings, anxious, obviously in distress, and so on? Does the child have any obvious major injuries or major bleeding? These observations will help you prioritize the child.

Level of Consciousness While Stabilizing the Cervical Spine

The initial approach to the child should be nonthreatening. Because the incidence of cervical spine injuries in children is greater with head trauma cases, it is particularly important to maintain spinal motion restriction in these patients. You must stabilize the cervical spine of any child with an altered mental status. Even with a febrile child with no history of trauma, prolonged seizure activity may be a sign of an occult head injury (e.g., shaken baby syndrome).

You may quickly assess a child's level of consciousness by using the AVPU system (A, alert; V, responds to verbal stimuli; P, responds to painful stimuli; and U, is unresponsive). If the child has an abnormal level of consciousness, record the score for the modified GCS after you finish the ITLS Primary Survey (Table 10.1).

PEARLS

Assume that any child with an altered mental status has a head injury.

PEARLS

Prolonged seizure activity, even without a history of trauma, may be a sign of an occult head injury. Consider stabilization of the cervical spine. This will also help maintain neutral positioning of the airway.

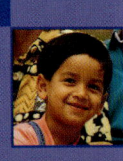

Table 10.1: Pediatric Glasgow Coma Scale

	Patient < 2 years	Patient > 2 years	
Eye Opening	Spontaneous	Spontaneous	4
	To speech	To voice	3
	To pain	To pain	2
	None	None	1
Verbal Response	Coos, babbles	Oriented	5
	Cries irritably	Confused	4
	Cries to pain	Inappropriate words	3
	Moans to pain	Incomprehensible	2
	None	None	1
Motor Response	Normal movements	Obeys commands	6
	Withdraws to touch	Localizes pain	5
	Withdrawal-pain	Withdrawal-pain	4
	Abnormal flexion	Flexion-pain	3
	Abnormal extension	Extension-pain	2
	None	None	1

Total = Eye + Verbal + Motor

Airway

Whenever uncertainty exists as to what has happened to the child, protect the cervical spine. Ensure that the child has an open airway as manual control of the cervical spine is established. Sometimes children with head injuries will lose their gag reflex and will be unable to control their own secretions. Opening the airway via the modified jaw-thrust maneuver and suctioning may be all that is needed for adequate airway control. A child who is unconscious and has lost the gag reflex may need help to protect the airway. If the child is experiencing apneic episodes, immediately begin bag-valve-mask ventilations. To prevent the development of a secondary injury from hypoxia, early administration of 100 percent oxygen is essential, even in conscious patients. If intubation is necessary, monitor the end-tidal CO_2 once intubation is completed.

Breathing

Assess the child's respiratory status, checking the rate and quality. It is important to keep in mind that irregular respirations are a sign of increased intracranial pressure. Be proactive in assisting the child's ventilations if they are not adequate. The patient should be ventilated at the normal respiratory rate for the child's age unless there are obvious signs of herniation (e.g., unequal pupils, extensor posturing, progressive neurologic deterioration), in which case you should hyperventilate the child. Maintain spinal motion restriction throughout any manipulations of the airway.

Circulation

After securing the airway, ensuring effective ventilations and applying oxygen, assess the child's circulatory status. Shock rarely occurs following an isolated head injury, but it may be present with multisystem injury. It is necessary to evaluate the rate, rhythm, and quality of pulses, as well as the capillary refill. Control all active bleeding immediately with careful attention to any deformities noted on the skull. Hypotension will markedly worsen the outcome of a severe head injury so you must be proactive in the treatment of shock and in shock prevention. After controlling any external hemorrhage, manage the blood pressure to within normal ranges for the child's age. Bradycardia is an ominous sign and may be indicative of hypoxia or very high intracranial pressure. You may see Cushing's triad (bradycardia, hypertension, and irregular respirations) in children with very high intracranial pressure; this indicates a severe head injury. Because children with bradycardia may experience respiratory problems (inadequate oxygenation, esophageal intubation), it is important to ensure that the airway is secure and to administer 100 percent oxygen. Remember that it is vital to maintain adequate oxygenation and adequate circulation.

Rapid Trauma Survey

A rapid head-to-toe examination is imperative in the patient with a head injury. Often, head-injured patients are unable to communicate the presence of other life-threatening injures due to their altered levels of consciousness.

After the head-to-toe exam, obtain baseline vital signs (blood pressure, pulse, and respiratory rate) and also obtain the SAMPLE history if possible. If a load-and-go situation is present (see the Critical Interventions and Transport Decisions section that follows), transport now and obtain the vital signs during transport.

If the child has an abnormal level of consciousness, perform a brief neurological exam including the GCS score. In the modified GCS, any score less than 13 implies a serious head injury, and any score less than 9 indicates a profound, life-threatening neurological dysfunction. Any child with an altered mental status requires rapid package and transport. If a child has seizures after a head injury, he must be managed carefully. Although a single short seizure following a head injury may be benign, multiple seizures can be indicative of a severe head injury.

Critical Interventions and Transport Decisions

If any signs of an unstable airway, respiratory distress, shock, or an altered mental status are present, package and transport the child rapidly following the Rapid Trauma Survey. The keys to a successful outcome following a head injury are early recognition and rapid management. Because head trauma accounts for 80 percent to 90 percent of pediatric trauma deaths, early, proactive management makes a tremendous difference in the child's outcome. When making transport decisions, remember that children with severe head injuries have a greater chance of survival if they are treated in trauma centers equipped to handle pediatric patients. If the child has sustained a penetrating injury to the head, carefully assess the child. Do not remove any object impaled in the child's head. Stabilize the object in the position in which it was found.

Airway and Cervical Spine

Completely restrict spinal motion with appropriately sized equipment before the child is moved. Any child with an altered mental status requires cervical spine control to protect the spine during transport. If the child is not in shock and has an isolated head injury, elevate the head of the backboard slightly to lower intracranial pressure. If unable to effectively ventilate via bag-valve-mask ventilation, intubation may be indicated, but its use should be rare. The Brain Trauma Foundation states that there is no evidence to support the superiority of prehospital endotracheal intubation over bag-valve-mask ventilation in

Pediatric Trauma Life Support

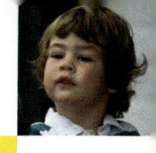

pediatric patients with traumatic brain injury. Suctioning equipment should be easily accessible, as emesis is a frequent problem in the head-injured child, particularly with airway manipulation.

Breathing

Every head-injured child should receive 100 percent oxygen. Monitor oxygen saturation (pulse oximetry) and end-tidal CO_2 (capnography) with appropriately sized equipment, especially if the child is intubated (Fig. 10.6). If the child's ventilations are inadequate (hypoxia [pulse oximetry < 95 percent] or hypercapnia [etCO$_2$ > 45]), support ventilations via bag-valve-mask technique.

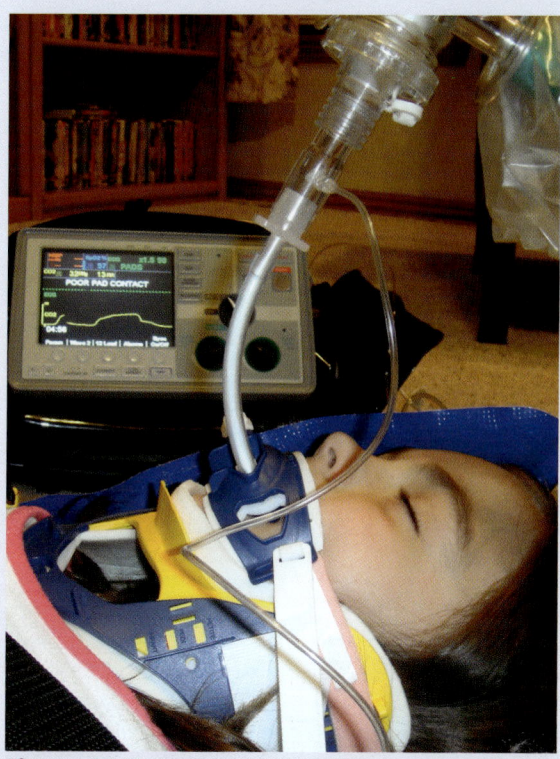

Figure 10.6 *Capnography should be used to monitor end-tidal CO_2, especially if the child is intubated.*

Circulation

If the child shows signs of shock, establish IV/IO access and administer the standard 20 mL/kg bolus of normal saline or other medically approved crystalloid (see Chapter 7). In order to maintain cerebral perfusion, the child must have an adequate circulating blood volume. It is critical to administer fluids to a child with head injury and shock. In the absence of hemodynamic instability, establish IV access and administer fluid at a rate that will keep the vein open.

Seizures

Because seizures increase intracranial pressure and decrease oxygenation, stop them as soon as possible. Follow local protocol, but remember that diazepam (administered via IV, IO, or rectal routes), or another benzodiazepine is usually effective.

Pediatric Head Trauma

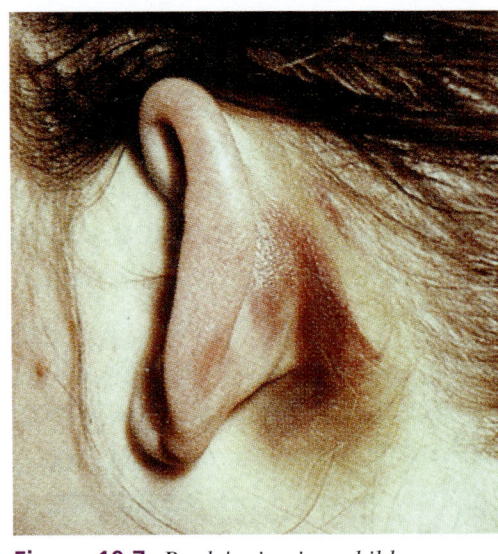

Figure 10.7 *Battle's sign in a child.*

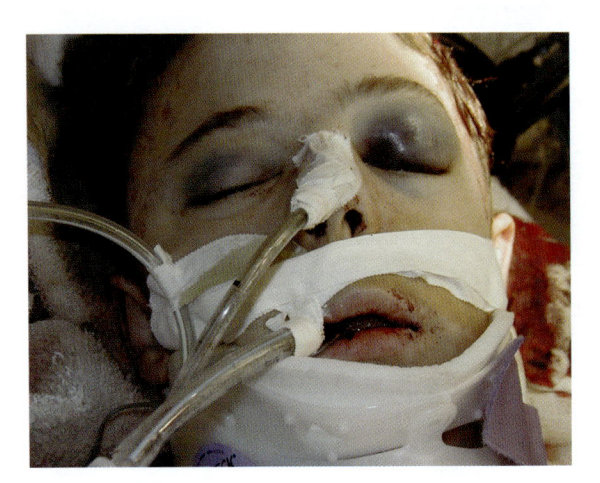

Figure 10.8 *Raccoon eyes in a child.*

ITLS Secondary Survey

Have a team member repeat the vital signs while you perform the ITLS Secondary Survey. Perform a fingerstick glucose test on all patients with altered mental status.

Head Examination

During the head examination, look for signs of a serious injury. Carefully examine the head for lacerations, hematomas, depressions, and cerebrospinal fluid leaks. Note the depth and location of lacerations. Also note any fractures underneath lacerations; carefully stop bleeding and palpate the wound for subtle fractures. Note the location and size of any swelling on the child's head. Be particularly careful if the hematoma is over the middle meningeal artery, as some children with this injury may develop epidural bleeds. Depressions can be palpable immediately following an injury; note their depths and locations. Note any fluid or blood draining from the nose or ears, and look for postauricular or mastoid ecchymosis (Battle's sign) or raccoon eyes (Figs. 10.7, 10.8).

In children less than one year of age, a fontanel is present in the anterior portion of the skull. You must assess the fontanel of these patients. While bulging or tenseness may be noted in a normal crying infant, any bulging in a quiet, upright baby may be indicative of increased intracranial pressure.

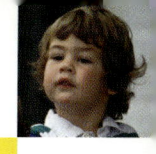

Complete Neurologic Examination

This examination should address the following areas:

1. Repeat the Glasgow Coma Scale score. Report any change to medical direction.
2. Pupillary examination should note the size and reactivity of the pupils. Unequal or fixed and dilated pupils are indicative of severe trauma to the brain.
3. Motor and sensory examination should note the child's ability to move the extremities. Check the motor strength and sensation in each extremity. In severe head injuries, a variety of abnormal muscle movements, referred to as posturing, may be noted (Fig. 10.9). In decerebrate posturing, all extremities extend and rotate inward. Decorticate posturing is recognized by the presence of extended legs and flexed arms. Progression from decorticate (flexion) posturing to decerebrate (extension) posturing is an ominous sign.

Careful reassessment is important in children with a head injury. With severe head trauma, the alterations in behavior and vital signs are usually present at the time of the initial evaluation. With mild-to-moderate head injuries, the changes may be ongoing, and early recognition and transport are critical in these patients.

Behavioral changes following a head injury may be progressive, subtle changes that indicate an internal injury. Information from parents or caregivers may alert prehospital personnel to subtle changes in the child's behavior that may indicate an underlying head injury. Always ask what the child is "normally" like.

Treatment Medications

As mentioned earlier, seizures may occur with a head injury. Although most seizures will be short and not cause complications, some head-injured children may have prolonged seizures that require pharmacologic therapy as mentioned in the Critical Interventions section earlier.

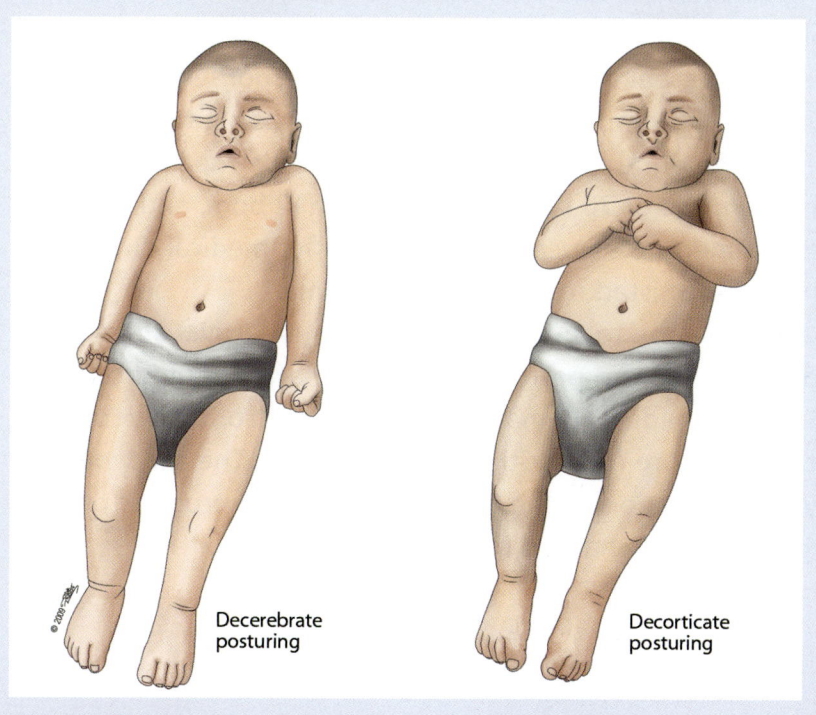

Figure 10.9 *Posturing in an infant.*

Pediatric Head Trauma

Case Study continued

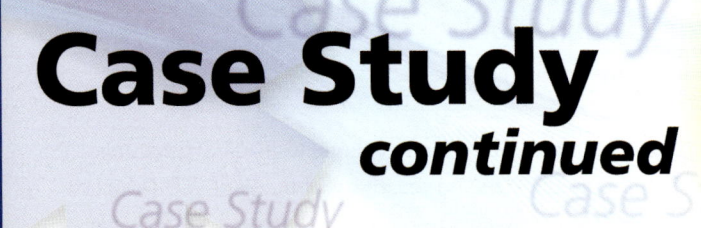

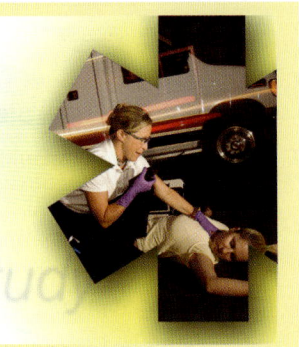

Susan and the team complete the scene size-up. As they approach, they see a child lying motionless on the ground. The general impression is not good. Bob provides spinal motion restriction to the child's head as Susan determines a level of consciousness. The child opens his eyes and localizes pain on applying pressure over the forehead (supraorbital ridge). He appears disoriented. His airway is clear (absent of foreign matter, blood, and secretions). His respiratory rate is normal (18 breaths per minute) but irregular. John initiates ventilatory assistance with a bag-valve mask and 100 percent oxygen as Susan assesses the child's circulation. His radial pulse is 80 beats per minute and slightly irregular. The rate is normal, and his skin is pale, cool, and dry with no obvious bleeding. Susan decides this is a load-and-go patient as he has signs of shock and has decreased level of consciousness.

Because of the mechanism, a Rapid Trauma Survey is performed. A bruise to the right temple and bleeding from his right nostril are noted. Pupils are 4 mm in size and react to light. Examination of the neck, chest, abdomen, pelvis and extremities are normal.

A cervical collar is applied and the child placed onto a backboard with spinal motion restriction maintained while examining the back. En route to the hospital, an IV is established, and vital signs are obtained.

As there was altered mental status, Susan does a neurological exam. The patient opens his eyes to verbal stimuli and localizes in response to pain. He does not speak but makes incomprehensible sounds. He has a gag reflex. His GCS is 10 (E3, V2, M5). The right pupil dilates to 6 mm while the left remains at 4 mm. Vital signs are pulse of 70 bpm, respiration of 12 bpm, and BP of 100/60 mmHg. Pulse oximetry is 95 percent. Susan notifies medical direction of the situation and starts assisted respiration at 20 bpm.

The trauma team meets the team at the ambulance on arrival at the pediatric trauma center. A CT scan performed promptly after intubation and ventilation reveals a right epidural hematoma, underlying frontal cerebral contusion and a stable fracture of the 6th cervical vertebra. The child went straight to surgery for evacuation of the clot. He made good progress on the neurosurgical ward and was discharged home in two weeks.

Case Study *wrap-up*

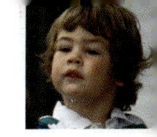

Bicycle accidents are a significant cause of head trauma in children 5 to 15 years of age. The use of bicycle helmets is of paramount importance in preventing head injuries and their long-term complications. However, motor vehicle collisions remain the leading cause of head injuries in children as well as adults. Because of the variance in growth and developmental stages that children go through, the mechanism of injury also varies with each age group. In this case scenario, the rescuer should approach the scene by noting the lack of a helmet and the location of the child in relation to the bicycle. The priorities of assessment are airway with spinal motion restriction, breathing, and circulation. Susan suspected a basal skull fracture and took appropriate action when the signs of increased intracranial pressure developed en route to the pediatric trauma center. The mechanism was also suspicious of a spinal injury and the boy indeed has a 6th cervical vertebral fracture, which fortunately was stable.

SUMMARY

1. Head trauma is the leading cause of traumatic death in the pediatric population.
2. The large size of the head and weak neck muscles of children predispose them to serious head injury.
3. Careful assessment and appropriate interventions such as oxygenation, appropriate ventilation, and maintenance of cerebral blood flow are necessary to prevent secondary brain injury and to control intracranial pressure.
4. All serious head injuries should be considered life-threatening and require aggressive management of the ABCs.
5. Rapidly package any child with an altered mental status and transport to the nearest appropriate facility.
6. Currently, the only indication for hyperventilation is in the child with impending cerebral herniation.

Recommended Reading

Ackerman, Alice D. "Current Issues in the Care of the Head Injured Child." *Current Opinions in Pediatrics* 3 (1991): 433–38.

Altimier, Leslie B. "Pediatric Central Neurologic Trauma: Issues for Special Patients." *AACN Clinical Issues* (February 1992): 31–40.

American College of Surgeons. "Head Trauma." In *Advanced Trauma Life Support for Doctors*, 8th ed. Chicago: Author, 2008.

Bouma, Gerrit J., et al. "Blood Pressure and Intracranial Pressure-volume Dynamics in Severe Head Injury." *Journal of Neurosurgery* 77 (1992): 15–19.

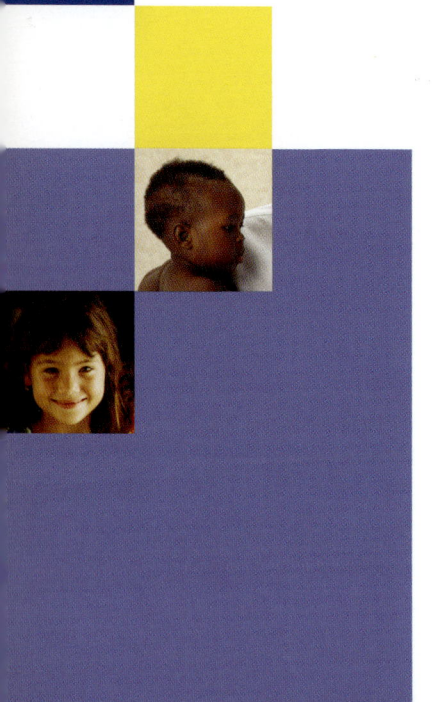

Brain Trauma Foundation. *Guidelines for the Prehospital Management of Severe Traumatic Brain Injury*, 2nd ed. New York: Author, 2007.

Bruce, Dennis A., et al. "Diffuse Cerebral Swelling Following Head Injuries in Children." *Journal of Neurosurgery* 54 (1992): 170–178.

Campbell, John Emory, ed. "Head Trauma." In *International Trauma Life Support for Prehospital Care Providers*, 6th ed., 141–59. Upper Saddle River, N.J.: Pearson/Prentice Hall, 2008.

Dean, J. Michael. "Cerebral Protection and Neurologic Outcome Following Closed Head Injury in Children." *Current Opinions in Pediatrics* 2 (1990): 514–18.

Easton, A. "Respiratory Involvement in Pediatric Head Injury." *Jems-Pediatric Notebook* (April 1993): 63–66.

Fisher, M. D. "Pediatric Traumatic Brain Injury." *Critical Care Nursing Quarterly* 20 (May 1997): 36–51.

Ghajar, Jamshid and Robert J. Hariri. "Management of Pediatric Head Injury." *Pediatric Clinics of North America* 39 (1992): 1093–1125.

Grubbs, Thomas C., et al. "Hypotensive Closed Head Injuries in Children: Case Report." *Air Medical Journal* 16 (October-December 1997): 108–112.

Inaba, Alson S. and P. N. Seward. "An Approach to Pediatric Trauma." *Emergency Medical Clinics of North America* 9 (1991): 523–548.

Johnston, Michael V. and Joan P. Gerring. "Head Trauma and Its Sequelae." *Pediatric Annals* 21 (1992): 362–68.

Langlois, Jean A., Wesley Rutland-Brown, and Karen E. Thomas. *Traumatic Brain Injury in the United States: Emergency Department Visits, Hospitalizations, and Deaths*. Atlanta: Centers for Disease Control and Prevention, National Center for Injury Prevention and Control, 2006.

Mayer, Thom A. and Marion L. Walker. "Pediatric Head Injury." *Annals of Emergency Medicine* 14 (1985): 1178–84.

Nichols, David G., Myron Yaster, Dorothy G. Lappe, et al. *Golden Hour: The Handbook of Pediatric Life Support*. 289–309. St. Louis: The CV Mosby Co., 1991.

Simon, Joseph. E. and Aron T. Goldberg. *Prehospital Pediatric Life Support*. St. Louis: Mosby-Year Book, 1989.

Tepas III, Joseph J., Mary E. Fallat, and Thomas M. Moriaty. "Trauma" In *APLS: The Pediatric Emergency Resource*, 4th ed., edited by Susan Fuchs, Marianne Gausche-Hill, Loren Yamamoto, et al., 269–323. Sudbury, M.A.: Jones and Bartlett, 2007.

11

CHAPTER 11
Pediatric Spinal Trauma

Ann Hoffman, RN, CPN
Sherri Kovach, RN, EMT-B
Francis R. Mencl, MD, FACEP

Objectives

Upon completion of this chapter, you should be able to:

1. Describe how trauma and pediatric spinal anatomy and physiology poses specific concerns.

2. Describe acceptable equipment and steps for spinal motion restriction.

3. Identify the criteria for removing a child from a car seat.

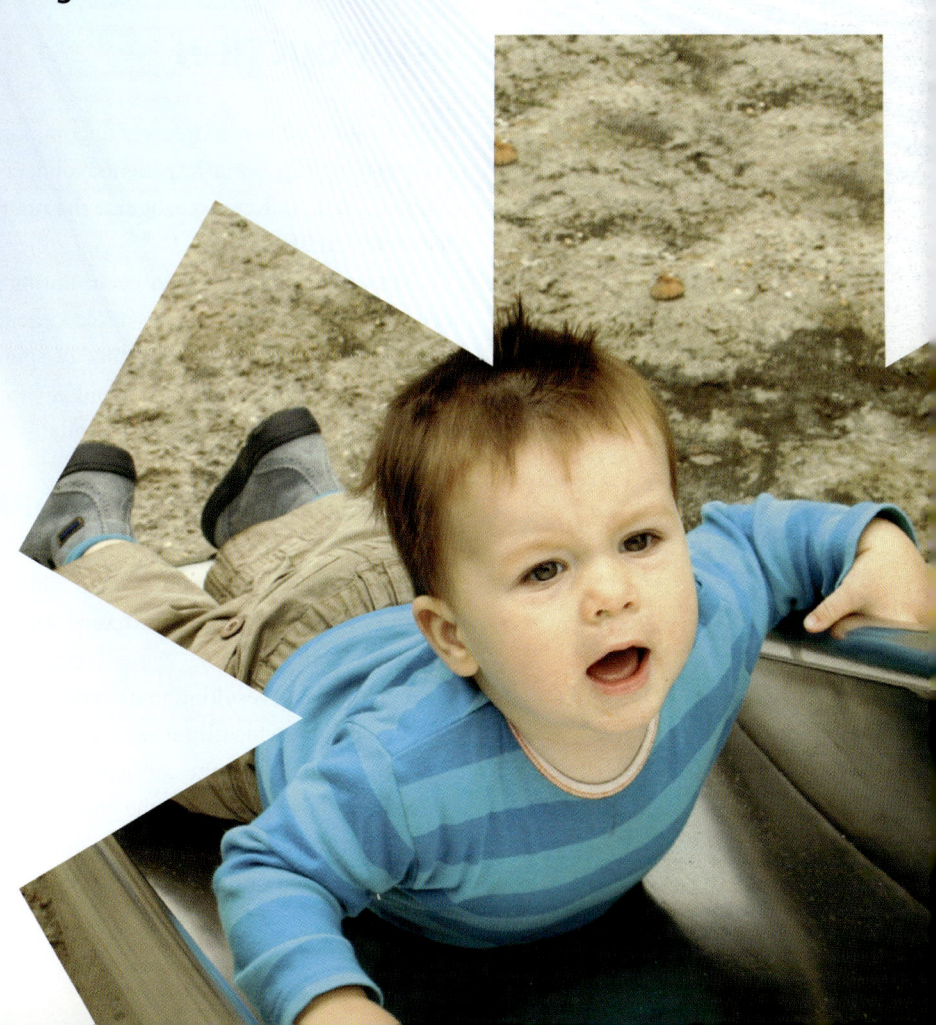

Case Study

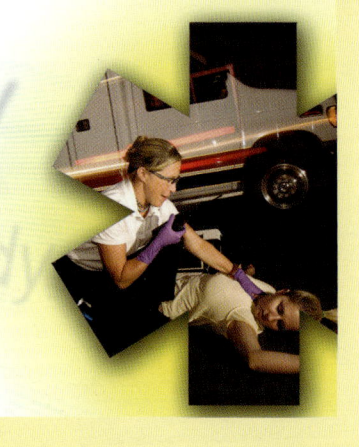

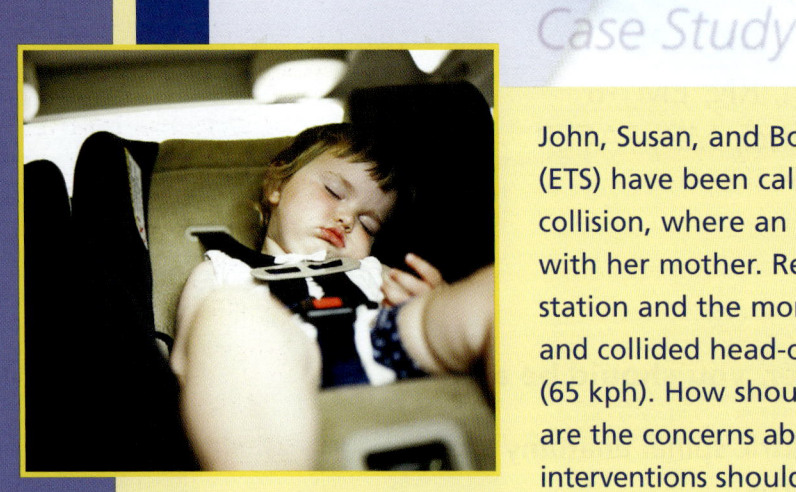

John, Susan, and Bob of the Emergency Transport System (ETS) have been called to the scene of a motor vehicle collision, where an 18-month-old child was riding in a car with her mother. Reportedly, they were going to the gas station and the mom swerved to avoid hitting an animal and collided head-on with a tree at approximately 40 mph (65 kph). How should the team approach this child? What are the concerns about the mechanism of injury? What interventions should they perform for this child in the field? When is it appropriate to use spinal motion restriction for infants and children in their car seats? Keep these questions in mind as you read the chapter. Then, at the end of the chapter, find out how the rescuers completed this call.

INTRODUCTION

Spinal cord trauma is extremely uncommon in preadolescent children. Only five percent of all spinal injuries occur in patients younger than 16 years of age. Although spinal cord trauma is rare, failure to recognize the injury may result in devastating consequences for the child and his family.

Most acute spinal injuries occur during a motor vehicle collision (MVC) or a sporting event. As the child approaches adolescence, more motorcycle and automobile crashes occur, leading to a higher incidence of spinal trauma with a pattern similar to that in adults. The prehospital provider must avoid any injury to the child's spinal cord from the time of the injury until treatment at the hospital is complete.

ANATOMY AND PATHOPHYSIOLOGY

A child's spine is not simply a small adult spine. The child's anatomy, physiology, and response to trauma are very different. The child's head is relatively large compared to the rest of the body. This may cause a force that is directed at the head to be transmitted through the neck, resulting in a cervical spine injury. The child's neck is short compared to that of an adult, which limits its mobility when undergoing stress from trauma. Finally, the ligaments that support the cervical spine in a child are relatively loose and may permit too much neck movement when the child is "thrown around," resulting in devastating injuries. Because of these anatomic factors, most cervical spine fractures in children will involve the upper portion of the cervical spine (Fig. 11.1).

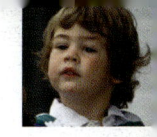

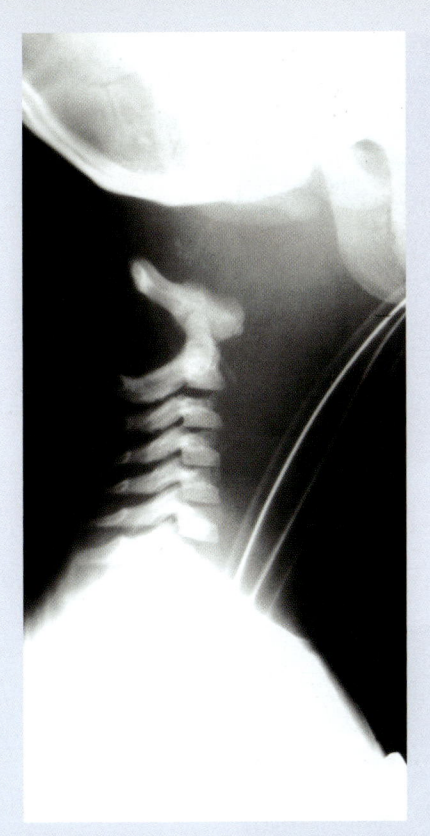

Figure 11.1 *The upper portion of the child's cervical spine is more susceptible to injury due to anatomy factors.*

> ### PEARLS
> Most spinal injuries that occur in children ages 10 and younger involve the cervical region. However, remain suspicious of potential thoracic and lumbar spinal injuries in a child as well.

Although most spinal injuries that occur in the first decade of life involve the cervical region, children also may sustain thoracic and lumbar spinal injuries. These injuries usually will occur at the level of T11–L2 because this is where the relatively rigid thoracic elements adjoin the more mobile lumbar segments. In an MVC involving a frontal impact, a child restrained in a standard rear seat lap belt may sustain a lumbar spinal fracture. External belt-shaped abrasions to the child's lower abdomen are important clues to a possible lumbar spine injury. It is important to note that there is a high association of bowel injury in a child with seat belt abrasion and a lumber fracture ("Chance" fracture).

PATIENT ASSESSMENT

Follow the standard approach for assessment of the pediatric trauma patient:

1. ITLS Primary Survey
   A. Scene Size-up
   B. Initial Assessment
   C. Rapid Trauma Survey or Focused Exam
   D. Critical Interventions and Transport Decisions
   E. Contact medical direction as needed.
2. ITLS Secondary Survey and/or Ongoing Exam

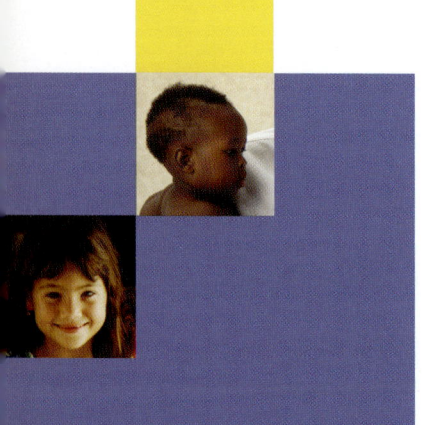

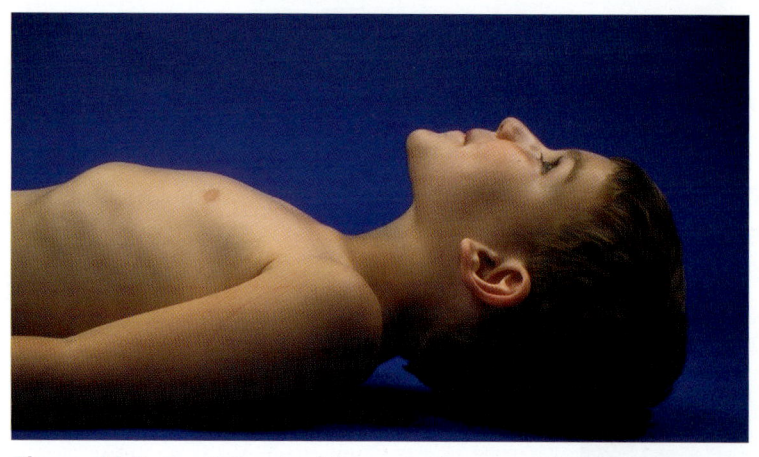

Figure 11.2 *Providers should assume that any child who suffers a traumatic injury that could injure the spine to have a spinal injury until proven otherwise.*

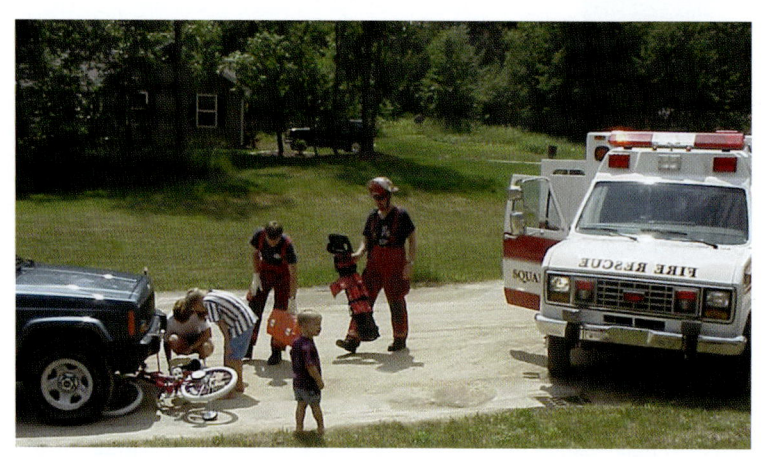

Figure 11.3 *Motor vehicle-pedestrian collisions and bicycle accidents are scenarios in which neck injuries are commonly seen.*

ITLS Primary Survey

Scene Size-Up

Consider any child who suffers a potential traumatic injury that could injure the spine to have a spinal injury until proven otherwise (Fig. 11.2). Situations in which neck injuries are more likely to occur include motor vehicle–pedestrian collisions, falls from heights, bicycle accidents, and sports injuries (Fig. 11.3).

Children with head trauma or an altered mental status (drugs or alcohol) are particularly likely to have a coexistent cervical spine injury. Take extra care to protect their spines.

Initial Assessment

General Impression

Particularly with infants and young children, general appearance is very important, often giving vital clues to the child's stability. Components of the general appearance include alertness, distractibility or consolability, speech or cry, skin color, respiratory efforts, and eye contact.

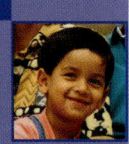

> **PEARLS**
>
> Suspect cervical spine injury in children with head trauma or altered mental status.

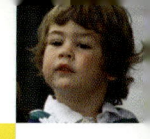

Airway and Cervical Spine
While maintaining spinal motion restriction, assess the airway. Use your hands for the initial stabilization. Speak calmly to the child as you hold the neck firmly in the neutral position. If the child has sustained a severe neck injury, you may be able to palpate a step-off on the back of the neck during the examination. Assess the child's airway. If the airway is unstable and you are unable to ventilate with a bag-valve mask, proceed as directed in Chapter 4, but remember to maintain spinal motion restriction.

Breathing
Carefully assess the child's breathing. Remember, any trauma patient with an upper cervical spine injury may lose the ability to breathe (apnea). This usually occurs if the injury is above the level of C5, which results in the loss of function of the phrenic and intercostal nerves. A child who is not breathing must be rapidly assisted with bag-valve-mask ventilation as discussed in Chapter 4. All patients with any suspected spinal injury should receive 100 percent oxygen (to keep the brain, spinal cord, and other vital organs well oxygenated). Continue to maintain spinal motion restriction.

Circulation
As discussed in Chapter 7, assess the child's pulse rate and other signs of perfusion to determine if the patient is showing signs of shock. The most common cause of shock in any trauma patient is hypovolemia. Treat all shock as hypovolemic shock. Occasionally, a child with an upper cervical spine injury develops neurogenic shock, a special type of shock in which the patient is hypotensive, normothermic, and has a low heart rate. Because neurogenic shock is a diagnosis of exclusion, these children should be treated as if they are hypovolemic until a definitive diagnosis can be made at the hospital.

Rapid Trauma Survey
The Rapid Trauma Survey is designed to identify all life-threatening injuries and may provide information related to the suspected spinal injury and neurological exam.

The Rapid Trauma Survey consists of a brief, targeted examination from head to toe. In assessing for spinal injury, look for the inability to feel or move any of the four extremities or the presence of any mechanical breathing deficit.

Brief Neurologic Assessment
The likelihood of a cervical spine injury increases with a head injury. The unconscious trauma patient carries a 15 percent to 20 percent risk of spinal column damage. Carefully maintain spinal motion restriction on any child with an altered mental status until a definitive evaluation is done at the hospital. If the child has altered mental status, the neurological exam conducted at the end of the Rapid Trauma Survey should include an age-appropriate Glasgow Coma Scale (GCS) score. Maintain spinal motion restriction on any awake and alert child who complains of neck pain.

PEARLS

A pediatric trauma patient with a cervical spine injury may lose the ability to breathe. Be prepared to assist ventilations.

PEARLS

Children with spinal trauma may develop a special type of shock with hypotension, normothermia, and low heart rate. However, treat the child for hypovolemic shock until a definitive diagnosis can be made at the hospital.

Critical Interventions and Transport Decisions

Any child with an unstable airway, obvious respiratory insufficiency, shock, or an altered mental status requires rapid package and transport to the nearest facility able to give adequate pediatric care.

Airway and Cervical Spine

Recent studies have indicated that oral endotracheal intubations can be performed safely in patients with spinal injuries as long as manual in-line stabilization is maintained throughout the procedure; however, there is no evidence that prehospital endotracheal intubation improves survival in pediatric patients. As indicated in Chapter 4, if a child can be effectively oxygenated and ventilated using a bag-valve mask, you may delay intubation until arrival at the hospital. Always supply the patient with 100 percent oxygen.

Perform spinal motion restriction before moving the child. A cervical collar may be used as long as the appropriate size is available. Place it carefully on the child. Because collars alone do not effectively stabilize a child's neck, you must use additional supplemental devices. If an appropriately size collar is not available (especially in children less than 1 year of age), towels may be used to restrict the child's neck motion while maintaining the neutral position. Secure the child to a rigid spine board. If an appropriately sized collar is available, apply it to the child's neck. Secure the torso and lower body while continuing manual spinal motion restriction. Once you have secured the body, stabilize the head using a head motion restriction device, towel rolls, or whatever is available.

As mentioned earlier, a child has a larger head than an adult as compared to the rest of the child's body. To correct for this difference, use a pediatric backboard (Fig. 11.4). If a pediatric backboard is not available, you may create a modified backboard by placing padding under the child's shoulders to place the neck in the "neutral" position (Fig. 11.5). Place the padding on the board before placing the child on the board.

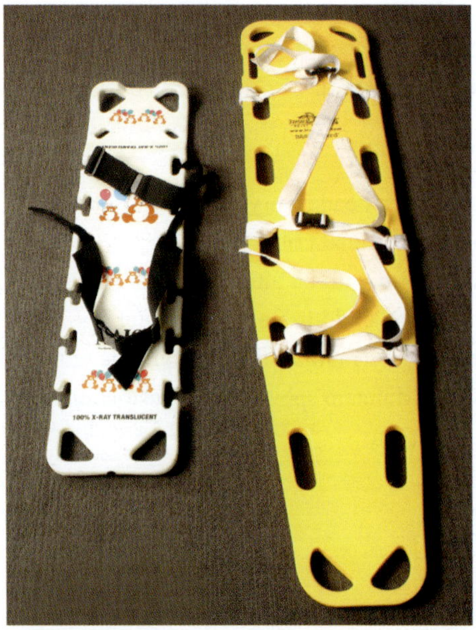

Figure 11.4 *Use a pediatric backboard if one is available to correct for the larger head of a child compared to the rest of the child's body.*

PEARLS

Prehospital providers are skilled at spinal motion restriction and should extricate children from child safety seats whenever possible. One rescuer should stabilize the neck from above, while the other helps move the child from below. Continue to maintain spinal motion restriction while removing the child from the seat.

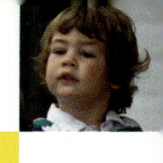

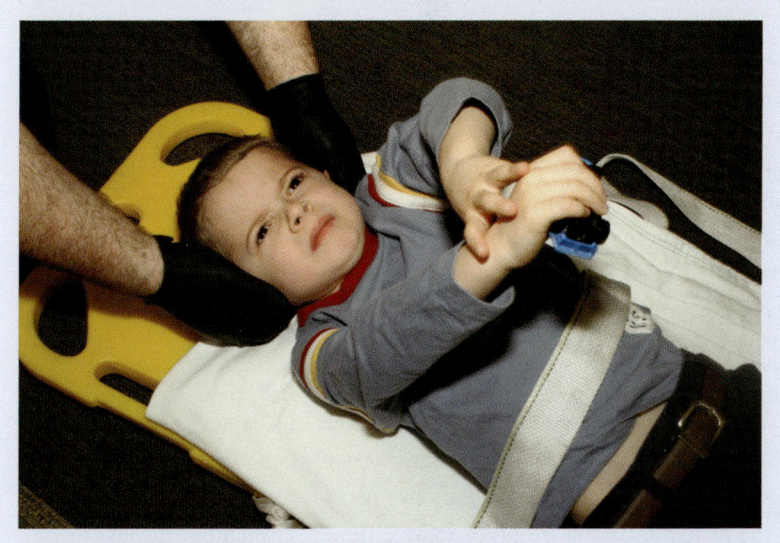

Figure 11.5 *Modify an adult backboard for a child by placing padding under the child's shoulder to maintain the neutral position of the neck.*

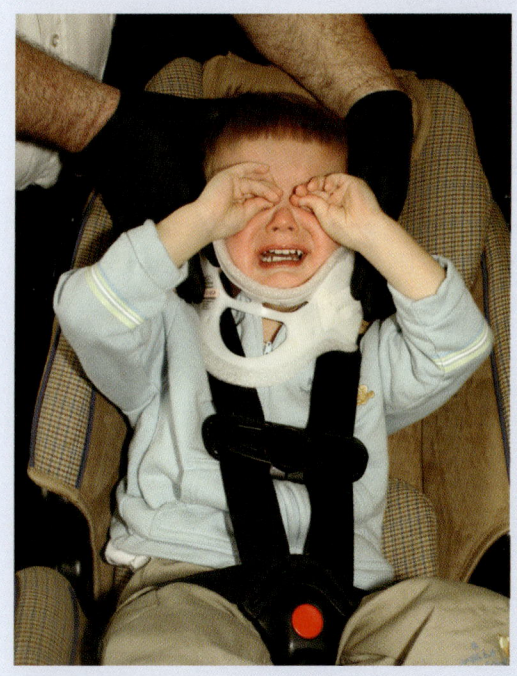

Figure 11.6 *If a child in a car seat shows no signs of injury and the seat was appropriately restrained and undamaged, you may transport the child in the car seat.*

Car Seats

Children in car seats must be managed cautiously. Perform the Initial Assessment, or at least the general impression, with the child in the car seat. If there is any concern for potential injury or compromise in the level of consciousness or ABCs, or if there is any damage to the car seat, extricate the child to a rigid pediatric backboard. One rescuer should stabilize the neck from above, while the other helps move the child from below. Maintain spinal motion restriction while removing the child from the seat. Restrict motion with a cervical collar or other cervical device (e.g., towel rolls), and secure to a rigid pediatric backboard using padding to offset any possible cervical spine flexion. Always ensure that the child's neck is in the neutral position, regardless of how the child is secured. If the car seat is not damaged, was appropriately restrained, and the child has no signs of injury, you may transport the child in the car seat (Fig. 11.6).

Pediatric Spinal Trauma

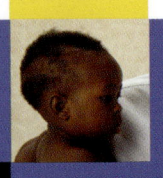

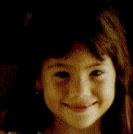

Breathing

A significant number of children with spinal injuries will have associated head injuries. If using a bag-valve mask, ventilate the child at the normal rate for age unless there are signs of brain herniation. As discussed in Chapter 10, hyperventilation may cause further brain damage in a child with head trauma and should be reserved for the child with a unilaterally dilated pupil, extensor posturing, or progressive neurologic deterioration.

Circulation

If the child shows signs of shock, follow the recommendations in Chapter 7. If possible, start two IV lines en route to the facility. An intraosseous (IO) infusion may be considered for children in full arrest or those critical patients who have no IV access after two attempts or 90 seconds. For the pediatric patient in shock, initiate fluid resuscitation en route to the hospital.

ITLS Secondary Survey

The purpose of the ITLS Secondary Survey is to discover and document all apparent injuries. Perform the ITLS Secondary Survey en route to the hospital for patients with compromised ABCs. You may perform a thorough ITLS Secondary Survey prior to transporting stable children in car seats. It includes a careful history, vital signs, a more thorough neurological exam, and a careful head-to-toe exam. The following specific areas are of particular importance to evaluate in the child with a potential spinal injury.

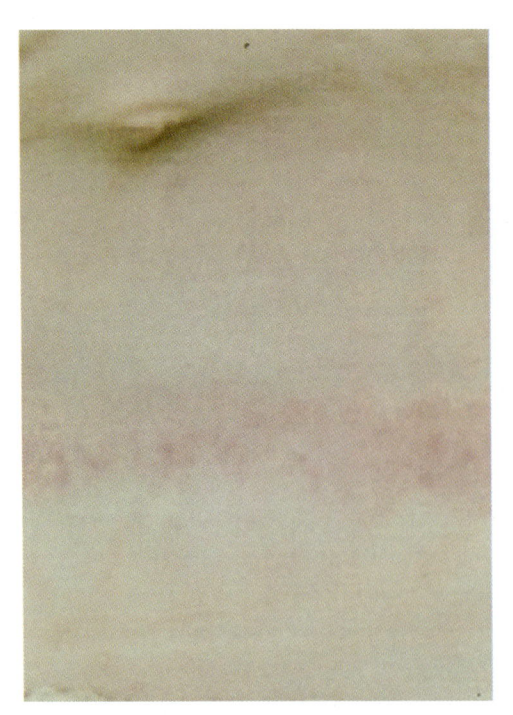

Figure 11.7 *Abdominal trauma, such as that caused by a seat belt, suggests possible lumbar spinal trauma.*

PEARLS

Assume that any child with an altered mental status has a head injury.

PEARLS

Prolonged seizure activity, even without a history of trauma, may be a sign of an occult head injury. Consider stabilization of the cervical spine. This will also help maintain neutral positioning of the airway.

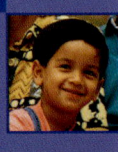

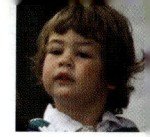

Abdominal Examination

Carefully evaluate the abdomen for any DCAP BTLS. This should not only raise the suspicion of a visceral injury, but also suggest possible lumbar spinal trauma (Fig. 11.7).

Neurologic Examination

Conduct a complete neurological assessment, appropriate for the child's age, as part of the ITLS Secondary Survey. Include muscle tone and function, and sensory status. Carefully note the position of both the upper and lower extremities. If the child is awake and alert, ask him to move the extremities. If the child is not conscious, or too young to understand, note the level of function so that you can assess improvement or deterioration.

A loss of function in the lower extremities with preservation of the upper extremities suggests the presence of an injury at the thoracic or lumbar level. Children with a complete spinal cord lesion (i.e., no sensory or motor function below the level of the injury) have a very poor prognosis for recovery of function. However, children with incomplete lesions (i.e., preservation of some function) may have complete recovery. Therefore, it is necessary to carefully examine the sense of position, deep pain, light touch, pinprick, and hot/cold, if time allows. Reflexes are preserved above and absent below the level of the injury.

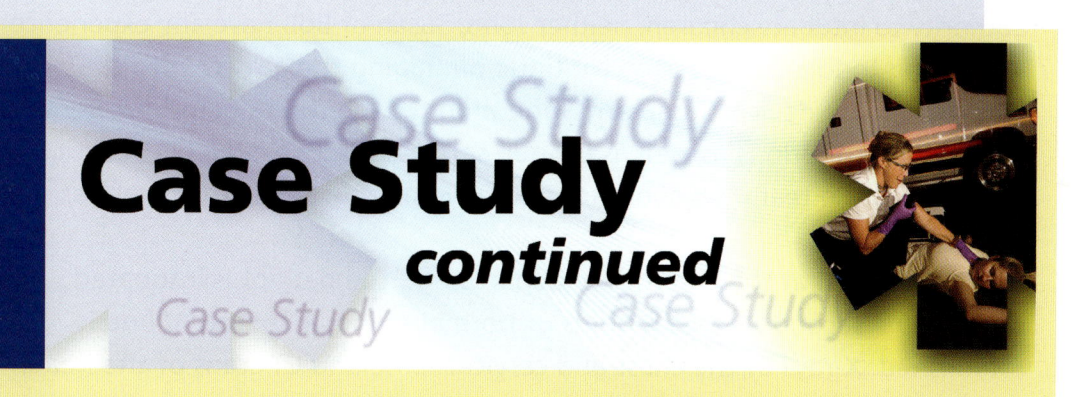

Case Study continued

John, Susan, and Bob of the Emergency Transport System (ETS) have been called to the scene of a head-on motor vehicle collision into a tree. En route, Susan has opted to be the team leader. As they approach the scene, they perform a scene size-up and don't identify any hazards. Upon their arrival, they notice moderate to severe front-end damage to the mid-sized car. Susan approaches the child and initiates the Primary Survey. She notes the child is unbelted and slumped over in her infant car seat, dressed in a sleeper. The car seat is facing forward and not secured to the car. The child is apneic, pale, and unresponsive. Susan directs John to stabilize the child's cervical spine with simultaneous opening of the airway by modified jaw thrust maneuver. The airway is patent and clear, but the child remains apneic. John initiates positive-pressure ventilations using a bag-valve-mask ventilation device with 100 percent oxygen. Symmetrical chest excursion is noted with the bagging. Susan continues with her Rapid Trauma Survey and notes the patient has a hematoma of the forehead, pupils are fixed and dilated, and is unresponsive to painful stimulation. The child's skin is cool, and her brachial pulse is very fast and weak. The chest wall is stable to palpation. The abdomen is soft, flat and doesn't elicit a pain response with palpation. The pelvis is stable to compression. Susan quickly auscultates the chest and notes clear and equal breath sounds bilaterally. No movement of the extremities is noted.

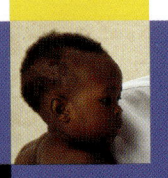

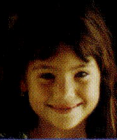

Bob has prepared for spinal precautions, and the child is extricated from the car seat onto a pediatric spinal motion restriction device while bag-valve-mask ventilation with 100 percent oxygen is continued. The child is quickly secured to the spinal motion restriction device, moved to the ambulance and immediately transported to a pediatric trauma facility.

En route to the hospital, one IV is established and she is given a 20 mL/kg fluid bolus of normal saline based on the significant findings of a weak, thready, rapid brachial pulse on scene. Though the crew has the authority to intubate children, neither John, Susan or Bob have any experience intubating toddlers and opt to continue managing the airway with the bag-valve-mask device. Susan and John monitor the child's blood pressure, pulse and respirations as well as oxygen saturations. End-tidal CO_2 is not available to the team. No spontaneous movement of the extremities has been noted.

Upon arrival at the emergency department, the patient is intubated and given a second 20 mL/kg bolus of normal saline. A second IV line is established. X-rays of the chest and cervical spine and CT scans of the head, chest and abdomen are performed.

Fluid resuscitation is continued using crystalloids and packed red cells, and the child is taken to the operating room.

Later, feedback from the pediatric trauma center informs the team that the child had a fracture/dislocation of C4/C5, an epidural hematoma, and free blood in the abdomen. After a complicated hospital course, she was transferred to a rehabilitation unit.

Case Study *wrap-up*

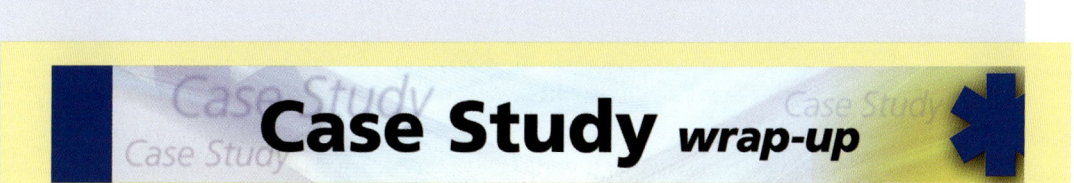

Though spinal injury in children is relatively rare in children, the consequences of not using spinal motion restriction in a potential spinal injury could be devastating to the child and family for a lifetime. As in this case, where there were already signs of potential spinal cord injury, you should carefully package the patient to prevent secondary injuries and give the child the best chance of a good recovery.

SUMMARY

1. Spinal cord damage is not always predictable. Trauma patients who are unconscious or who have experienced a dangerous mechanism of injury affecting the head, neck, or trunk deserve spinal motion restriction.
2. It can be very difficult to "clear" the spine in young children due to their varying communication skills, so these patients may require a lower threshold for spinal motion restriction.
3. Once spinal motion restriction is performed, the patient loses some ability to control his airway, so you must remain vigilant, prepared at all times to intervene in the event of airway compromise.
4. According to the National Highway Traffic Safety Administration (NHTSA), approximately one-third of all children in the United States under the age of 12 years are improperly restrained while riding in a motor vehicle. Therefore, you must carefully evaluate all scenes for the position and restraint devices used for each infant or child in the motor vehicle.

Recommended Reading

American College of Surgeons. "Spine and Spinal Cord Trauma." In *Advanced Trauma Life Support for Doctors*, 8th ed. Chicago: Author, 2008.

Bohn, Desmond et al. "Cervical Spine Injuries in Children." *Journal of Trauma* 30 (1990): 463.

Campbell, John Emory, ed. "Spinal Trauma." In *International Trauma Life Support for Prehospital Care Providers*, 6th ed., 160–82. Upper Saddle River, N.J.: Pearson/Prentice Hall, 2008.

Fesmire, Francis and Robert Luten. "The Pediatric Cervical Spine: Developmental Anatomy and Clinical Aspects." *Journal of Emergency Medicine* 7 (1989): 133.

Herzenberger, John, Robert Hensiger, Dale Dedrick, et al. "Emergency Transport and Positioning of Young Children Who Have an Injury of the Cervical Spine." *Journal of Bone and Joint Surgery* 71A (1989): 15–22.

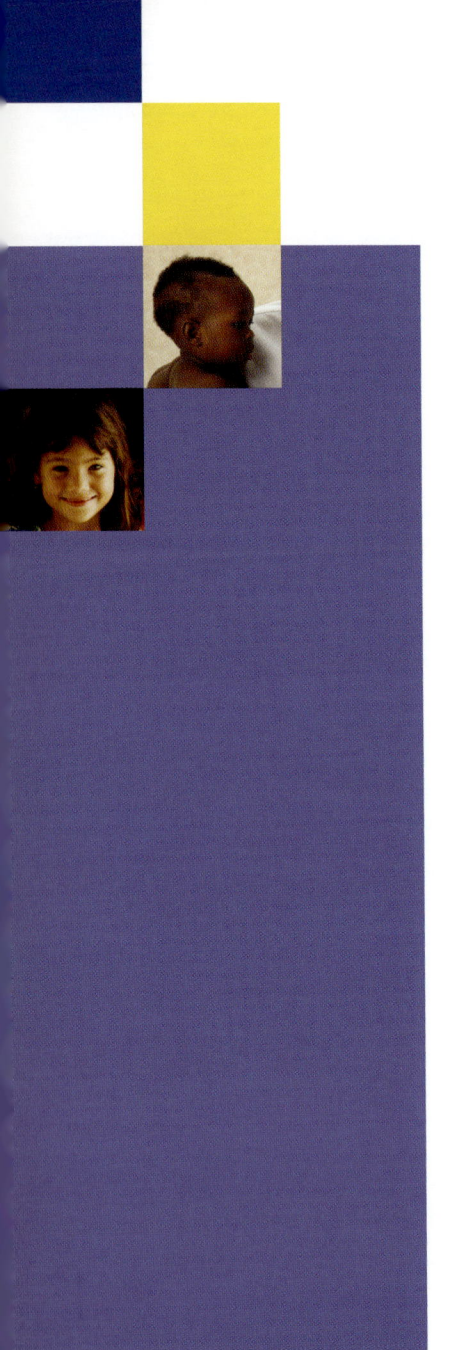

Marx, John A., ed. *Marx: Rosen's Emergency Medicine: Concepts and Clinical Practice Part 5*, 6th ed. St. Louis: Mosby, 2006.

Ralston, Mark, Mary Fran Hazinski, Arno L. Zaritsky, Stephen M. Schexnayder, and Monica E. Kleinman, eds. *Pediatric Advanced Life Support Provider Manual*. Dallas: American Heart Association, 2007.

Stauffer, Shannon and John Mazur. "Cervical Spine Injuries in Children." *Pediatric Annals* 11 (1982): 6.

Young, Wise. *Pediatric Spinal Cord Injury*. Piscataway, N.J.: Rutgers University Press, 2003.

12

CHAPTER 12
Spinal Motion Restriction and Extrication Skills

Ann Marie Dietrich, MD, FACEP, FAAP
Debi Hastilow, EMT-P, RN

Objectives
Upon completion of this skills chapter, you should be able to:

1. Demonstrate application of an appropriately sized cervical collar.
2. Demonstrate log-rolling a patient onto a spinal motion restriction device.
3. Secure a pediatric patient to a spinal motion restriction device.
4. Identify which patients should be extricated from a child passenger restraint device in a motor vehicle.
5. Perform an extrication of a child from a child passenger restraint device while maintaining spinal motion restriction.

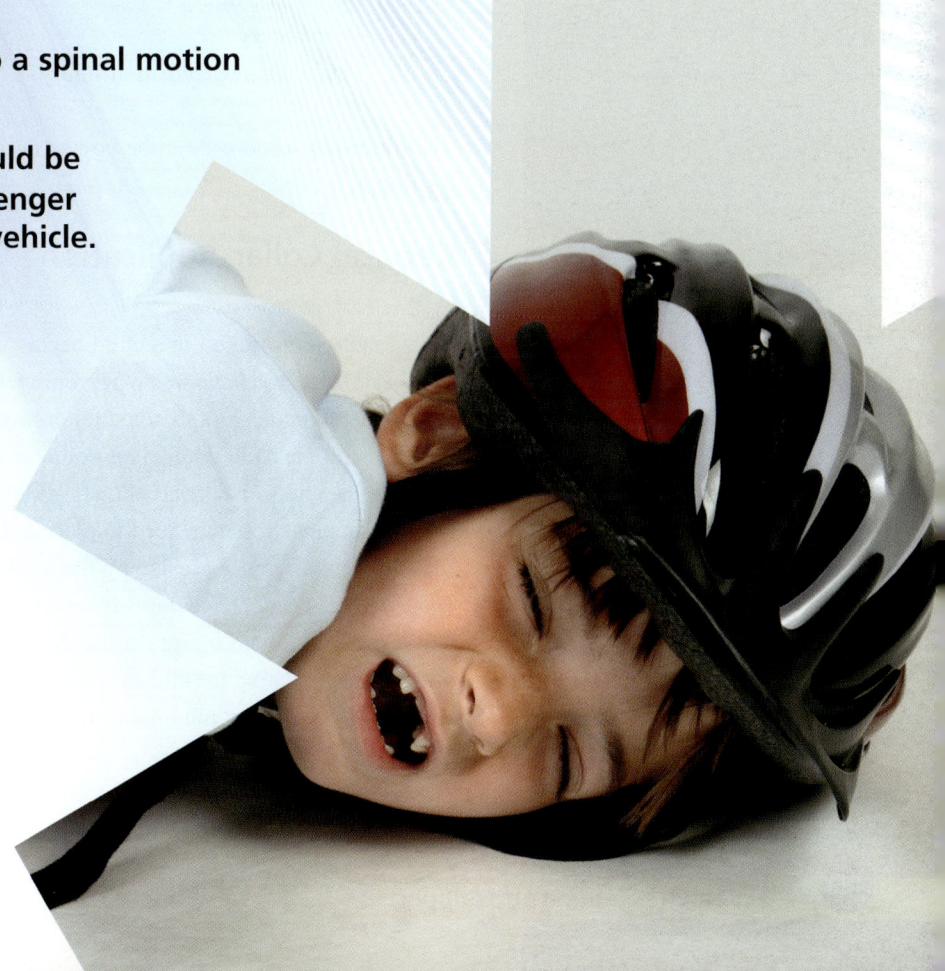

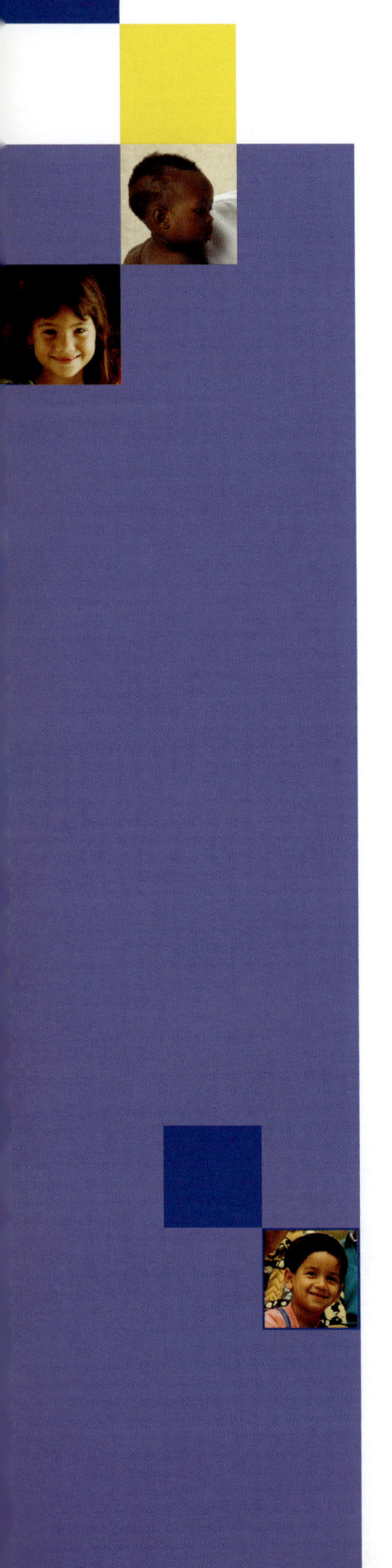

INTRODUCTION

While relatively uncommon, a spinal injury in the pediatric patient can be a life-altering event. Appropriate assessment and proper management techniques can greatly improve the chances for a successful outcome for the victim of such an injury. High-force mechanisms, such as a motor vehicle collision (MVC) or falls, greatly increase the risk of such injuries. Therefore, you should maintain a high index of suspicion for spinal injuries in the presence of such mechanisms. While much attention has recently been given to "clearing" the cervical spine in the field setting, this may be difficult in the pediatric patient due to age-related difficulties in communication. Therefore, you should have a low threshold for motion restriction of pediatric patients.

Initial spinal motion restriction and the ITLS Primary Survey, including the Initial Assessment and Rapid Trauma Survey, literally go "hand in hand." If the scene size-up and the child's general appearance suggest the need for spinal motion restriction, you must initiate immediate manual control of the cervical spine.

SPINAL MOTION RESTRICTION

Following are situations that require spinal motion restriction:

1. Mechanism of injury—motor vehicle collision, fall, sports
2. Significant injury above the nipple line
3. Head injury
4. Altered mental status
5. Distracting injuries
6. Poor history
7. Unknown mechanism of injury

The following sections describe how to ensure maximum stabilization when spinal motion restriction is needed.

Cervical Collar Application

Spinal motion restriction of a child begins with manual stabilization. After completing the ITLS Primary Survey, apply an appropriately sized cervical collar (Fig. 12.1). Maintain the neck in a neutral position before and during application.

Log-roll the child onto an appropriate spinal motion restriction device. Remember to examine the child's back and allow for the space under the shoulders created by placing the child supine. You may need to place a folded sheet, towel, or padding on the board to make up the difference created by the head. The smaller the child, the more padding is needed. If you cannot accomplish log-rolling, pull the child onto a backboard using a long axis–type drag. Avoid lifting the child, if possible. It is extremely difficult to lift a child without manipulating the spine. The main goal is to place the child on a spinal motion restriction device with minimal spinal movement.

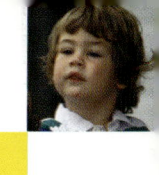

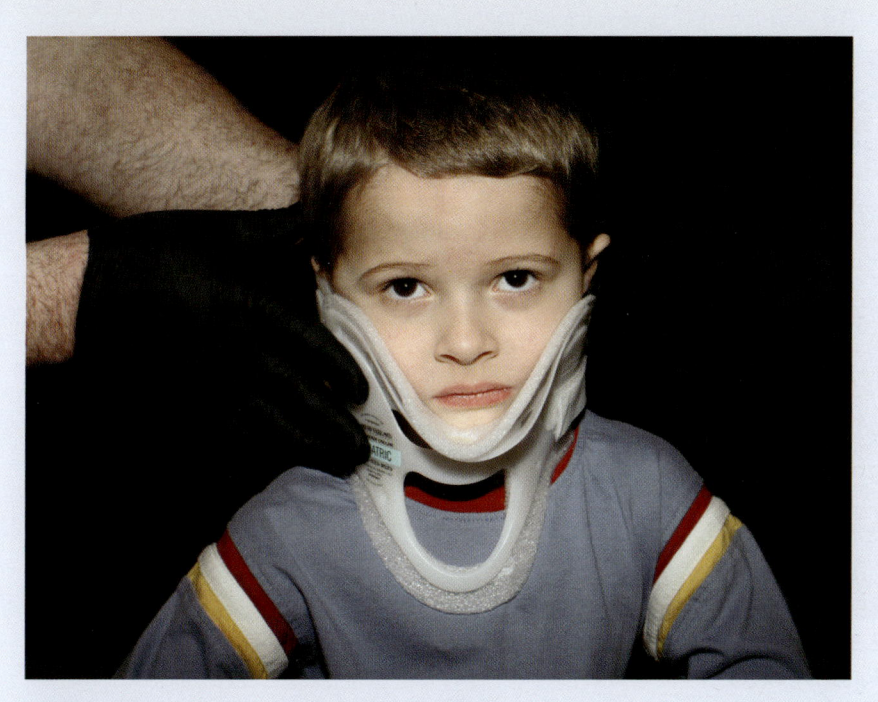

Figure 12.1 *Apply an appropriately sized cervical collar to the pediatric patient after completing the ITLS Primary Survey.*

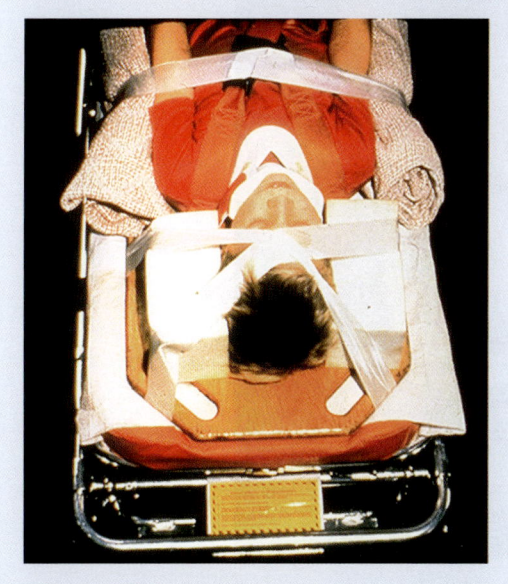

Figure 12.2 *Final spinal motion restriction of a patient on a backboard includes securing the head to prevent lateral movement.*

Secure the child to the spinal motion restriction device. It is necessary to use straps or other restraining devices to limit the child's movement. Because this can be a very frightening procedure, especially for younger children, involve the parent or guardian as much as possible to comfort the child. It is okay for children to be scared. Do not discourage the child or tell him to "be quiet." Comfort the child and explain what you are doing. Secure the child's body first, then his head.

Secure the head to the spinal motion restriction device using a cervical immobilization device or towel rolls and tape. Secure the head to prevent lateral movement of the cervical spine (Fig. 12.2).

Spinal Motion Restriction and Extrication Skills

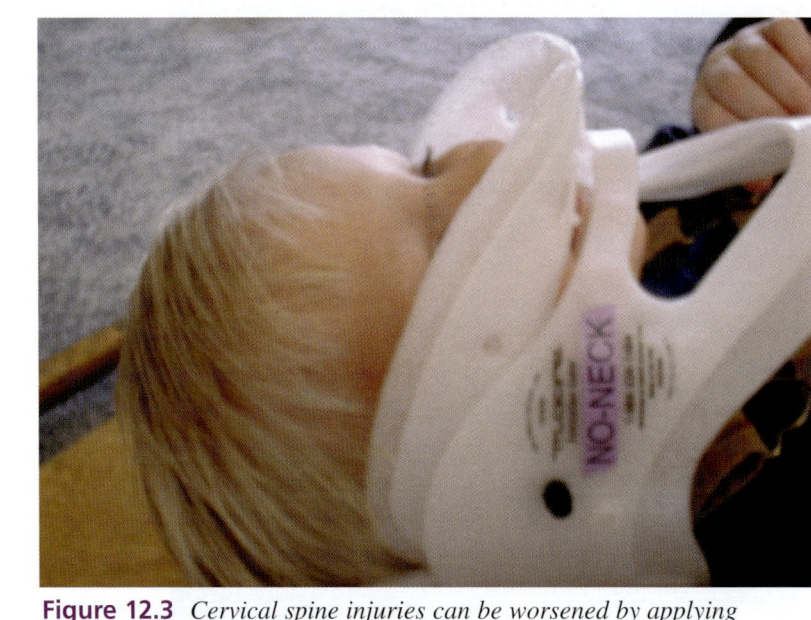

Figure 12.3 *Cervical spine injuries can be worsened by applying a collar that is too large or too small.*

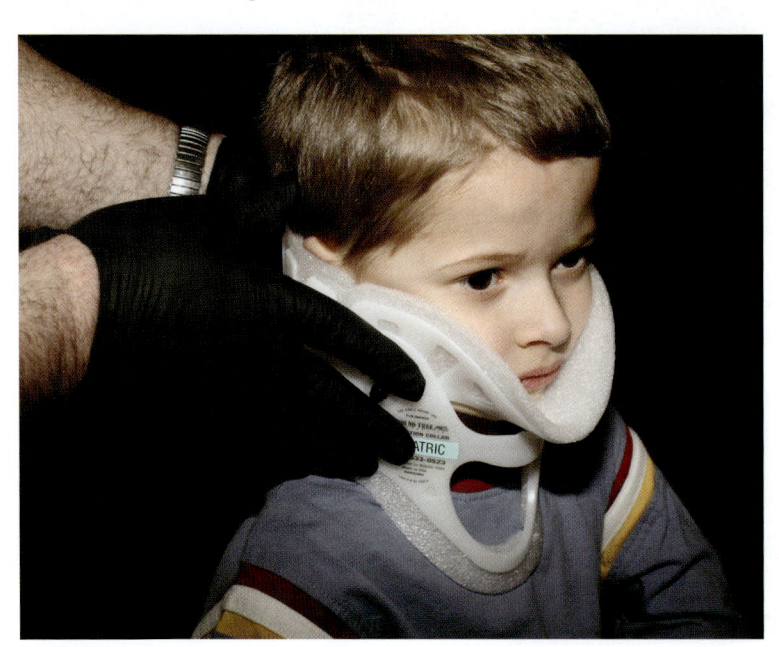

Figure 12.4 *An appropriately sized cervical collar keeps the neck and spine in neutral position.*

Selecting Appropriate Equipment

Cervical Collar

Ensure that the cervical collar fits the child properly. A collar that does not fit correctly may actually worsen a cervical spine injury (Fig. 12.3). An appropriately fitted cervical collar will position the child in the "neutral" position, which will decrease any pressure on the spinal cord (Fig. 12.4).

Backboards/Pediatric Boards and Straps

After selecting an appropriately sized cervical collar, secure the child on a rigid device. The device may be a backboard or other customized pediatric spinal motion restriction device (Fig. 12.5). No matter what device is used, you must use it properly. Secure the child in a

Pediatric Trauma Life Support

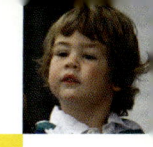

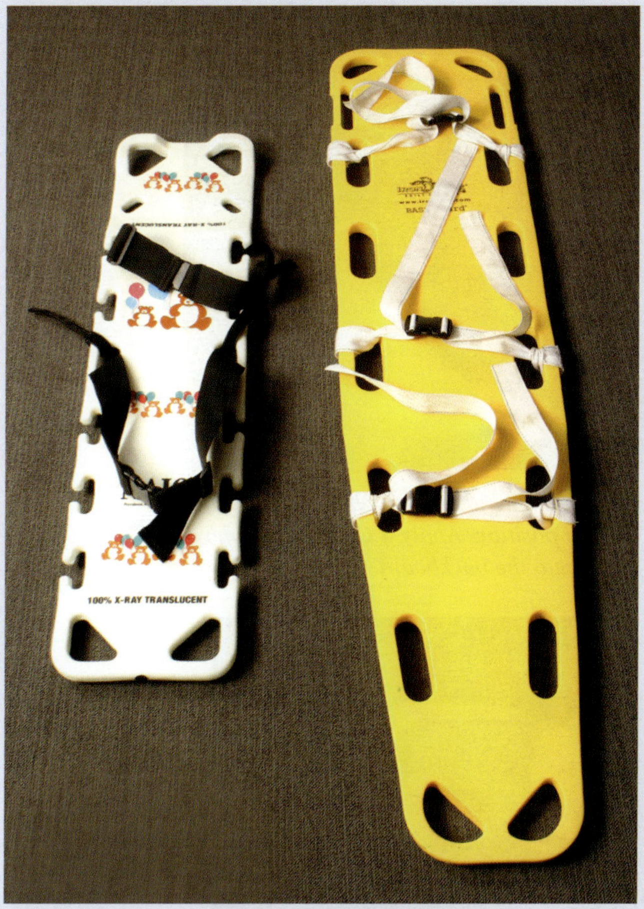

Figure 12.5 *Children can be secured to a specialized pediatric board or to an adult backboard with padding to correct for the smaller size and anatomical difference of a child.*

neutral position. When working with a small child, place a "filler" such as a blanket or foam pad under the child's shoulder area to align the neck properly (Fig. 12.6). The child should "fit" the board or device so that the child will not move when the board is tilted. Secure the child to the board with straps or other securing devices to prevent movement. Usually, a minimum of three straps is needed to accomplish this task. Secure the chest (above the nipple line), pelvis, and lower extremities (above the knees) to prevent movement (Fig. 12.7).

Head Motion Restriction Device

After the cervical collar is in place and you have secured the child's torso to the board, secure the head. You may accomplish this with commercially available devices, cardboard, plastic, or foam (Fig. 12.8). If these are not available, you may use a rolled blanket or other lightweight bolsters to secure the head. The head motion restriction device must prevent lateral and anterior movement of the cervical spine.

CHILD PASSENGER RESTRAINT DEVICES

Assess a child found in a car seat while still in the seat. The results of your assessment will determine whether the child should be extricated from the car seat before further examination or interventions.

Spinal Motion Restriction and Extrication Skills

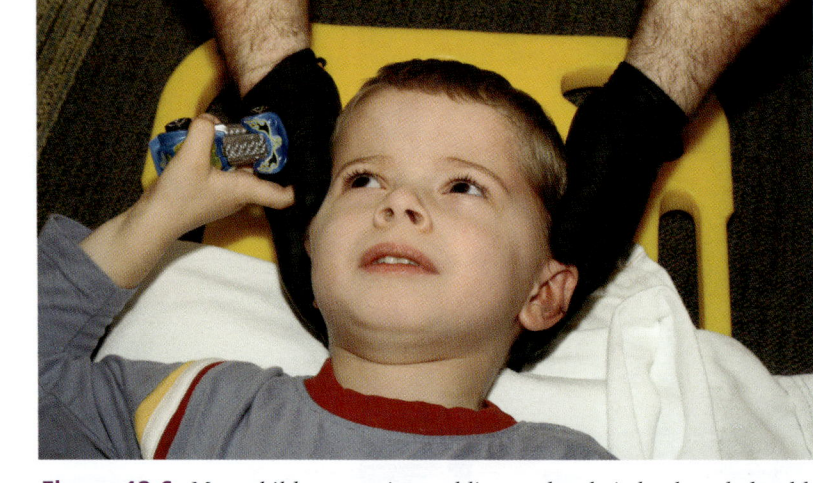

Figure 12.6 *Most children require padding under their back and shoulders to keep the cervical spine in a neutral position. Apply a C-collar whenever possible before log-rolling the child onto the backboard.*

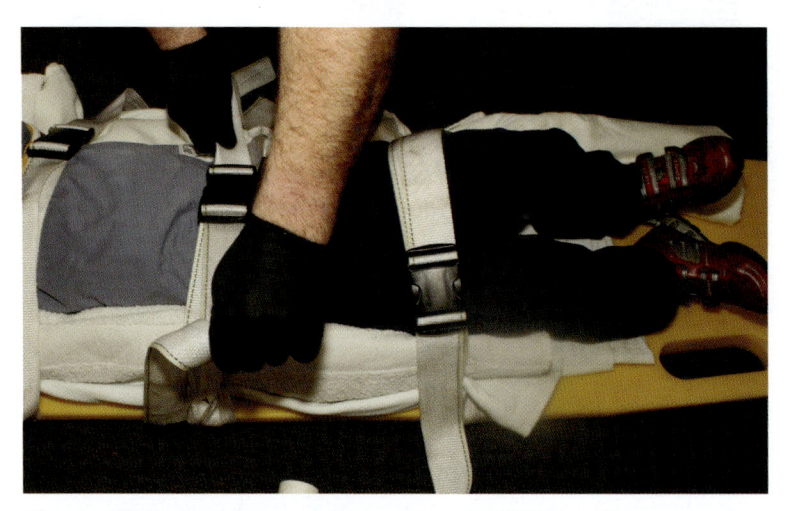

Figure 12.7 *A minimum of three straps should be used to secure the child to the backboard, securing the chest above the nipple line, the pelvis, and the lower extremities above the knees.*

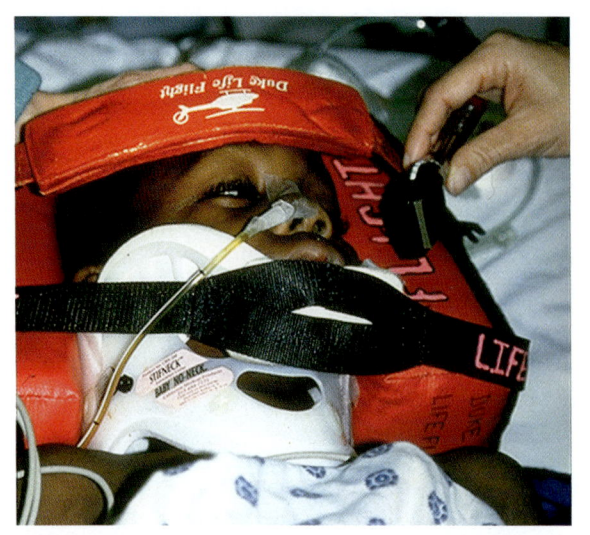

Figure 12.8 *Secure the head last, using commercially available device, foam, or rolled towels or blankets as available. Restriction of the head prevents lateral and anterior motion of the cervical spine.*

Pediatric Trauma Life Support

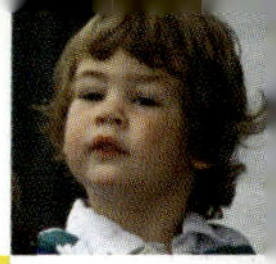

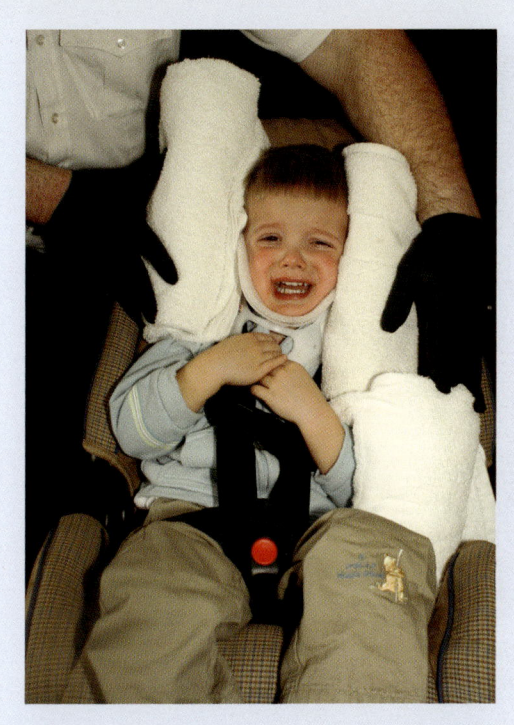

Figure 12.9 *When transporting a child in the car seat, apply a cervical collar and secure the head with towel rolls to further restrict motion of the cervical spine.*

Extrication for a Normal Assessment—No Abnormalities Found

If the car seat is not damaged, there are no abnormalities noted on a careful assessment, the child is not in distress, and you decide that the child should be evaluated in the emergency department due to the mechanism of injury, you may secure the child and transport him in the car seat. (The car seat must be removable and undamaged.)

Apply a cervical collar, if possible, and secure the head with towel rolls (Fig. 12.9). Although there are no scientific studies showing that motion restriction in a car seat is effective, this is an option if there are no noticeable injuries.

Extrication for an Abnormal Assessment—Injury Suspected

Manually restrict motion in the cervical spine and evaluate the child to determine if extrication is necessary (Fig. 12.10). If there is any compromise of the ABCs, the child has an altered mental status, or the car seat is damaged, remove the child from the car seat to facilitate further examination or interventions.

Continue manual motion restriction of the cervical spine and place a cervical collar on the child before extricating the car seat (Fig. 12.11). It is preferable to extricate the car seat if possible, because this preserves spinal protection. However, if it is inappropriate or impossible to remove the car seat from the vehicle, then proceed to extricate the child from the car seat, maintaining spinal motion restriction. The first rescuer should maintain manual stabilization of the cervical spine while a second rescuer positions himself beside the seat and inserts his hands down and under the child to grab the child's legs. The second rescuer should then lift the child up and out, while a third rescuer places a pediatric spinal motion restriction device under the child (Fig. 12.12). Secure the child to the backboard using appropriate technique as described earlier.

Spinal Motion Restriction and Extrication Skills

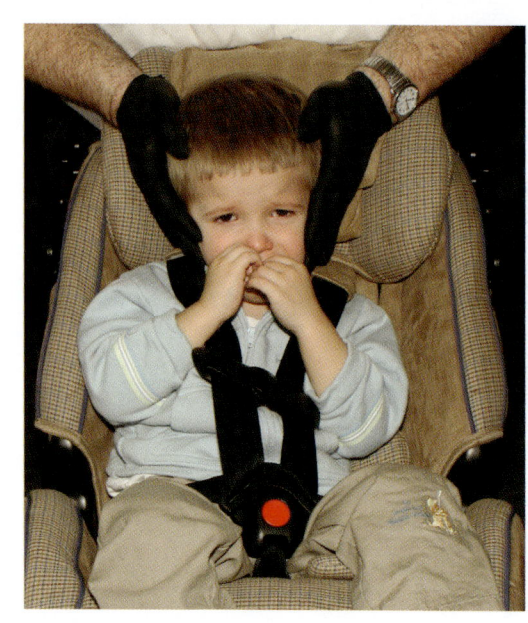

Figure 12.10 *Maintain manual control of the cervical spine while determining whether extrication of the child from the car seat is necessary.*

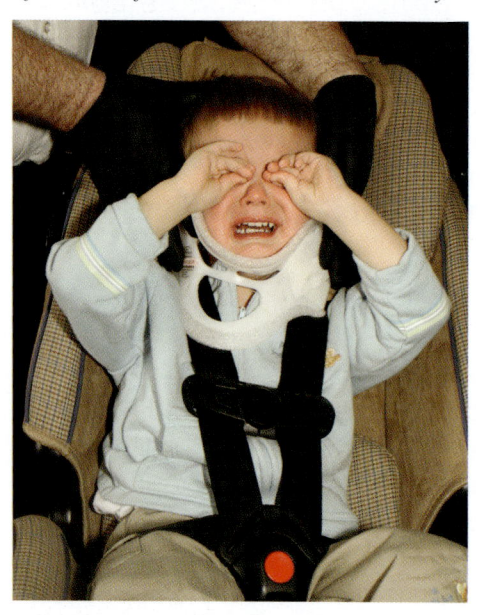

Figure 12.11 *Place a cervical collar on the child before extricating the car seat from the vehicle or the child from the car seat.*

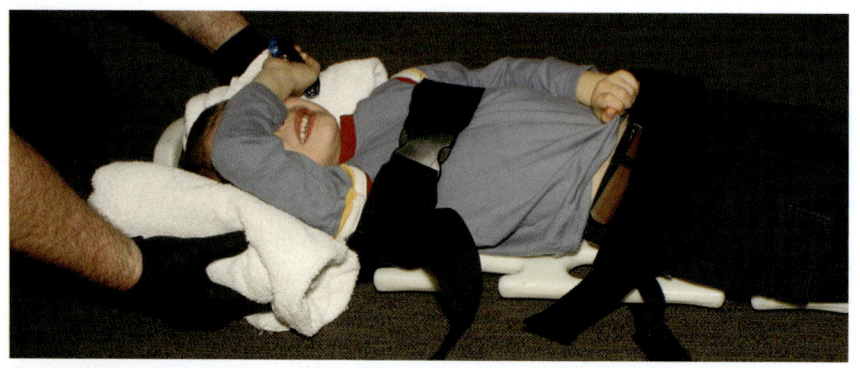

Figure 12.12 *After the child has been extricated from the car seat onto the backboard, continue motion restriction with towel rolls and straps.*

Pediatric Trauma Life Support

CHAPTER 13
Pediatric Extremity Trauma

William Cotton, MD
Ronald R. McWilliams, NREMT–P
Wendy J. Pomerantz, MD, MS

Objectives
Upon completion of this chapter, you should be able to:

1. Describe the signs and symptoms of extremity trauma in a child.
2. Discuss the treatment of specific extremity injuries.
3. Discuss the presentation and management of compartment syndrome and amputations in children.

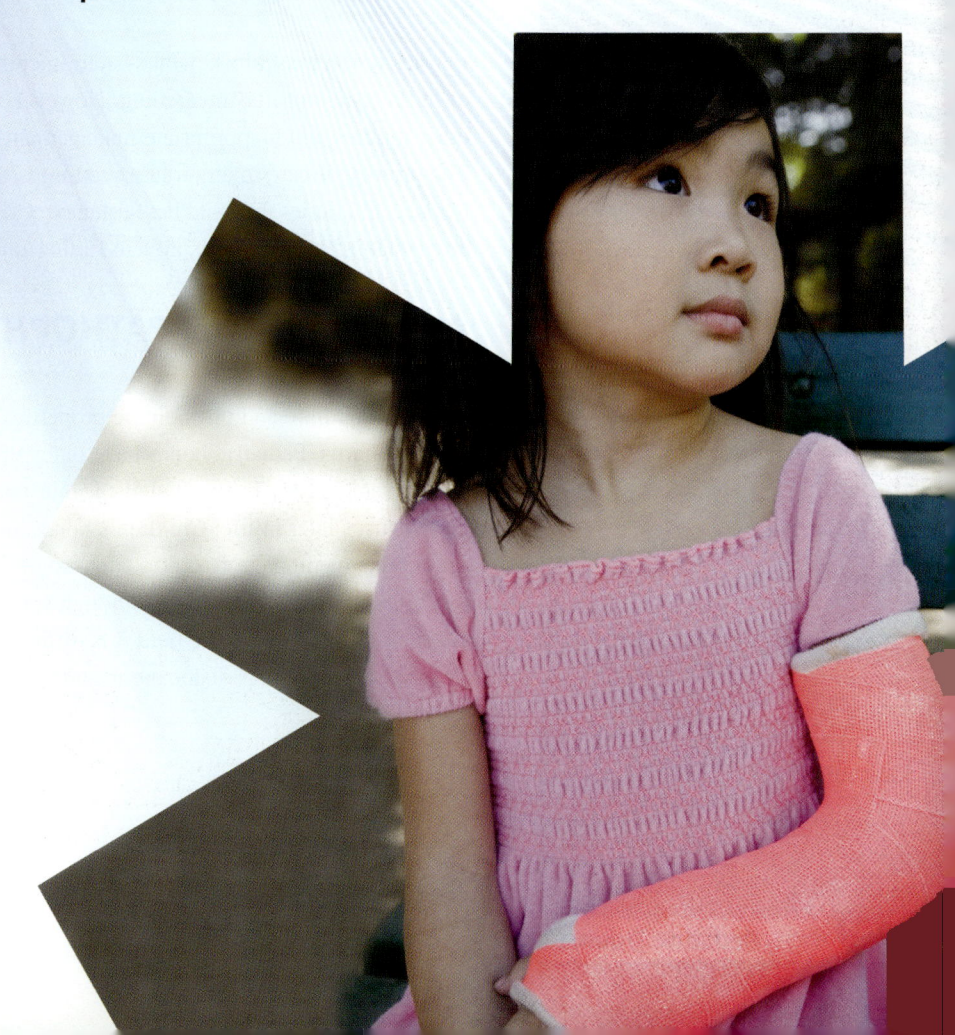

Case Study

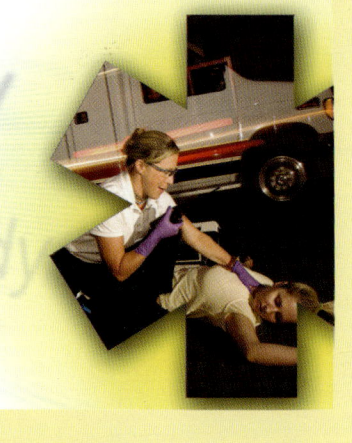

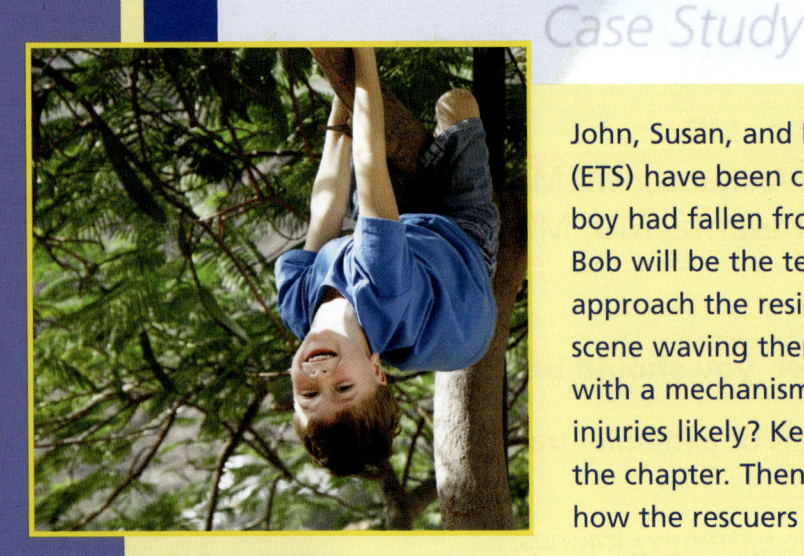

John, Susan, and Bob of the Emergency Transport System (ETS) have been called to the scene where a 6-year-old boy had fallen from a tree. En route, they decide that Bob will be the team leader when they arrive. As they approach the residence, law enforcement is already on scene waving them in. What injuries should they expect with a mechanism of this type? Are head and spinal injuries likely? Keep these questions in mind as you read the chapter. Then, at the end of the chapter, find out how the rescuers completed this call.

INTRODUCTION

Injuries to the musculoskeletal system in children are common; fortunately, the majority of injuries are not life-threatening. However, extremity injuries may be accompanied by other injuries and inappropriate management may result in a poor functional outcome. The priority of care in any trauma setting is to treat life-threatening injuries first, then manage all injuries the child has sustained. Goals for treating children with extremity trauma are to stabilize the patient, prevent further injury, and maximize functional outcome.

ANATOMY AND PATHOPHYSIOLOGY

Specific anatomic and physiologic properties of children's bones contribute to unique injury patterns. Pediatric bones have many unique characteristics, such as growth plates (epiphyses) that are frequent sites of injury. Injury to these sites may lead to growth disturbances later in life. Children's bones are resilient and elastic, and these qualities may create incomplete fractures such as greenstick and torus fractures. Children also exhibit rapid fracture healing. Although sprains and strains occur frequently in the pediatric population, in the field it is difficult to differentiate these injuries from fractures. Other injuries, such as dislocations and compartment syndromes, are not commonly seen in children.

PEARLS

The priority of care in any trauma setting is to treat life-threatening injuries first, then manage all injuries, including musculoskeletal, that the child has sustained.

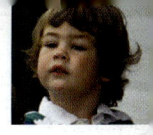

PATIENT ASSESSMENT

Assessment is of primary importance in the management of any patient. Just as in the adult patient, assessment of the pediatric patient should proceed in the following manner:

1. ITLS Primary Survey
    A. Scene Size-Up
    B. Initial Assessment
    C. Rapid Trauma Survey or Focused Exam
    D. Critical Interventions and Transport Decisions
    E. Contact medical direction as needed.
2. ITLS Secondary Survey and/or Ongoing Exam

ITLS Primary Survey

Scene Size-Up

The mechanism of injury provides important information. Significant force is required to cause certain fractures in children and such force may cause multisystem injury in children. Up to 90 percent of childhood injuries are caused by blunt trauma. Preventable trauma accounts for 25 percent of fractures in children less than three years of age. Besides motor vehicle collisions (MVCs), mechanisms likely to cause musculoskeletal injuries include falls and incidents with lawn mowers, farm equipment, bicycles, all-terrain vehicles (ATVs), and personal watercraft recreational vehicles (Fig. 13.1).

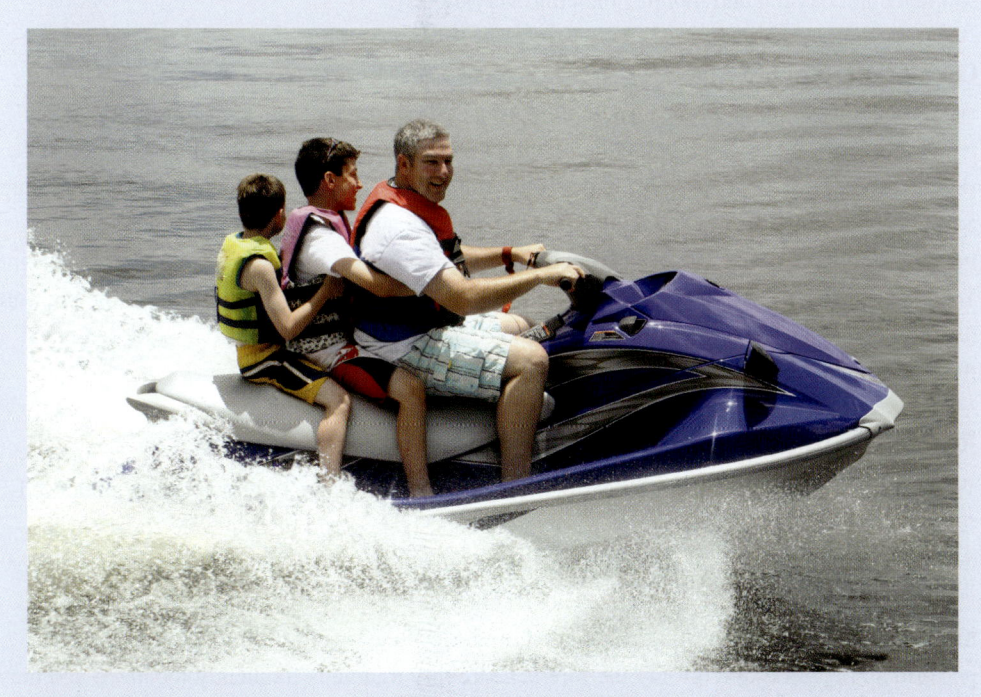

Figure 13.1 *Personal watercraft recreational vehicles often cause musculoskeletal injuries.*

Pediatric Extremity Trauma

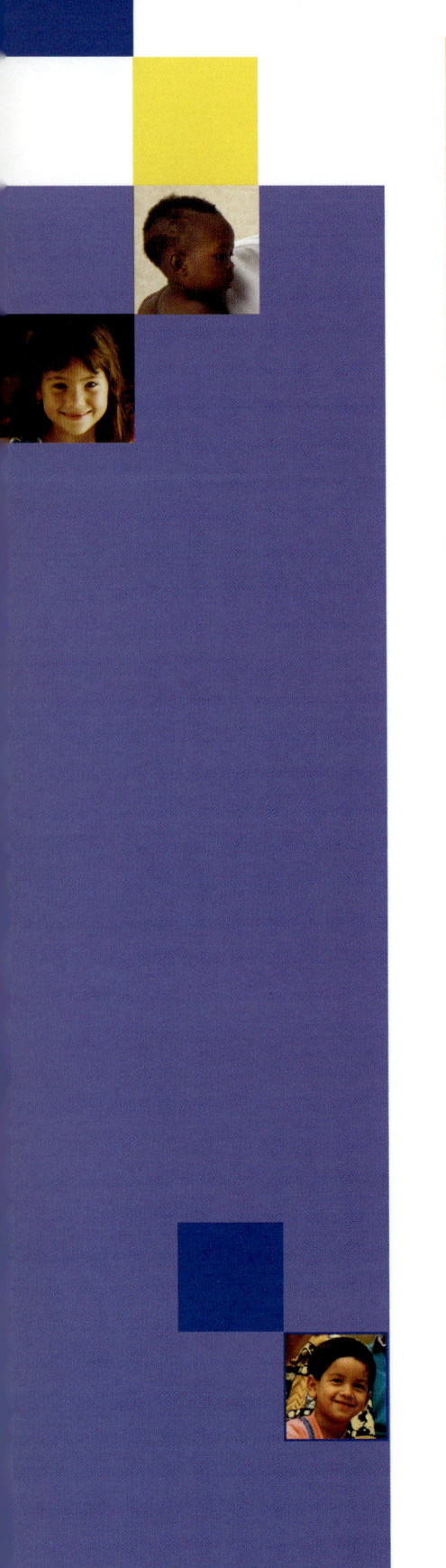

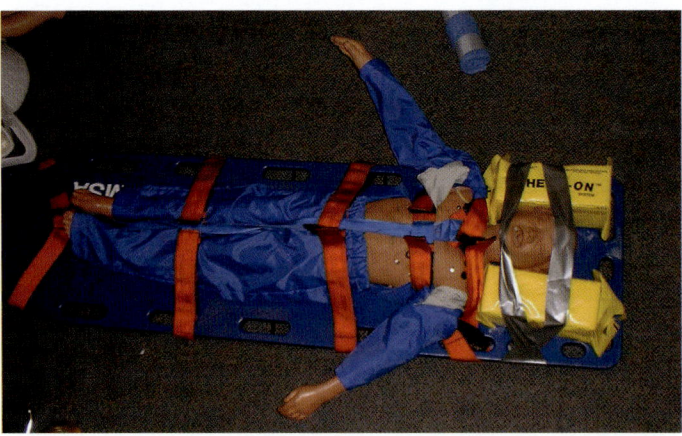

Figure 13.2 *Spinal motion restriction procedures demonstrated on a pediatric mannequin.*

Initial Assessment
Airway and Cervical Spine
Because pediatric patients with extremity injuries may have multisystem injury, carefully determine the need to perform spinal motion restriction (Fig. 13.2). Assess and manage the airway as discussed in Chapter 4.

Breathing
Assessment and management of breathing is discussed in Chapters 4 through 6. In addition, consider that when children are in pain, they might become tachypneic. Administer supplemental oxygen and monitor the child very closely.

Circulation
As indicated in Chapter 7, even small amounts of blood loss (e.g., an extremity injury) may result in hypovolemic shock in a child. Tachycardia and poor perfusion may indicate possible shock. Promptly stop all active bleeding. If the child has an amputation, focus care on the stump. Stump care is aimed at controlling bleeding by applying a pressure dressing. If the injury involves a major extremity or if the amputation is incomplete, the bleeding may be significant and result in shock. Early application of a dressing, and sometimes a tourniquet if the pressure dressing is not sufficient, will reduce blood loss. Rarely, you may need hemostatic agents if they are available.

Rapid Trauma Survey or Focused Exam
When dealing with extremity trauma, the need for a Rapid Trauma Survey versus a Focused Exam depends entirely on the findings in the Scene Size-Up and the Initial Assessment. If there is a dangerous generalized mechanism of injury (such as an MVC or significant fall) or the child is unconscious, perform a Rapid Trauma Survey. If there is a dangerous focused mechanism of injury suggesting an isolated injury (such as a stab wound to the groin), perform a Focused Exam of only the injury. Extremity trauma is frequently localized and may not require a head-to-toe exam. However, a fall in which the child has an obvious broken arm but also an altered level of consciousness requires a Rapid Trauma Survey to rule out other injuries such as head trauma.

Critical Interventions and Transport Decisions
Immediately transport all children with evidence of shock after the ITLS Primary Survey. In addition, rapid transport is indicated for any child with a major extremity amputation.

Pediatric Trauma Life Support

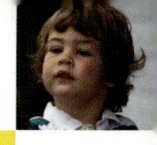

Airway and Cervical Spine
Provide care as discussed in Chapters 4 and 11.

Breathing
Provide care as discussed in Chapters 4 through 6.

Circulation
Assess the child's circulatory status and provide care as discussed in Chapter 7. Stop bleeding with pressure and, in rare cases, tourniquet and/or hemostatic agents. Obtain IV access en route to the hospital.

ITLS Secondary Survey

Extremity Assessment
A careful extremity assessment is part of the ITLS Secondary Survey. If a child is unstable, perform the ITLS Secondary Survey en route to the hospital. If the transport time is short, the ITLS Secondary Survey may not occur at all. This is why a rapid scan of the extremities for bleeding and obvious fractures is part of the Rapid Trauma Survey. Early application of a pressure dressing may prevent shock from developing and minimize ongoing fluid losses

During the ITLS Secondary Survey's assessment of an extremity injury, check the following items:

1. Soft tissue for ecchymosis, swelling, and breaks in the skin
2. Tenderness, instability, and crepitation (TIC)
3. Pulse, motor function (i.e., is the patient able to move the extremity on command?), and sensory function (pulse, motor function, and sensory function [PMS])
4. Skin color, condition, and capillary refill

Document the initial findings and carefully monitor the child for changes during transport. Document the PMS before and after applying a splint.

FRACTURES AND DISLOCATIONS

Most pediatric fractures are classified in a manner similar to that for adults. Decide whether the fracture is open or closed. Open fractures have a laceration over the site of trauma. They are more likely to become infected because of contamination. Therefore, it is important to note all lacerations and open areas prior to applying a dressing. Most fractures in children are simple fractures (one break in the bone) and not comminuted (broken into multiple pieces).

Two unique fractures of childhood are the greenstick and torus fractures. A greenstick facture results when a bone breaks on the outer surface but is maintained intact on the inner surface (Fig. 13.3). A torus fracture is caused by buckling of the outer surface (Fig. 13.4). Although dislocations occur infrequently in children, they can be a major cause of morbidity. It is important to check the neurovascular function (PMS) below any joint that is swollen or painful.

> **PEARLS**
>
> During the ITLS Secondary Survey, assess TIC and PMS of the extremities. Document these before and after splint application.

Pediatric Extremity Trauma

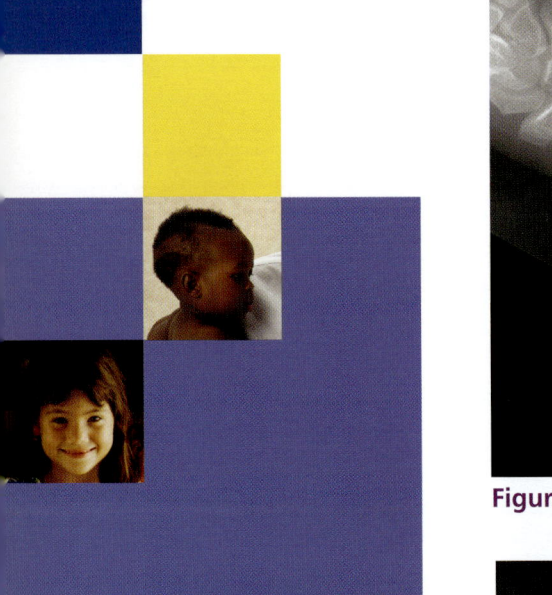

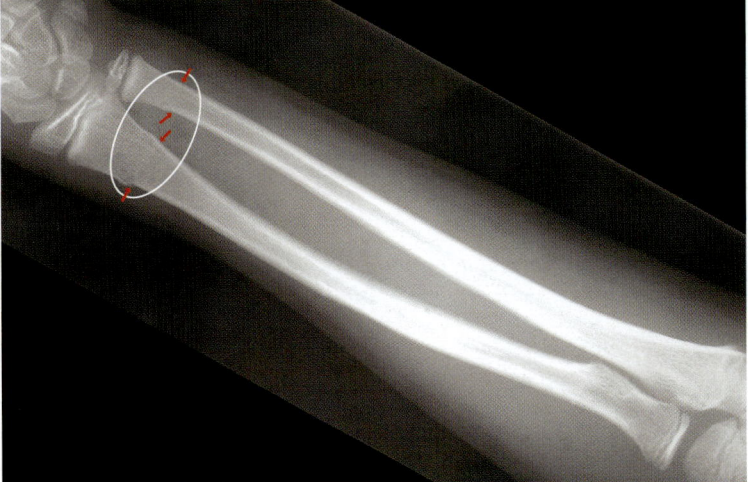

Figure 13.3 *Greenstick fracture in a child.*

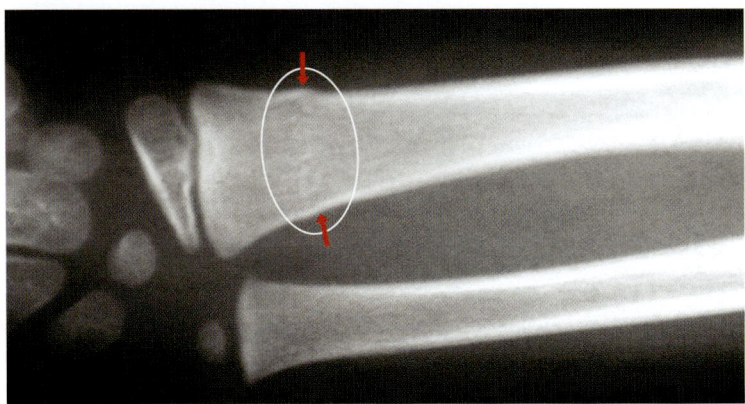

Figure 13.4 *Torus fracture in a child.*

Signs and Symptoms

In general, assess children with fractures in the same manner as adults. Usually, the child will have pain, swelling, and deformity at the site of the injury. Younger children may refuse to move or walk on the injured extremity. If there is uncertainty as to whether a fracture exists, *treat the injury as a fracture*. If the fracture involves a joint, the child may also exhibit decreased range of motion and possible vascular compromise.

Treatment

The goals of fracture management include stabilization, reduction of pain, and prevention of further injury. To accomplish these goals, ensure that proper equipment is available and be familiar with immobilization techniques. Incorrect immobilization techniques may result in loss of function in the extremity and serious long-term problems for the child.

Initially stabilize unstable pediatric patients on a backboard and transport. Perform other splinting en route to the hospital. If there is a break in the skin, a sterile pressure dressing must be applied. Once you control the bleeding and appropriately bandage the extremity, immobilize the extremity. When stabilizing a fracture or suspected fracture, immobilize the actual injury, the joint above, and the joint below the injury. Always check the PMS of the extremity before and after immobilization and document your findings. If a child has a dislocation, immobilize it in a position in which the patient is most comfortable and the neurovascular status is intact (Fig. 13.5).

PEARLS

If there is uncertainty as to whether a fracture exists, *treat the injury as a fracture.*

PEARLS

Your correct immobilization techniques can help prevent loss of function in the extremity and serious long-term problems for the child.

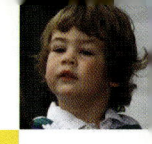

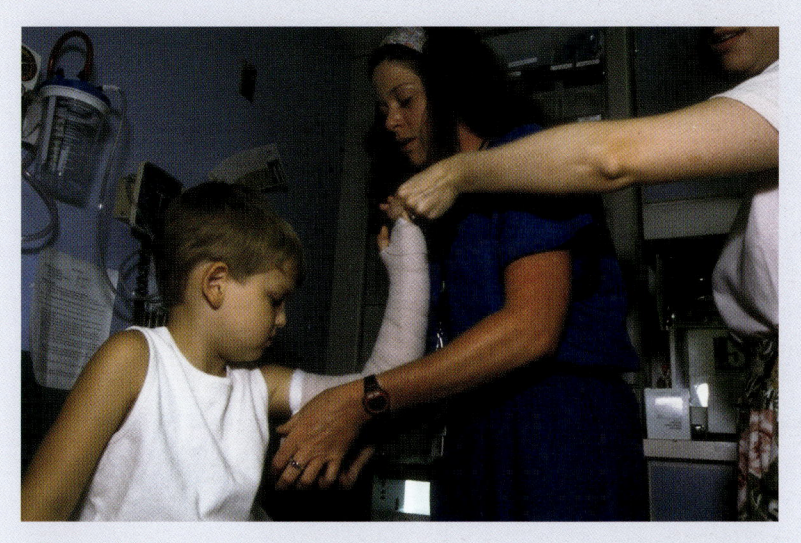

Figure 13.5 *When treating an elbow dislocation, avoid manipulation and splint in the position found.*

Swelling typically occurs with extremity injuries and may progress rapidly. Elevate the extremity when possible and remove any jewelry from the affected extremity. Cold (ice) application is useful in the acute stage of inflammation (injury) but may not be available in the field. Cold application causes local vasoconstriction, which decreases swelling and pain. Do not apply ice directly to the skin as it may cause frostbite and further tissue damage. Assess and appropriately manage pain in the field. Immobilization of injuries will reduce pain, but pain medications are frequently warranted. Transport to the nearest appropriate facility.

Specific Extremity Treatments

Shoulder: Sling and swathe. Elbow should be flexed at a 90-degree angle with some support between the elbow and the abdomen.

Elbow: Splint in the position found. Do not manipulate, as severe neurovascular complications may occur (Figs. 13.6, 13.7). Sling and swathe when possible.

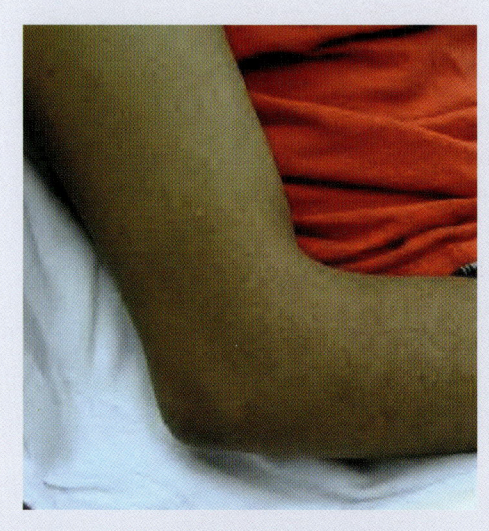

Figure 13.6 *Manipulation of an elbow dislocation may cause severe neurovascular complications.*

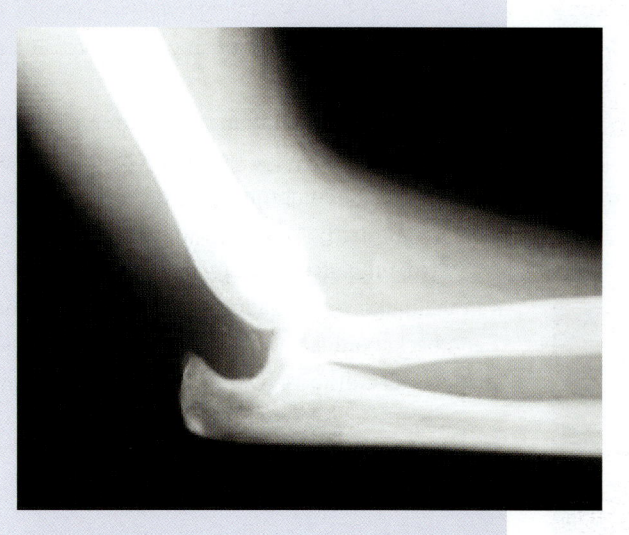

Figure 13.7 *X-ray of an elbow dislocation in a child.*

Pediatric Extremity Trauma

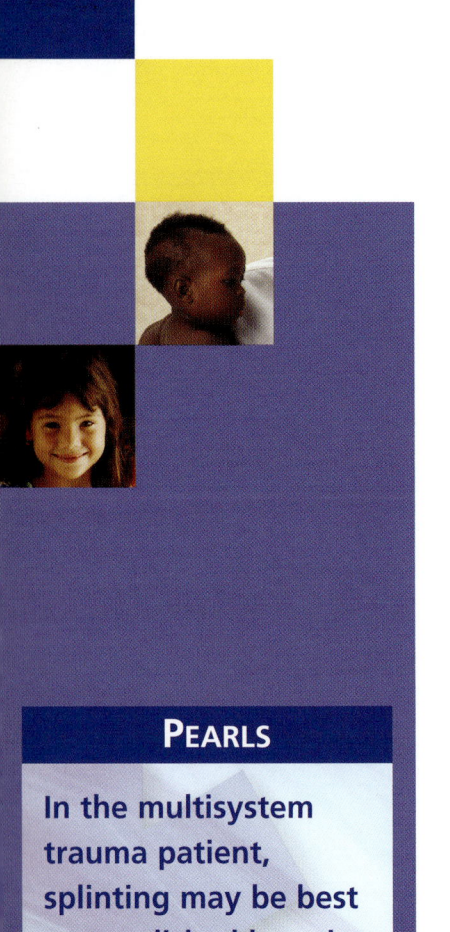

Humerus: If the fracture is in the upper part of the humerus, a sling and swathe is sufficient. Treat deformities in the lower part of the humerus as if they were elbow fractures.

Forearm: Utilize a rigid-type splint to immobilize the fracture site.

Wrist: Utilize a board splint with gauze placed between fingers, and support the hand on a board with roller gauze in the palm of hand.

Hand: Support the hand on a cushion or pillow. An alternative method is to insert a roll of gauze in the palm, place gauze pads between the fingers, and wrap the entire hand in a very bulky dressing.

Pelvis: You may consider pelvic wrap devices/splints in an adolescent child, based on the size of the child and equipment available. You may use a sheet or commercial device specifically sized for the pediatric patient to stabilize an unstable pelvic fracture. It is best to immobilize the full body to a backboard (and pad for comfort when appropriate).

Hip: Splint in the position found. Secure to the backboard. Do not use traction splints on hip fractures.

Femur: If a femur fracture is present (typically indicated by pain, deformity, instability, and angulation of the thigh), apply an appropriate splint and secure to the backboard. This is the only fracture in which a traction splint may be used.

Tibia/fibula: Utilize a rigid-type splint and secure to the backboard.

Knee: Immobilize in the position found. If distal pulse is absent, apply gentle longitudinal (in-line) traction to the limb. Secure to the backboard. A knee fracture or dislocation is frequently associated with vascular injury. This is a true orthopedic emergency. Patella dislocations are frequently mistaken for knee dislocations.

Ankle/foot: Splint using a compression dressing (pillow-type splint).

Do not take splinting of an extremity lightly, even though it is a basic skill. Several complications, including changing a closed fracture to an open fracture, causing neurovascular compromise, and creating a greater displacement of a joint, may occur if done improperly.

Not all pediatric trauma patients will—or should—be splinted as previously described. In the multisystem trauma patient, splinting may be best accomplished by using the body and backboard as the only splint until after you are en route. Remember, ABCs should always take priority over the extremities.

Pearls

In the multisystem trauma patient, splinting may be best accomplished by using the body and backboard as the only splint until after you are en route.

SPRAINS AND STRAINS

Sprains are ligamentous injuries that occur around the joint. Strains are tears of the muscle tendon junction and usually occur away from joints.

Signs and Symptoms

In the field, these injuries are not easily differentiated from fractures, with most children presenting with pain and swelling. Children have a greater tendency to fracture than do adults, so manage any injured extremity as a fracture.

Treatment

The initial treatment of a sprain or strain follows fracture management principles.

COMPARTMENT SYNDROME

Compartment syndrome results from increased pressure within a closed space, as a result of blunt or penetrating trauma. Compartment syndrome has many causes, including tight dressings, splints or casts, internal bleeding, or edema following an injury. Early recognition of this syndrome is crucial in preventing permanent nerve and vascular damage to the extremity. Unless you have long transport times, this is not usually a concern in the prehospital phase.

Signs and Symptoms

Signs and symptoms of this syndrome are severe pain, paresthesias, pallor, puffiness (swelling), and pulselessness. The symptoms usually develop over hours. Pulses may be present initially and then gradually disappear. The loss of a palpable pulse is a very late finding. Pain that seems out of proportion to the injury is usually the earliest sign.

Treatment

If unrecognized, compartment syndrome can lead to permanent loss of function in the extremity. Splint the extremity and notify the receiving facility of the possibility of compartment syndrome. Surgery will be necessary to relieve the pressure as quickly as possible to preserve function.

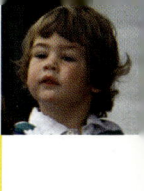

Pediatric Extremity Trauma

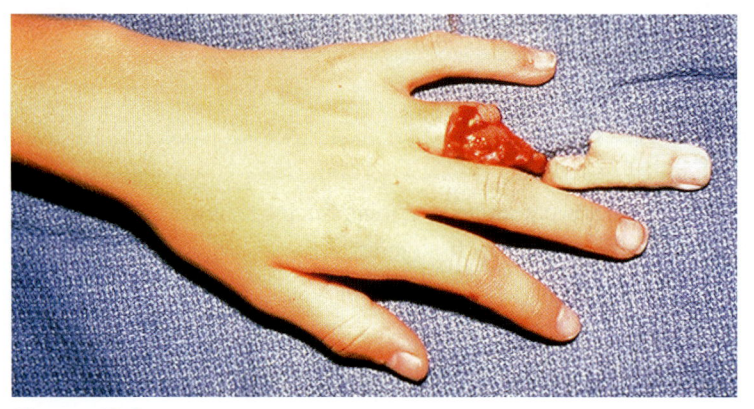

Figure 13.8 *Avulsion of the ring finger of a teen.*

AMPUTATIONS

Amputations are either complete or incomplete. The mechanisms causing an amputation are clean-cut injury (guillotine-type), crush injury, or avulsion injury (Fig. 13.8). The repair of an incomplete amputation is known as revascularization. The repair or reattachment of a completely amputated part is known as replantation.

A clean-cut amputation has the best rate of successful repair after microsurgery. The success rate for digit replants is lower in children, but when they succeed, the function is better than for adults. The small size of vessels in children makes the repair technically difficult. The decision about treatment is made after many considerations. Hand dominance, importance of the part for function, associated injuries, and nature of the injury are all considered. Never assure a patient that a digit or limb will be replanted.

Signs and Symptoms

Identify all areas of potential injury. Determine whether the amputation is partial or complete. If the child has had active bleeding from the site, this determination will have been made in the circulation portion of the assessment.

Treatment

Goals of treatment include control of bleeding and preservation of amputated parts. Although each individual facility will have a specific protocol for managing amputations, the following information should serve as a guideline for the care of both complete and incomplete amputations.

Complete Amputations

Care of the stump is addressed in the circulation portion of the assessment. Be sure to control the bleeding through the application of a pressure dressing. If pressure dressing is not adequate to control the bleeding, consider the application of a tourniquet, making sure it is not too tight. Retrieve amputated parts and rinse with sterile saline. This removes gross contaminants. Wrap the part in saline-moistened (not soaked) gauze and place in a plastic bag or container and seal. Place the sealed container in another container with ice (Fig. 13.9). The tissue should never contact the ice. Never use dry ice. The proper cooling of amputated parts slows metabolism and extends ischemic time, allowing the surgeon time for microsurgical repair or reconstruction.

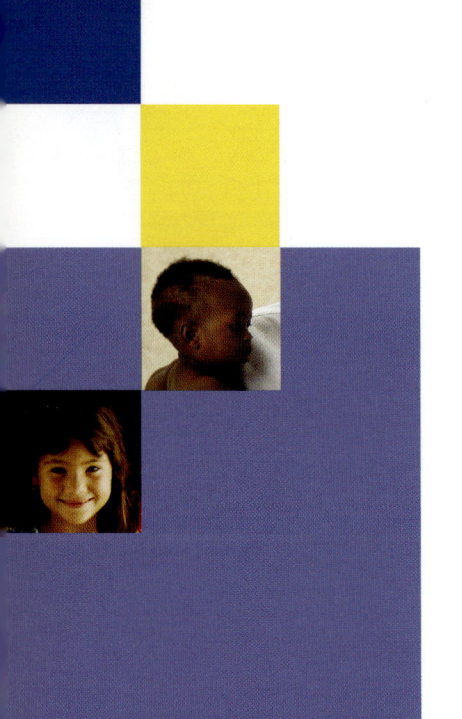

PEARLS

Goals of treatment in an amputation include control of bleeding and preservation of amputated parts.

Pediatric Trauma Life Support

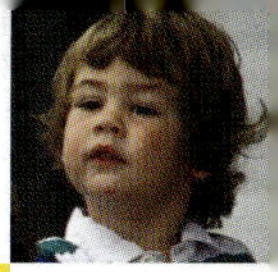

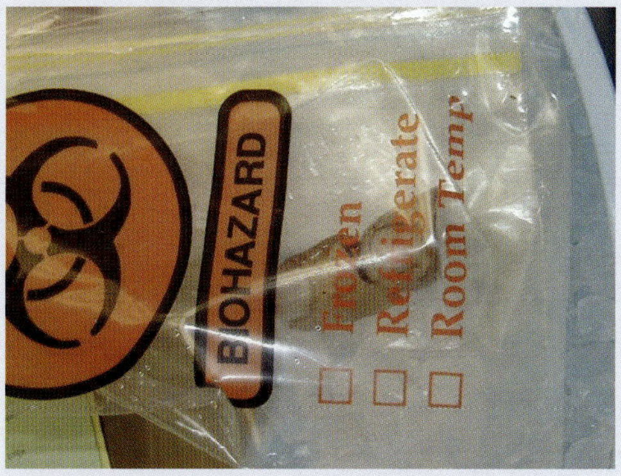

Figure 13.9 *The amputated part should be wrapped in saline-moistened gauze, sealed in a plastic bag or container, and placed on ice.*

Incomplete Amputations

Treatment of incomplete amputations is similar to that of complete amputations. Control bleeding, and then place a dressing moistened with saline over open tissue. Apply a pressure dressing and splint, if necessary, to stop the bleeding and stabilize the injury. Place ice packs over the area without blood flow. Place ice over a dressing, never directly on the skin.

Case Study continued

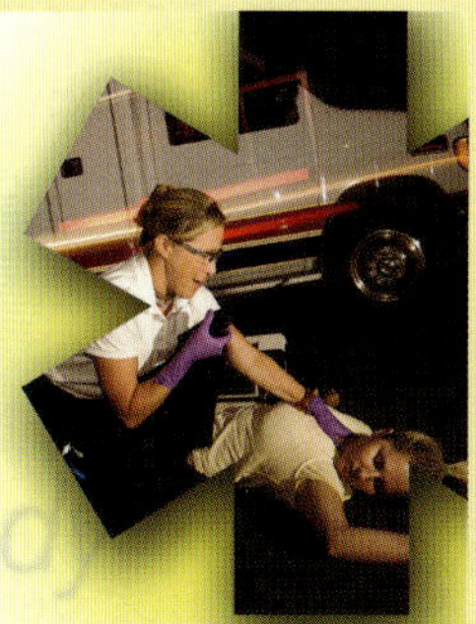

John, Susan, and Bob of the Emergency Transport System (ETS) have been called to the scene where a 6-year-old boy had fallen from a tree. On arrival, the scene appears safe. The team is led to the back yard where they see the child is lying on the ground. Bystanders state the boy was climbing a plum tree and fell approximately 12 feet (3 meters) onto the grass. He is crying and responding appropriately to the environment, but appears distracted by his leg injury. His skin is pale and cool. His mother saw him fall and reports that he started crying and complained of severe pain in his left leg. Susan approaches the patient, talking to him and telling him not to move and that she is going to support his head while her partner, Bob, "takes a closer look at that leg."

John begins to gather a SAMPLE history from the patient's mother and notes that the patient's past medical history is negative. He takes no medications and has no allergies, and he last ate at breakfast (5 hours ago). The mother also states that her son weighs approximately 60 pounds (27 kg).

Pediatric Extremity Trauma

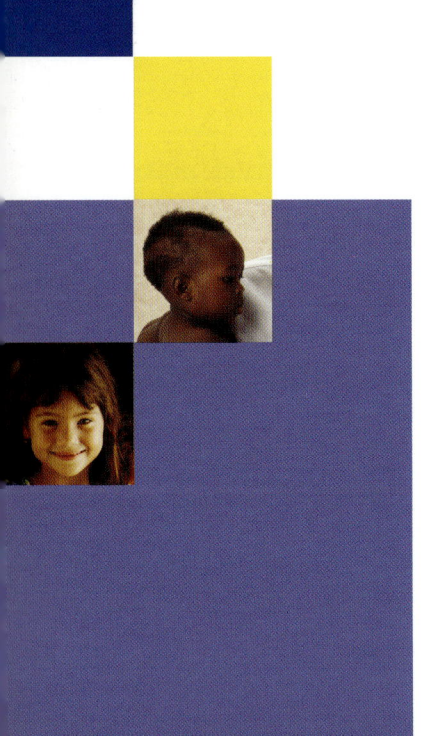

Because of the mechanism of injury (12-foot fall from a tree), Bob performs a Rapid Trauma Survey and notes that the child's airway is clear and his breath sounds are equal bilaterally with an adequate rate. His chest is stable and non-tender. His abdomen is soft and is not painful to palpation. His pelvis is stable and is non-tender. His heart rate is very rapid and his distal pulses are decreased. His left pant leg is soaked in blood. There is no obvious head trauma. The patient acts appropriately for his age and circumstances, though he is a little slow to respond to questions. His pupils are equal and reactive to light. Upon removing the child's clothes, there are no obvious injuries noted except for the left thigh, which appears angulated and swollen with an actively bleeding wound. The distal left leg pulse is decreased compared to the pulse in the right leg. Bob decides that it is a load-and-go situation.

Direct pressure is applied to the thigh wound and a pressure dressing is applied. The patient is given oxygen and placed on a spinal motion restriction device with cervical spine stabilization. Because of signs of hypovolemic shock, the child is immediately transported (load-and-go).

An intravenous line and a bolus of normal saline are initiated en route, and a traction splint is applied to the left leg. After splinting, the child appears to be in less distress, the thigh is less angulated, and the distal pulses are stronger. Analgesia is considered at this time.

Bob decides with 20 minutes left in the transport that a second IV bolus of 20 mL/kg of normal saline would be beneficial, given that the patient's heart rate is still tachycardic at 110 bpm, his mental status is still depressed, and his systolic blood pressure is only 90 mmHg. The patient's mental status, heart rate and blood pressure improve after the second IV bolus and he is alert upon arrival at the local hospital. The patient was also given analgesia prior to arrival at the hospital.

Following further assessment and investigation, it is confirmed that the patient had sustained an open left femoral fracture. The wound was photographed, covered with iodine soaks and redressed. A dose of intravenous antibiotic was given, and the patient was promptly taken to the operating room for wound debridement and fixation of the fracture. He made a good post-operative recovery and was discharged home with arrangements for an orthopedic follow-up.

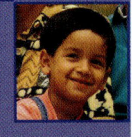

Pediatric Trauma Life Support

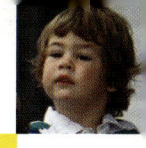

Case Study wrap-up

This child had a serious mechanism of injury, resulting in a distracting injury. Spinal motion restriction was initiated without startling the child, and then maintained given the child's age, distracting injury, and mechanism of injury. This child was recognized to be in shock, even without taking an initial blood pressure, because of his heart rate, mental status and estimated blood loss. Therefore, he was a "load-and-go" patient. Intravenous access was achieved en route, followed by a 20 mL/kg fluid bolus. Traction splinting was also initiated en route and analgesia was provided, all leading to a favorable outcome to the child's traumatic experience.

SUMMARY

1. While not typically life-threatening, extremity injuries are often disabling. These injuries are often more obvious than more serious internal injuries and can distract caregivers to defer the usual steps of the ITLS Primary Survey and attend to the non-life-threatening extremity trauma.
2. Pelvic and femur fractures can be associated with life-threatening internal bleeding, so patients with these injuries are in the load-and-go category.
3. Proper splinting is important to protect the injured extremity from further injury as well as to minimize pain.
4. Dislocations of the elbows, hips, and knees, while rare, require careful splinting and rapid transport to prevent severe disability to the affected extremity.

Recommended Reading

American College of Surgeons. "Musculoskeletal Trauma." In *Advanced Trauma Life Support for Doctors*, 8th ed. Chicago: Author, 2008.

Barkin, Roger and Peter Rosen. "Management Principles." In *Emergency Pediatrics*, 6th ed., 525. St. Louis: Mosby, 2003.

Campbell, John Emory, ed. "Extremity Trauma." In *International Trauma Life Support for Prehospital Providers*, 6th ed., 211–28. Upper Saddle River, N.J.: Pearson/Prentice Hall, 2008.

Cmiel, Peggy and Clare. E. Cavanaugh. "Digital Replantation in Children." *American Journal of Nursing* 9 (1989): 1158–61.

Gould, Barbara. *Pathophysiology for the Health Professions*, 2nd ed. Philadelphia: W. B. Saunders, 2002.

Limmer, Daniel, Michael O'Keefe, and Edward Dickinson. *Emergency Care*, 10th ed. Upper Saddle River, N.J.: Pearson/Prentice Hall, 2007.

Reff, Richard B. "Musculoskeletal Injury." In *Pediatric Trauma Care*, edited by Martin R. Eichelberger and Geraldine L. Pratsch, 133–44. Rockville, M.D.: Aspen Publishers, 1988.

Richards, Robin. R. and James R. Urbaniak. "The Surgical and Rehabilitation Management of Vascular Injury to the Hand." *Hand Clinics* 2 (1986): 171–77.

CHAPTER 14
Pediatric Burns

Howard A. Werman, MD, FACEP

Objectives
Upon completion of this chapter, you should be able to:

1. Describe the assessment priorities in children with burn injuries.
2. Integrate the concepts of burn management with the assessment and treatment of other traumatic injuries.
3. Discuss the unique treatment priorities in management of the burned child.
4. Describe the unique elements in caring for children with high-voltage electrical injuries and lightning strikes.

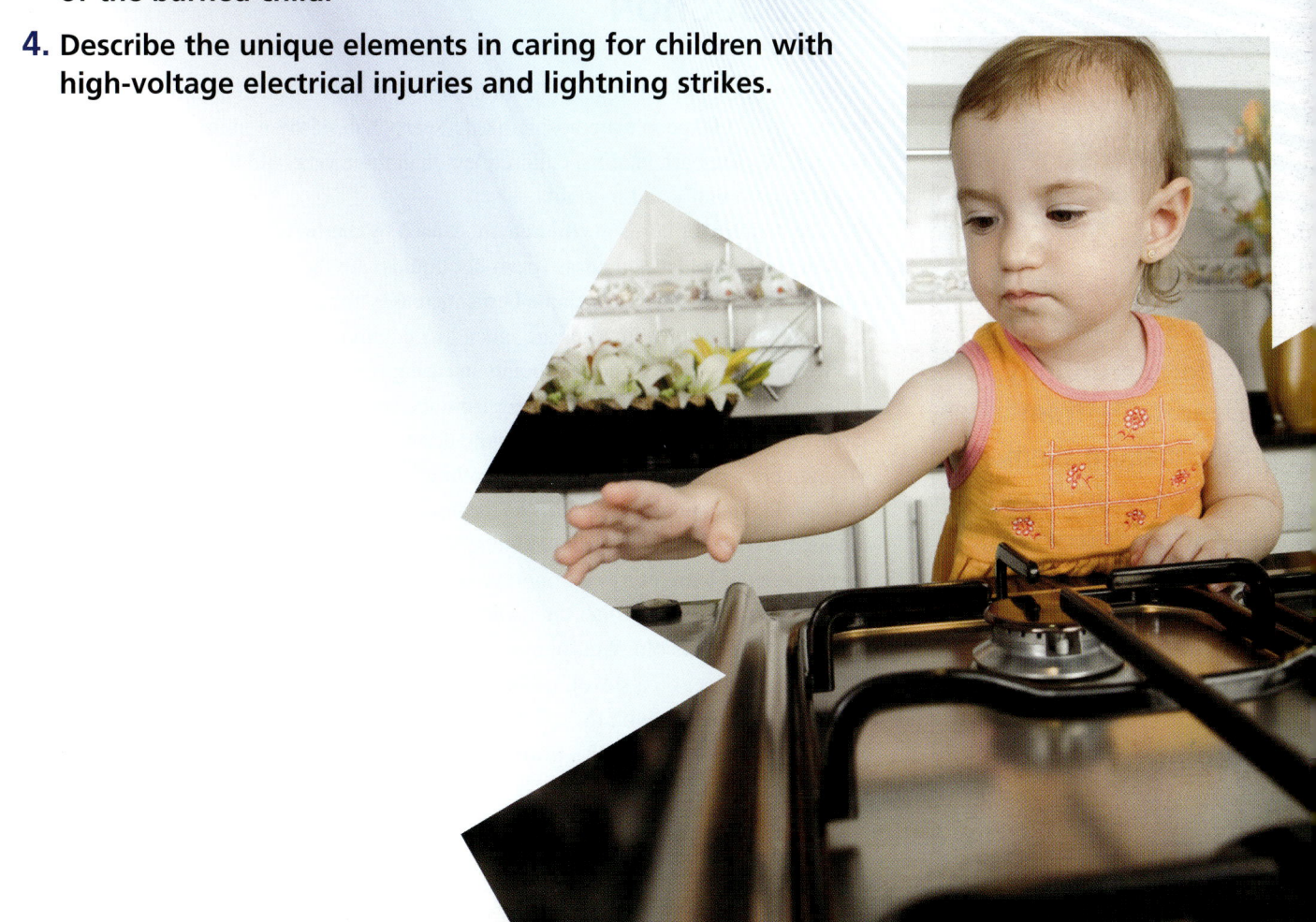

Case Study

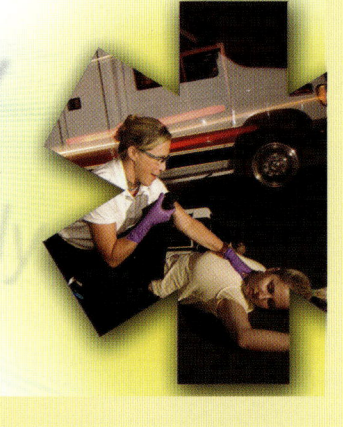

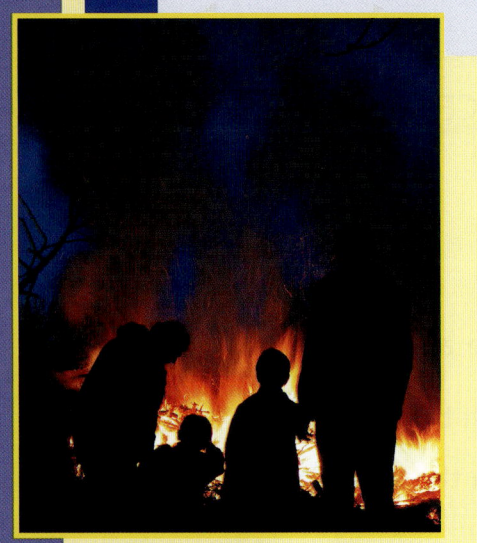

Susan, John, and Bob of the Emergency Transport System (ETS) have been called to the scene of a home fire in which a 4-year-old child is reported to be a victim. The team responds to the scene with fire suppression units. John agrees to be the team leader. How should the team approach this situation? How should their assessment and treatment priorities for the burned child differ from children with other traumatic injuries? Keep these questions in mind as you read the chapter. Then, at the end of the chapter, find out how the rescuers completed this call.

INTRODUCTION

Each year in the United States, 1.25 million people seek medical attention for treatment of burns, and 50,000 people are hospitalized. Nearly half of these injuries occur in pediatric patients. Among burn victims, children less than three years old have the greatest risk of long-term morbidity and mortality.

The majority of burns in children are caused by thermal injuries. In children less than three years old, scald burns (from hot liquids) are the most common cause of burns (Fig. 14.1). The incidence of flame burns increases after the age of two. Electrical, lightning, and chemical injuries are much less common in children.

Remember several important points in caring for the pediatric burn patient. The first priority is to safely remove the patient from the source of injury (fire, smoke, electricity, chemicals, and so on). Burns can be quite dramatic in appearance. However, first focus your attention on the child's airway, breathing, and circulation. Life-threatening injuries can develop in children with burns as the result of associated traumatic injuries from automobile collisions, falls from heights, or blast injuries. Aggressive resuscitation in the early phases of burn injury can improve the child's long-term prospects for a full recovery. Finally, remember to consider child abuse as a possible cause of scald burns in children less than three years old. Well-outlined burns of the buttocks, a contact burn outlining an object (e.g., burner on a stove), multiple burns of various ages, a history of mechanism of injury not compatible with the child's injuries or development, evasive answers, a delay in seeking medical attention, or a prior history of repeated trauma are suggestive of child abuse (Fig. 14.2).

> **PEARLS**
>
> **Children less than three years old have the greatest risk of long-term morbidity and mortality from burns, making them a target point for injury prevention initiatives.**

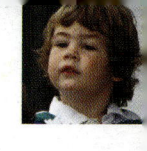

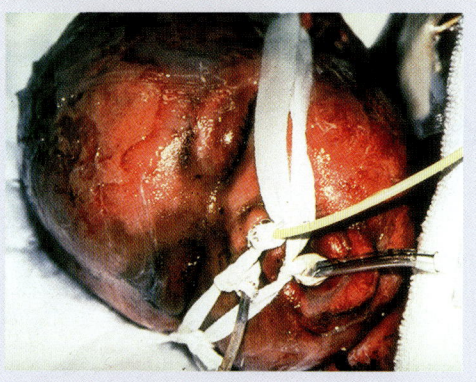

Figure 14.1 *Scald burns are the most common cause of burns for children under three years.*

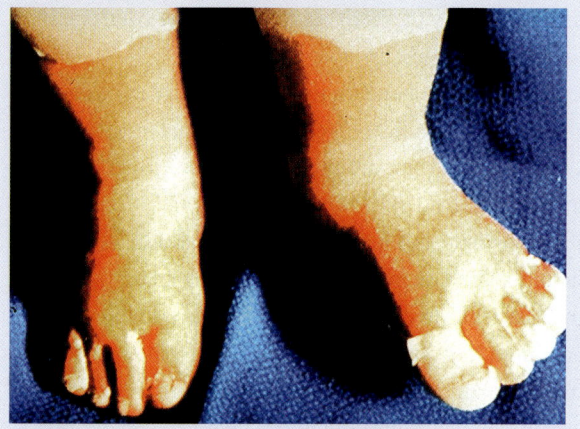

Figure 14.2 *A burn pattern of the feet as shown suggests child abuse.*

PEARLS

Remove the child from the source of burn injury; focus on the ABCs; consider abuse as a cause.

Partial Thickness Burns | **Full Thickness Burn**

Epidermis
Dermis
Hypodermis

Normal Skin Anatomy

First Degree
Epidermis only
Painful and red

Second Degree
Epidermis and Dermis
Painful, red, and blistered

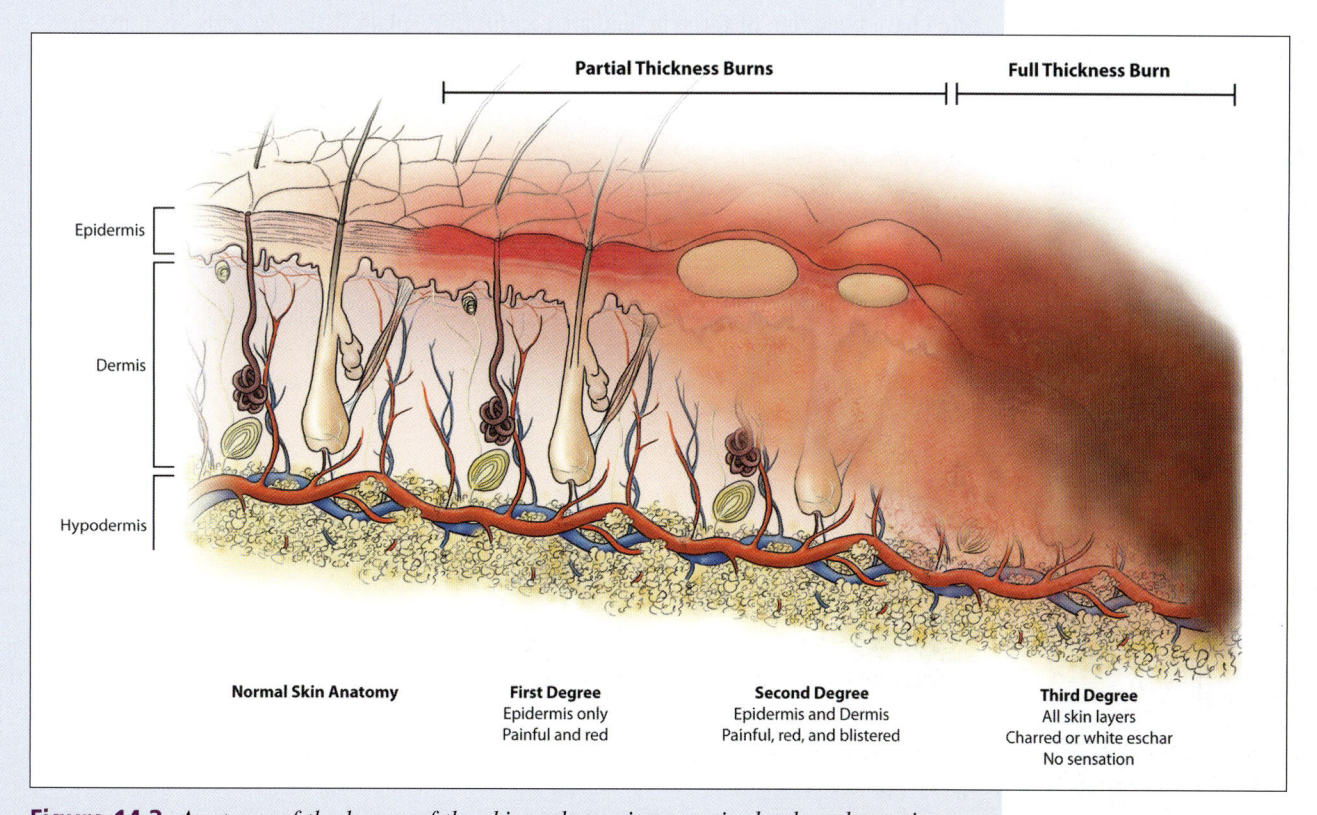

Third Degree
All skin layers
Charred or white eschar
No sensation

Figure 14.3 *Anatomy of the layers of the skin as burns increase in depth and severity.*

Pediatric Burns

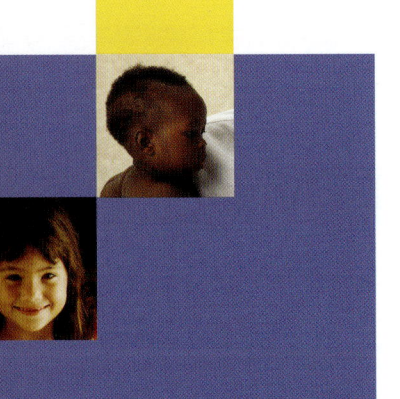

ANATOMY AND PATHOPHYSIOLOGY

Burns are caused by the application of heat to the skin and underlying structures. The amount of heat transferred and the length of time in contact are the major determinants of the extent of the burn.

Burn Depth

The skin is divided into two layers: the epidermis and dermis (Fig. 14.3). The epidermis is the most superficial area of the skin and consists of several thick layers of cells. The primary function of the epidermis is to protect the body against invasion from microorganisms and to prevent leakage of body fluids.

The dermis is a connective tissue layer that lies beneath the epidermis. It contains several important skin appendages, including hair follicles, sweat glands, nerve endings, and blood vessels. The dermis is crucial for several important skin functions, including temperature regulation and regeneration of damaged skin.

The depth of the injury is determined by inspection of the burn wound. Burns are characterized as superficial partial thickness (first degree), deep partial thickness (second degree), and full thickness (third degree) depending on the amount of injury to the dermis and epidermis (Table 14.1). Because children have thinner skin than adults, they tend to be burned more deeply when exposed to the same amount of heat. Superficial partial-thickness burns extend through the epidermis and occasionally into the upper layers of the dermis. These burns appear red and dry and are painful. Because the lower layers of the epidermis tend to be spared by the burn, these wounds are likely to heal on their own in 10 to 14 days. Deep partial-thickness burns extend deep into the dermis. They appear red and wet, often have blistering of the skin, and are painful (Fig. 14.4). These wounds often require some degree of skin grafting to heal completely.

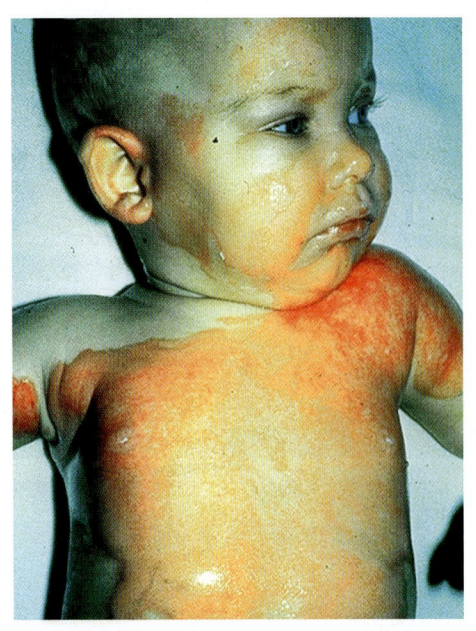

Figure 14.4 *An infant with a combination of second and third degree burns.*

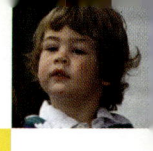

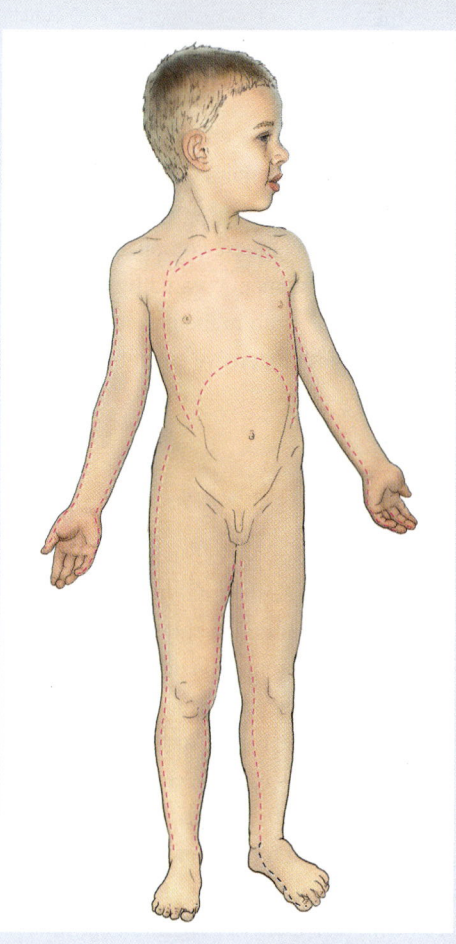

Figure 14.5 *Dotted lines indicate potential incision lines for performing an escharotomy to relieve the confinement created by the eschar in a burn patient.*

Table 14.1: Types of Burns

	Superficial partial thickness (1st degree)	Deep partial thickness (2nd degree)	Full thickness (3rd degree)
Layer	epidermis	epidermis, dermis	all layers
Color	bright red	pale red	white or charred
Blisters	none	large	dry
Pain	moderate	severe	none
Healing	3 to 5 days	1 to 3 weeks	never
Scarring	none	moderate	severe

Full-thickness burns extend through the dermis. These burns are white or charred in appearance due to the coagulation of skin and blood vessels (eschar). Because the nerve endings are destroyed, these burns are usually painless. Full-thickness burns do not heal without skin grafting and can be particularly troublesome when they extend around the chest, an extremity, or a joint.

Pediatric Burns

Swelling below the eschar in a limb can create a tourniquet-like effect, leading to neurovascular compromise. Circumferential full-thickness chest burns can cause respiratory compromise. Circumferential burns involving the extremities or chest often require a procedure called an escharotomy or fasciotomy to prevent these complications. An incision is made through the burned tissue to relieve the confinement created by the eschar (Fig. 14.5). This preserves the arterial and nerve supply to the limb in the case of an extremity burn and allows better ventilation of the patient with extensive chest burns. This is not a prehospital procedure.

Extent of Injury

In the adult, the extent of injury is determined using the "Rule of Nines," which assigns multiples of nine percent to certain areas of the body to calculate the total body surface area of the burn wound (Fig. 14.6). This simple rule is not accurate for children, however, because they have a proportionately larger head and proportionately smaller lower extremities than adults. As a result, the Lund Browder diagram is more useful in determining the body surface area of the burn in children (Table 14.2). Another helpful guideline is that the area defined by the child's palm and fingers is approximately one percent of the body surface area. For smaller burns, the extent of injury is estimated by determining how many of the child's palms and fingers are equal to the area of the burn.

Burns are classified as minor, moderate, and major. A moderate burn, in a child, involves 10 percent to 20 percent body surface area with less than 10 percent being full thickness. A major burn is more than 20 percent body surface burn or more than 10 percent being full-thickness injury. In addition, the burn is considered a major burn if the child has inhalation injury, evidence of significant electrical injury (including lightning strike), or associated trauma. Inhalation injuries and electrical injuries are discussed later in this chapter.

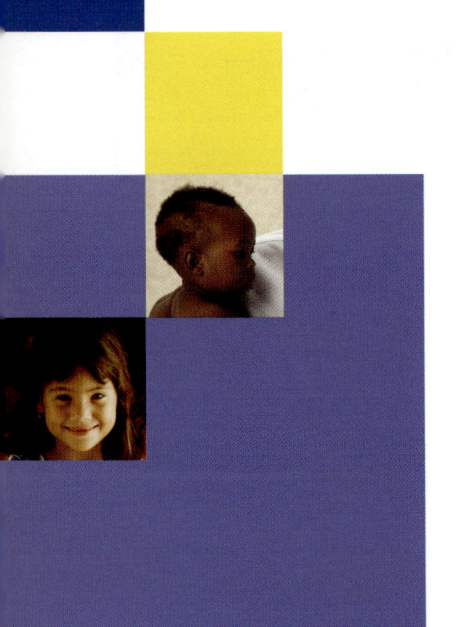

> **PEARLS**
>
> Pediatric burn surface area charts such as the Lund Browder chart can assist in determining fluid replacement calculations and should be standard tools.

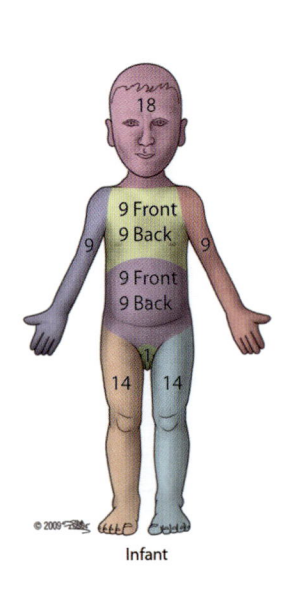

Figure 14.6a *The Rule of Nines demonstrated on an infant.*

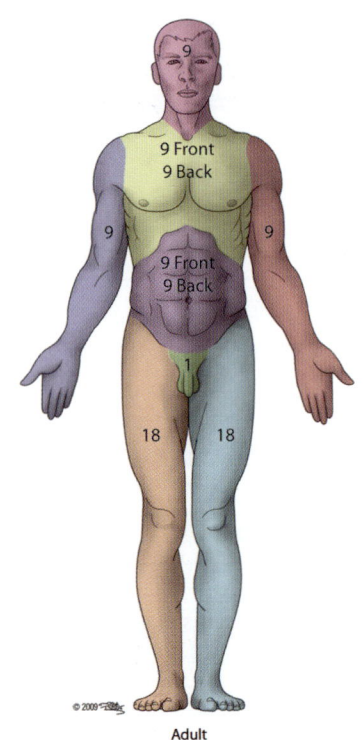

Figure 14.6b *The Rule of Nines demonstrated on an adult.*

Pediatric Trauma Life Support

Table 14.2: Lund Browder Chart

Area	0-1	1-4	Age (Years) 5-9	10-15	Adults	% 2nd Degree	% 3rd Degree	% Total
Head	19	17	13	10	7			
Neck	2	2	2	2	2			
Ant. Trunk	13	17	13	13	13			
Post. Trunk	13	13	13	13	13			
R. Buttock	2.5	2.5	2.5	2.5	2.5			
L. Buttock	2.5	2.5	2.5	2.5	2.5			
Genitalia	1	1	1	1	1			
R.U. Arm	4	4	4	4	4			
L.U. Arm	4	4	4	4	4			
R.L. Arm	3	3	3	3	3			
L.L. Arm	3	3	3	3	3			
R. Hand	2.5	2.5	2.5	2.5	2.5			
L. Hand	2.5	2.5	2.5	2.5	2.5			
R. Thigh	5.5	6.5	8.5	8.5	9.5			
L. Thigh	5.5	6.5	8.5	8.5	9.5			
R. Leg	5	5	5.5	6	7			
L. Leg	5	5	5.5	6	7			
R. Foot	3.5	3.5	3.5	3.5	3.5			
L. Foot	3.5	3.5	3.5	3.5	3.5			
					Total			

Weight: _____

Height: _____

PATIENT ASSESSMENT

Assess and manage all children with burns and related injuries in the same manner as all trauma victims.

1. ITLS Primary Survey
    A. Scene Size-Up
    B. Initial Assessment
    C. Rapid Trauma Survey or Focused Exam
    D. Critical Interventions and Transport Decisions
    E. Contact medical direction as needed.

2. ITLS Secondary Survey and/or Ongoing Exam

Pediatric Burns

ITLS Primary Survey

Scene Size-Up

When approaching a burn victim, survey the scene to determine if there is a safe approach to the child. Also determine if any special equipment is required. The immediate priority in caring for the burn victim is to remove the child from the burning source. Be careful, however, not to also become a victim. Safely remove the child from the source of heat. This often requires the aid of fire personnel. Remove loose burned clothing and any constricting jewelry from the child. In addition, briefly irrigate the wounds with cool water so that the burns do not continue to act as a heat source and increase the underlying injury. Never directly apply ice to a burn injury. Do not perform prolonged irrigation with cool water because of the risk of producing hypothermia.

In the case of electrical injuries, remove the child from any live electrical source. Experienced rescue personnel and the power company may be required for a safe extrication. If there are chemicals involved, only approach the child when it is determined that there is no risk to the rescuer. Thoroughly irrigate the burns after brushing any dry chemicals from the skin.

Initial Assessment

General Impression and Level of Consciousness

A badly burned victim can be terrifying to examine. The overall seriousness of the situation is influenced by many factors including the child's body position, the surroundings, and the work of breathing. It is important to remember that the initial care of the burn patient should focus on the basic ABCs. Begin your Initial Assessment with your general impression and level of consciousness. Your approach will be the same as with the adult patient.

Airway and Cervical Spine

As with any other trauma victim, if there is concern about the mechanism of injury or the patient has altered mental status, initiate manual cervical spine control as soon as possible. The ABCs are the priorities in assessment and management.

You must keep in mind special considerations when assessing the ABCs of a pediatric burn patient. While assessing the child's airway, remember that children rescued from an enclosed area are at particularly high risk for airway compromise. Clues suggesting possible airway injury include severe facial burns, singed eyebrows and nares, oral or pharyngeal burn, sooty sputum, hoarseness, or stridor. Focus close attention on the status of the airway in these children. Because of the smaller cross-sectional area of a child's trachea, even a small amount of swelling can significantly obstruct the airway. While preparing to urgently intubate the child, immediately reposition any child with an obstructed airway, suction the airway, and use bag-valve-mask ventilations to support their ventilation. Although children usually do not need to be intubated in the field, you may have to consider early intubation if you are unable to ventilate in spite of various airway maneuvers or if the child exhibits stridor.

Breathing

Assess the child's efforts at breathing next. Determine the depth and rate of respiration. Any sternal or intercostals retractions, cough, wheezing, grunting, stridor, drooling, or hoarseness are troublesome signs in a burned child. Hypoventilation, respiratory distress,

---

PEARLS

Consider early intubation if airway injury is suspected: severe facial burns, singed eyebrows and nares, oral or pharyngeal burn, sooty sputum, hoarseness, or stridor.

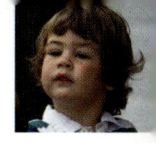

and respiratory arrest are common in patients with burns complicated by inhalation injury. Respiratory arrest is also seen in patients exposed to high-voltage electrical injuries and lightning strikes. You may also see pulmonary injuries in children burned after an explosion.

All children should receive 100 percent oxygen. In addition to correcting the hypoxemia the child may have been experiencing, this will begin to decrease the child's carbon monoxide level. Remember that the pulse oximeter is unreliable after smoke inhalation, so every child gets 100 percent oxygen.

Circulation

Next, address the circulatory status. Compare pulses in the neck and wrist to assess the child's circulation. As discussed in Chapter 7, consider the child's level of consciousness, skin color, and temperature in addition to the pulse rate and quality of the pulses. Shock is rare in the early stages after a burn. Generally, shock from burns takes several hours to develop and is caused by a shifting of fluids from the vascular system into the burned tissue. If it is determined that a child is in shock shortly after a burn injury, look for other possible sources including internal bleeding as the result of a fall or motor vehicle collision, neurogenic shock caused by high-voltage electrical injuries (more than 600 V), or myocardial damage resulting from electrical current.

The absence of pulses indicates a child in cardiac arrest. If the child has no detectable pulse, initiate immediate CPR. Cardiopulmonary arrest may occur with severe inhalation injury, high-voltage electrical injury, and lightning strikes. Once cardiac arrest is recognized, apply a monitor/defibrillator. Children with electrical injuries may present in ventricular fibrillation. Those injured by lightning may develop asystole secondary to a prolonged respiratory arrest. Follow standard ACLS/PALS protocols in this setting. Remember that children are usually healthy patients who will respond to resuscitation efforts if the duration of the cardiac arrest has not been too long. There are reports of survival after prolonged resuscitation.

Rapid Trauma Survey

Quickly complete the Rapid Trauma Survey looking for any life-threatening injuries. After the head-to-toe exam, perform a brief neurologic assessment if the child has altered mental status. Stabilize the ABCs as quickly as possible, and package and transport. In children with an altered level of consciousness after an inhalation injury, high levels of both carbon monoxide and cyanide may be present. The presence of these substances cannot be determined in the prehospital setting. Initiate treatment prior to confirming the presence of these agents. Prehospital treatment of carbon monoxide includes 100 percent oxygen delivered by a tight-fitting nonrebreather mask. This hastens elimination of carbon monoxide from the body.

Critical Interventions and Transport Decisions

As discussed, the initial concern in pediatric burn patients is the child's airway, breathing, and circulation. If any signs of an unstable airway, obvious respiratory insufficiency, shock, or an altered mental status are present, package and transport the child as quickly as possible.

Airway and Cervical Spine

Monitor children carefully for such signs of upper airway obstruction as tachypnea, stridor, or drooling. Establish endotracheal intubation early because airway problems can develop suddenly in a child with even a small degree of airway obstruction. Children with trouble handling their secretions, an altered mental status, or extensive facial and oral burns also should have their airways secured with an endotracheal tube. In this case, perform intubation at the scene prior to transfer to the hospital. Intubation should be performed in the usual manner, except you may need a smaller endotracheal tube (0.5 mm to 1.0 mm smaller than would normally be inserted). Avoid prolonged and difficult attempts at intubation to prevent further damage to the child's airway. Consider a rapid sequence induction technique or sedation-assisted intubation to reduce the possibility of laryngoscopy-induced airway injury. However, evaluate the benefits of providing sedation against the risk of the child losing spontaneous efforts at breathing.

Breathing

Monitor the child's respiratory status very carefully during transport. Give 100 percent oxygen and watch for signs of respiratory distress or failure.

Circulation

If the child presents with a thready, rapid pulse and signs of shock, seek another cause for the shock other than burns. In addition to oxygen therapy, IV access is essential for all burn patients. Children with burns suffer massive fluid losses during the early hours after their injuries. This is particularly true for children with electrical injuries where the extent of the external burns will grossly underestimate the child's fluid requirements.

Ideally, two large-bore IV lines should be established in peripheral veins, preferably in areas uninvolved by burns. Establish IV access during transport and do not delay removing the patient from the scene of the burn injury. In addition, prolonged attempts to establish access are not warranted and may be delayed until arrival at the hospital, particularly if transport times are less than 30 minutes or it is anticipated that venous access sites may be limited. Intraosseous (IO) access is an option for critical burns and shock. Insertion through a burn area is a relative contraindication for IO placement; therefore, use other locations first, if available, especially if ACLS medications or fluid resuscitation are indicated. However, IO is an effective alternative in a critical situation. Begin aggressive fluid resuscitation as discussed in Chapter 7 if the patient shows any evidence of shock. The initial bolus should be 20 mL/kg of normal saline or other medically approved crystalloid. It is reasonable to consult medical direction about the fluid rate.

Cardiac Monitoring. Conduct continuous cardiac monitoring on children in shock or those with high-voltage electrical injuries or lightning strikes because of the high incidence of cardiac dysrhythmias.

Thermoregulation

Keep the child warm during evaluation and transport. Because of their large surface area and small muscle mass, young children do not conserve body heat efficiently. When they suffer burns, their ability to conserve body heat is compromised even further, and hypothermia can develop. Remember, after making sure burning is not still taking place, patients should be covered with a dry sheet and kept warm. Finally, although children with burns may complain of thirst, do not give them anything by mouth.

PEARLS

Children with burns suffer massive fluid losses during the early hours after their injuries. Consider IV placement but do not delay transport to establish.

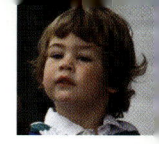

Table 14.3: American Burn Association Guidelines for Transfer to a Burn Center

1. Partial-thickness burns of greater than ten percent of the total body surface area
2. Burns that involve the face, hands, feet, genitalia, perineum, or major joints
3. Third-degree burns in any age group
4. Electrical burns, including lightning injury
5. Chemical burns
6. Inhalation injury
7. Burn injury in patients with preexisting medical disorders that could complicate management, prolong recovery, or affect mortality
8. Any patients with burns and concomitant trauma (such as fractures) in which the burn injury poses the greatest risk of morbidity or mortality. In such cases, if the trauma poses the greater immediate risk, the patient's condition may be stabilized initially in a trauma center before transfer to a burn center. Physician judgment will be necessary in such situations and should be in concert with the regional medical control plan and triage protocols.
9. Burned children in hospitals without qualified personnel or equipment for the care of children
10. Burn injury in patients such as children who will require special social, emotional, or rehabilitative intervention

Transport Considerations

Transport the vast majority of pediatric burn patients to the closest available emergency department for initial stabilization. You only need to transport to a specialty care center those children who have significant traumatic injuries associated with their burns. The American Burn Association has developed guidelines for children who should be transported to a pediatric burn center (Table 14.3).

ITLS Secondary Survey

Once a thorough assessment of the ABCs has been conducted, perform the ITLS Secondary Survey. Again, you should examine the patient from head to toe and attempt to identify any injuries that may have complicated the burn injury. Head, neck, chest, lungs, and abdominal injuries are seen as the result of falls, collisions, explosions, and high-energy currents that complicate the burn injury. Remember that injuries from explosion due to primary air blast are almost exclusive to air-containing organs (auditory, lungs and gastrointestinal system).

BURN WOUND MANAGEMENT

Once you have addressed the immediate life threats, you should attend to the burn wound itself. Assess the extent and depth of the burn in the burned child. Remember that in the prehospital setting, measurements of the extent and depth of the burn wound on any patient are only estimates and can change over the course of the patient's illness.

It is appropriate to cover the child with a clean, dry sheet. Any prehospital provider who handles the child should wear both gloves and a mask to prevent contaminating the burn wounds by microorganisms. Do not apply antibiotic ointment during the prehospital phase of care.

Pediatric Burns

Fluid Resuscitation

Aggressive fluid therapy is important in the early stages of a burn, but if the transport time is less than 30 minutes, it is not necessary to begin fluid resuscitation in the field for an isolated burn injury. However, initiate fluid resuscitation on any patient with signs or symptoms suggestive of shock as discussed in Chapter 7. For thermal burns, you may give normal saline or other medically approved crystalloid at an initial rate estimated by multiplying 0.25 by the child's weight (in kilograms) by the percent of the body burn. As an example, the initial infusion rate in a 10 kg child suffering a 20 percent body burn is 50 mL/hr (0.25 x 10 kg x 20%). This formula is not appropriate for victims of high-voltage electrical burns because the surface burn cannot accurately determine the underlying tissue damage. Fluid infusion of 20 times the child's body weight, in kilograms, may be used. In the example above, an initial infusion of 200 mL/hr would be initiated for an electrical burn.

Pharmacologic Therapy

Children who are victims of smoke inhalation may have been exposed to certain toxins such as carbon monoxide and cyanide. The initial therapy for carbon monoxide consists of supplying the patient with 100 percent oxygen to hasten eliminating carbon monoxide from the body.

Local protocols may allow prehospital administration of pain medications such as narcotics. Where allowed, adequately address the child's pain. Use narcotic agents with caution in patients with respiratory compromise, underlying head injury, or shock from other causes.

In the hospital, cyanide poisoning is treated safely using sodium thiosulfate solution. Sodium thiosulfate is available as a 50 mL vial of a 25 percent solution. You may give a a 30 mL (8 g) dose to a child under 12 years of age; in a child 12 years or older, you may give 50 mL (12.5 g), according to protocol. Recently, intravenous hydroxocobalamin in a dose of 70 mg/kg has been used for cases of suspected cyanide toxicity in children. At this time, the FDA has not yet authorized its use for children in the United States.

Special Problems in Burn Management

Inhalation Injuries

Inhalation injuries occur when heated air, smoke, and toxic products of combustion are inhaled. Children with inhalation injury can have serious airway and pulmonary complications, often without any external signs of a significant burn. Half of the deaths from burns are the result of inhalation injuries.

The effects of the inhalation are caused by the direct effect of heat on the airway and bronchial tree (airway obstruction and wheezing) as well as toxic effects of smoke, carbon monoxide, chlorine gas, and cyanide. Carbon monoxide is an odorless, colorless byproduct of incomplete combustion of many common compounds. Carbon monoxide prevents the binding of oxygen on hemoglobin in the bloodstream and prevents oxygen from being used efficiently by cells. Chlorine gas is a product of burning some common plastic materials. Cyanide acts in a similar fashion. Recent studies have shown that cyanide is often found in toxic levels in patients with significant inhalation injury.

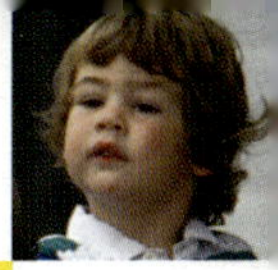

Electrical Injuries

Electrical injuries have a very different clinical picture. They are often divided between high-voltage (>1000 V) and low-voltage (<1000 V) injuries. The burns from the entrance and exit of the current in high-voltage injuries are often unimpressive, unless the child's clothing was ignited. However, there is often extensive damage of the nerves, blood vessels, and muscles in the path of the current as it passes through the child's body. Current that passes through the heart can cause cardiac dysrhythmias, especially ventricular fibrillation or asystole. In addition, release of myoglobin from damaged muscle can deposit in the kidneys and cause long-term renal failure if not treated aggressively. High-voltage electricity injuries are often accompanied by violent contraction of the skeletal muscles, leading to fractures and dislocations involving the long bones and spine. In addition, secondary injuries can result when the child falls following contact with a high-voltage wire.

The most common type of low-voltage electrical burns involves oral burns that occur when a child bites into a live electrical wire (Fig. 14.7). Although bodily injury is unlikely, the child requires a careful evaluation with particular attention to the extent of oral damage. Delayed bleeding approximately one week after oral burns is often seen with such injuries.

Lightning Injuries

Lightning injuries are also seen in children. Although these injuries involve high-voltage electricity, they produce much higher currents (10 million to 2 billion V) over a very brief period (milliseconds). Such injuries result in little internal injury and few surface burns. Instead, the majority of these pediatric patients present with profound respiratory arrest that leads to asystole. These patients may often respond to CPR if it is initiated soon after the lightning exposure.

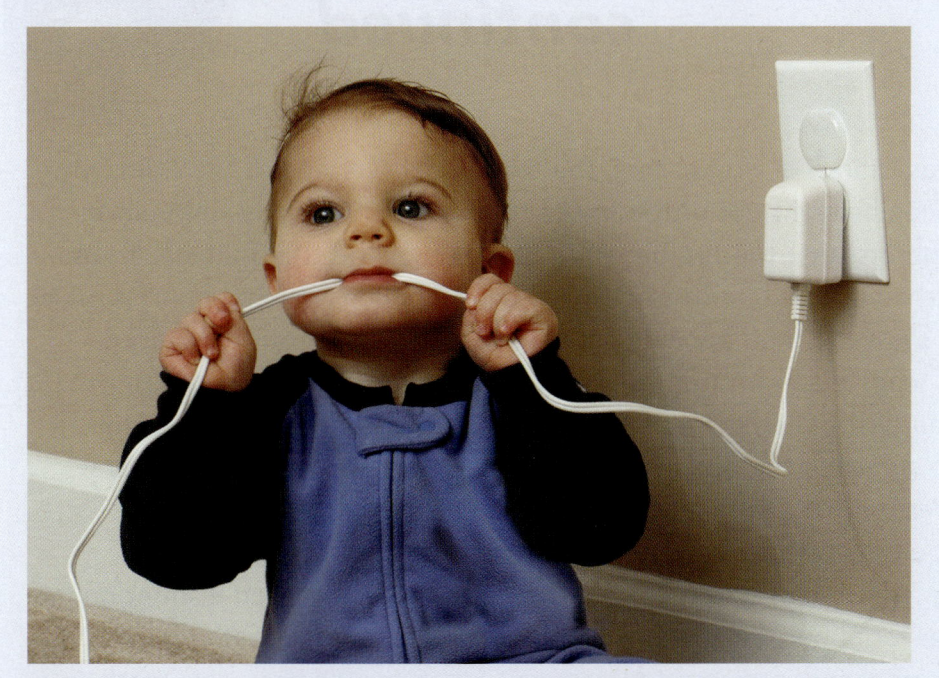

Figure 14.7 *Biting into a live wire causes oral burns and is a common cause of low-voltage electrical burns in children.*

Pediatric Burns

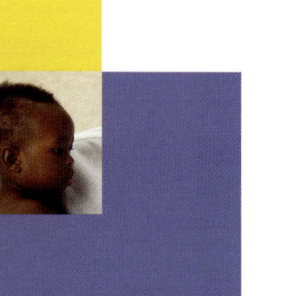

BURN PREVENTION

Many factors place a child at unnecessary risk for burn injury. These include overcrowding, inadequate child supervision, and failure to promptly notify the local fire department.

Smoke Detectors

Smoke detectors are among the most effective interventions available for reducing smoke inhalation and burn injury. When used correctly, detectors are thought to reduce the potential for serious injury by up to 66 percent. Provide ongoing education regarding the effectiveness of smoke and fire detectors and their use.

Education

Instruct children about the dangers of electrical injury. Instruct parents to minimize a child's access to electrical plugs and wires, including forbidding the child to enter any area that has electrical wires. Climbing trees and flying kites in these areas are particularly dangerous. Teach children that, during lightning, they should seek shelter inside and avoid high places and open areas. Teach them to also avoid metal fences during electrical storms.

Case Study continued

With the assistance of firefighters, the team makes its way to the child, who has just been brought out of the house to a safe place by the ambulance. The firefighters state the fire began in the kitchen and the child was found on the kitchen floor. There was no explosion. The team's general impression is not good since the child appears unconscious with stridorous respiration. John, the team leader on this call, begins the Initial Assessment. Susan removes all of the child's clothing as some edges are actively smoldering while Bob stabilizes the neck. The firefighters assist them in cooling several burned areas on the extremities, face, chest, and back.

John quickly assesses the child's level of consciousness, airway, and breathing. The child is unconscious with stridor noted on each inspiration. John notes facial burns and singed eyebrows. The child is breathing very fast and has sternal and intercostal retractions. Susan begins bag-valve-mask ventilation with 100 percent oxygen, supporting the child's respiratory

Pediatric Trauma Life Support

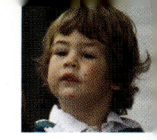

effort in preparation for endotracheal intubation. While Susan continues bag-valve-mask ventilation, John prepares for endotracheal intubation. In addition to a 5.0 mm endotracheal tube (normal for a 4-year-old child), he prepares 4.5 mm and 4.0 mm tubes because of concerns about the airway narrowing as the result of the burn. John is able to complete the oral intubation on the first attempt, passing a 4.5 mm tube through the vocal cords that are markedly swollen.

After addressing the child's airway and breathing, John reassesses the circulation. The child has strong radial and carotid pulses. The skin is warm and dry. Because the child is unconscious and already demonstrates compromised airway and breathing, John decides that immediate transport is warranted. A Rapid Trauma Survey assessing the neck, chest, abdomen, pelvis, and extremities fails to reveal any secondary trauma. Bob covers the child in a dry, clean sheet and places several blankets on the child to conserve body heat. The child is packaged on a pediatric backboard, then loaded and transported immediately.

During transport, Susan secures a single intravenous line in an unburned area in the left antecubital space. The child has burns involving the anterior torso, neck, face, and both upper extremities including the hands. The back, genital region, and most of the lower extremities are uninjured. Most of the burned areas are red, moist, and appear painful to the touch. There is some blistering noted. The impression is that these are deep partial-thickness burns. The burns on the anterior chest appear whitish and leathery, suggesting full-thickness burns. John estimates that the child has sustained deep partial-thickness and full-thickness burns over 40 percent of the body surface area. Rapid calculations suggest an initial IV fluid rate of (0.25) x (20 kg) x (40% BSA) or 200 mL/hr. The child is placed on a cardiac monitor and pulse oximeter.

John calls medical direction and give a brief update regarding his findings and interventions. The medical direction physician asks that the team maintain the infusion at 200 mL/hr and continue ventilation with 100 percent oxygen via the endotracheal tube. The physician requests that John give morphine sulfate 2 mg intravenously for pain control and sedation, and suggests that the ambulance proceed to the closest local emergency department for further stabilization, where arrangements will be made to transport the child to a pediatric burn center.

The patient has a long complicated course in the burn intensive care unit at the regional pediatric center. He develops pulmonary edema as the result of the inhalation injury and remains on the ventilator for about a week. John visits the patient two days after transport and finds that he appears diffusely swollen from the burns and has massive fluid requirements. The team later

Pediatric Burns

learns that the child required extensive skin grafting for the full-thickness burns and needed extensive physical therapy for the extremity burns. However, rehabilitation was progressing, and the patient is expected to be released from the hospital in the next few days.

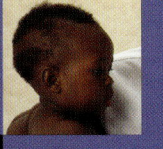

Case Study wrap-up

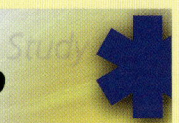

Fire in an enclosed space, as in this case, is likely to cause inhalation injury associated with upper airway burns. To allow assessment and treatment, it was imperative that the firefighters removed the child immediately from the home to a place of safety away from the blaze.

Burn wounds can be dramatic in appearance but the focus of attention should be on airway, breathing and circulation, which are assessed in the ITLS Primary Survey.

Once the immediately life-threatening conditions are addressed, the Rapid Trauma Survey will identify the associated and incidental injuries, especially if there has been an explosion.

It is important to remember that 50 percent of the deaths in burn victims are from inhalation injuries. The child in this study was at risk of losing his airway in due course; aggressive management in securing his airway and oxygenation with 100 percent oxygen was a life-saving procedure. The additional treatment comprised of intravenous fluid resuscitation and intravenous analgesia en route to hospital further enhanced his chances of a good recovery from this unfortunate incident.

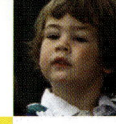

SUMMARY

1. The first priority in a pediatric burn patient is to separate the child from the source of the burn. Remove all loose burned clothing and take off anything constrictive (jewelry, belts, etc). Cool the burn injury with a small amount of cool fluid to avoid inducing hypothermia. Brush off any solid chemicals and use generous irrigation for all chemical injuries. Do not become a victim!
2. As with other trauma patients, first assess the child's airway, breathing, and circulation. Significant traumatic injuries are often associated with burn injuries. Do not overlook these injuries because of the dramatic appearance of the burns.
3. Be aggressive in managing the child's airway if signs of respiratory distress are present. Airway problems may suddenly worsen in children with upper-airway injury.
4. Shock in the early stages of a burn is not caused by the burn injury. Look for other sources of shock.
5. Initiate fluid resuscitation early if you have a transport time of more than 30 minutes. The rate of infusion is based on the child's weight and extent of burns. Provide more aggressive fluid resuscitation than suggested by the surface burns to children with high-voltage electrical injuries.
6. Consider child abuse in scald burns of patients less than three years of age.

Recommended Readings

American Academy of Pediatrics. "Trauma." In *Pediatric Education for Prehospital Professionals*, 2nd ed., edited by Ronald A. Dieckmann. Sudbury, M.A.: Jones & Bartlett Publishers, 2006.

American College of Surgeons. "Injuries Due to Burns and Cold." In *Advanced Trauma Life Support for Doctors*, 8th ed. Chicago: Author, 2008.

Antoon, Alia Y. and Mary K. Donovan. "Burn Injuries." In *Nelson Textbook of Pediatrics*, edited by Robert Kliegman, Richard E. Behrman, and Hal B. Jenson, 450–57. St. Louis: W.B. Saunders, 2004.

Brown, David F. M. "Lightning Injury." In *Harwood-Nuss' The Clinical Practice of Emergency Medicine*, 4th ed., edited by Allan B. Wolfson, Gregory W. Hendey, Phyllis L. Handry, Christopher H. Linden, and Carlos L. Rosen. Philadelphia: Lippincott, Williams and Wilkins, 2005.

Campbell, John Emory, ed. "Burns." In *International Trauma Life Support for Prehospital Care Providers*, 6th ed., 237 Upper Saddle River, N.J.: Pearson/Prentice Hall, 2008.

Gomez, Ruben and Leopoldo C. Cancio. "Management of Burn Wounds in the Emergency Department." *Emergency Medicine Clinics of North America* 25 (2007): 135–146.

Guidotti, Tee. "Acute Cyanide Poisoning in Prehospital Care: New Challenges, New Tools for Intervention." *Prehospital Disaster Medicine* 21 (March-April 2006, 2 Suppl 2): s40–8.

Hall, Lois M. and Robert M. Sills. "Electrical and Lightning Injuries." In *Pediatric Emergency Medicine: Concepts and Clinical Practice*, 2nd ed., edited by Roger M. Barkin, et al., 335–54. St. Louis: Mosby, 1997.

Holland, Andrew J. "Pediatric Burns: The Forgotten Trauma of Childhood." *Canadian Journal of Surgery* 49 (August 2006): 272–77.

Reed, Jennifer L. and Wendy J. Pomerantz. "Emergency Management of Pediatric Burns." *Pediatric Emergency Care* 21 (February 2005): 118–29.

Rudkin, Scott E. and Jennifer A. Oman. "Electrical Injuries." In *Harwood-Nuss' The Clinical Practice of Emergency Medicine*, 4th ed., edited by Allan B. Wolfson, Gregory W. Hendey, Phyllis L. Handry, Christopher H. Linden, and Carlos L. Rosen. Philadelphia: Lippincott, Williams and Wilkins, 2005.

Scalzo, Anthony J. "Inhalation Injuries." In *Pediatric Emergency Medicine: Concepts and Clinical Practice*, 2nd ed., edited by Roger M. Barkin, et al., 335–54. St. Louis: Mosby, 1997.

15

CHAPTER 15
Pediatric Submersion Injuries

Mary Jo Bowman, MD, FAAP
Richard N. Nelson, MD, FACEP

Objectives
Upon completion of this chapter, you should be able to:

1. List the various categories of drowning.

2. Describe the ITLS Primary Survey and how it relates to the priority plan.

3. Describe the critical transport decisions and the transport interventions that are important in providing the patient with the best neurological outcome.

4. Describe how the prehospital provider is in a unique position to gather historical and environmental information.

5. Describe the prognosis and outcome of submersion injuries.

6. Discuss how prevention is the key to avoiding submersion injuries.

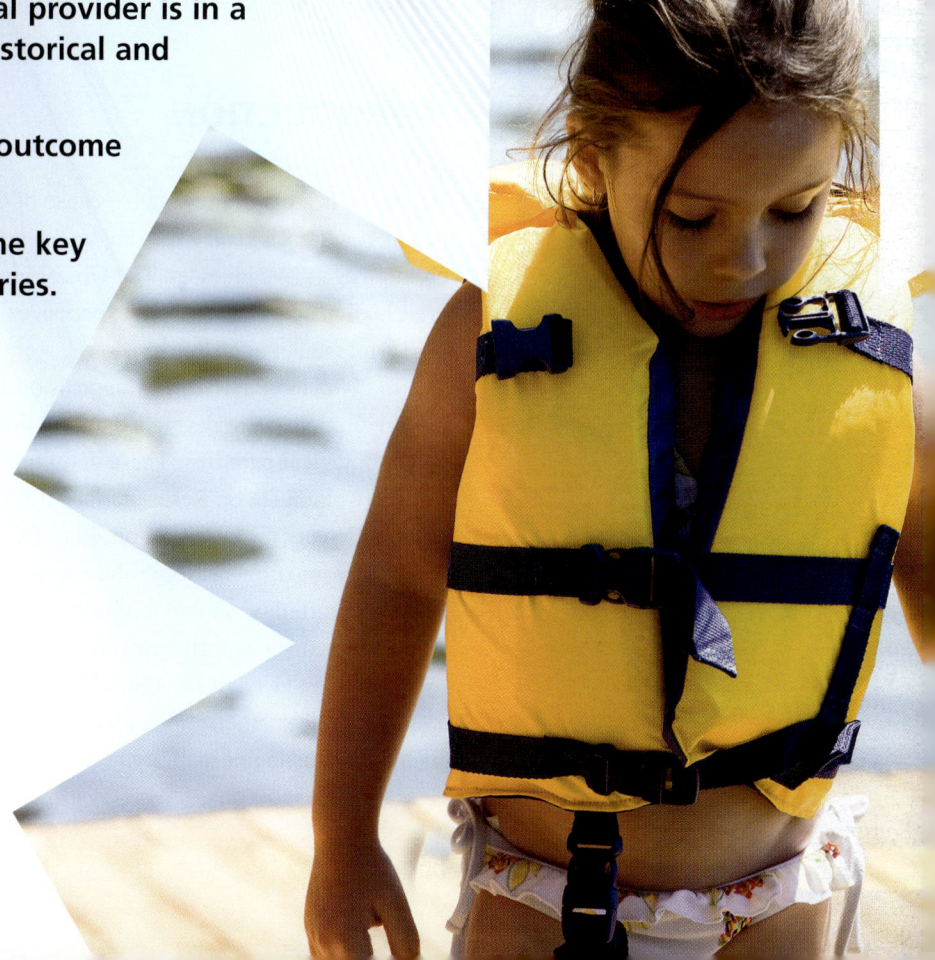

Case Study

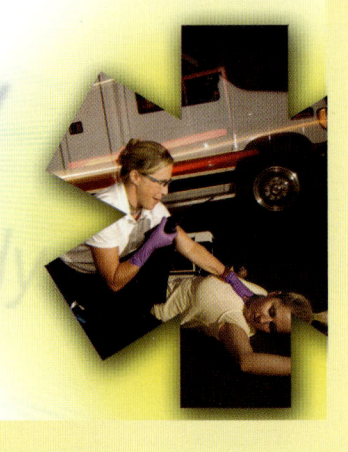

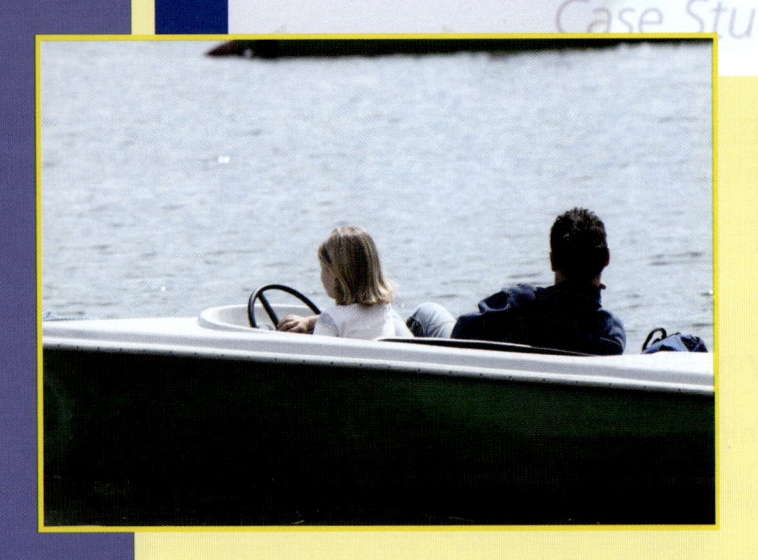

One warm summer day, Susan, John, and Bob from the Emergency Transport System (ETS) are called to a lake where a 6-year-old female was involved in a boating crash. The child, who was not wearing a personal floatation device (PFD), was thrown from the boat after it struck another boat. Bystanders report that the victim was rescued from the water after being "under" for approximately 30 minutes. CPR was performed by lay rescuers. John is the team leader for this call and the team arrives 10 minutes after CPR was started. What injuries should they expect with a mechanism of this type? What other emergency may be associated with the possible injuries? Keep these questions in mind as you read the chapter. Then at the end of the chapter, find out how the rescuers completed this call.

INTRODUCTION

Drowning is a major preventable cause of death. Worldwide, 140,000 to 150,000 drowning deaths occur each year. Drowning is the second leading cause of accidental deaths in children ages 14 and under. The typical profile of the pediatric drowning victim is a preschool male swimmer who experiences the submersion incident in a home swimming pool while under adult supervision.

In 2002, the First World Congress on Drowning was held in Amsterdam, Netherlands. New definitions were developed during this conference to facilitate data collection for epidemiological purposes. These definitions have been accepted by the International Liaison Committee on Resuscitation (ILCOR), the World Health Organization (WHO), and the Centers for Disease Control (CDC). Drowning is the process of experiencing respiratory impairment from submersion/immersion in a liquid. Outcomes are classified as death, morbidity, and no morbidity. The immersion syndrome is a form of drowning caused by sudden exposure to very cold water (less than 68° F [20° C]) that may be due to a vagally induced dysrhythmia.

While the submersion incident may occur as a result of readily explainable factors such as exhaustion or inability to swim, a precipitating event or associated condition is often present. There is a four-fold increase in submersion incidents for individuals who have a history of seizure disorders. It is important to recognize preexisting conditions, for example seizures or diabetes, to properly guide prehospital and emergency department management.

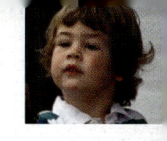

ANATOMY AND PATHOPHYSIOLOGY

Submersion Injury

Wet Drowning

Wet drowning occurs when water is aspirated into the lungs as a result of the victim losing protective airway reflexes or because of inability to suppress respirations. Freshwater aspiration constitutes the majority of drowning incidents. Because fresh water is less concentrated than plasma, water aspirated into the lungs is quickly absorbed into the circulation via simple osmotic forces, resulting in hypervolemia. Thus, a child pulled from the water after aspirating fresh water may have little water left in the lungs by the time resuscitation is started. Of more importance is the damage that freshwater aspiration causes to the lung tissue. Water disrupts surfactant activity, washing this important surface-active material from the alveolar membranes. As a result, alveolar surface tension is increased and lung compliance is decreased, leading to poor ventilation and oxygenation. Later, alveolar capillary membrane leakage occurs and causes pulmonary edema and further hypoxia.

Salt water is three to four times more concentrated than plasma. Thus, when salt water is aspirated into the lungs, fluid from the circulation is actually drawn into the lungs through the alveolar capillary membranes, resulting in hypovolemia and pulmonary edema.

Children who have aspirated salt water may have large amounts of water still in the lungs at the time of initial resuscitation. Surfactant in the alveolar capillary membranes is similarly affected with saltwater aspiration, and severe hypoxemia is common.

Polluted water aspiration compounds the problems previously discussed. Chemical irritation of the alveolar membranes produces an inflammatory response in addition to direct damage to the alveoli and surfactant. In addition, children who have aspirated polluted water are more prone to later infections.

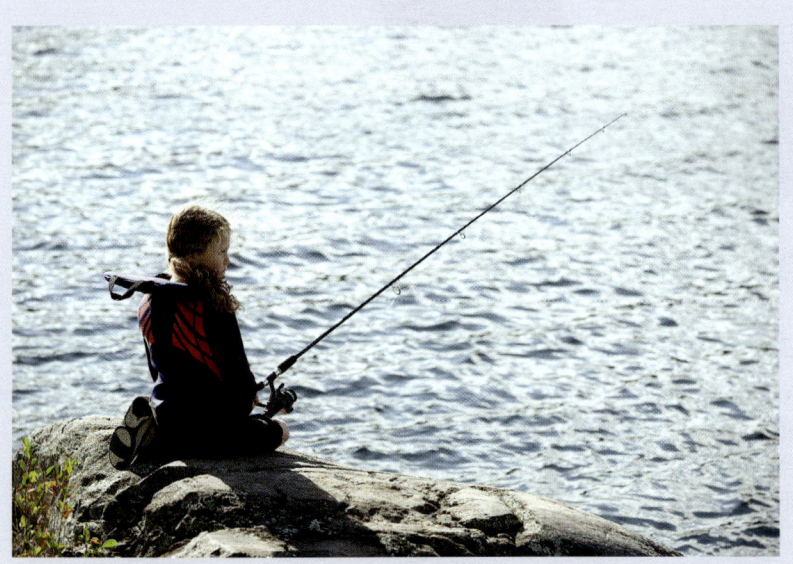

> **PEARLS**
>
> In the prehospital setting, the focus should be on oxygenation and ventilation rather than on the mechanism of drowning.

Dry Drowning

Approximately two percent of drowning occurs without aspiration. Apparently, laryngospasm prevents water from entering the lungs, resulting in death by airway occlusion or asphyxiation rather than by aspiration. Theoretically, these patients have a better chance of successful resuscitation because the lungs are spared direct damage. In the prehospital setting, wet drowning cannot be differentiated from dry drowning.

Immersion Syndrome

Sudden death that occurs as a result of contact with water, usually cold, is known as immersion syndrome. This poorly defined syndrome is probably the result of vagal-induced cardiac arrest or bradycardia with loss of consciousness. Alcohol ingestion is considered a predisposing factor.

PATIENT ASSESSMENT

All pediatric patients involved in a drowning incident should be considered multiple-trauma patients. Follow the standard pediatric ITLS approach.

1. ITLS Primary Survey
    A. Scene Size-Up
    B. Initial Assessment
    C. Rapid Trauma Survey or Focused Exam
    D. Critical Interventions and Transport Decisions
    E. Contact medical direction as needed
2. ITLS Secondary Survey and/or Ongoing Exam

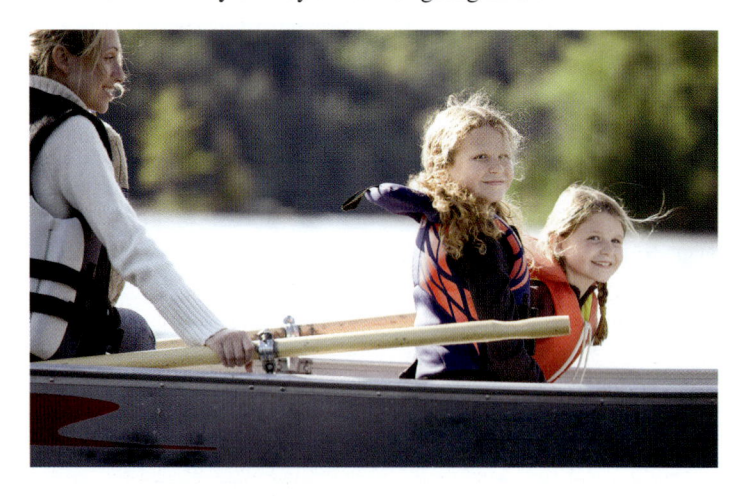

ITLS Primary Survey

Scene Size-Up

Determine whether the scene is safe. If the child is still in the water, determine whether there are any dangers in getting the child out. Rescuing children who have fallen through ice is particularly treacherous, and each year many would-be rescuers become victims themselves after being submerged in ice water.

> **PEARLS**
>
> It may be difficult to "wait" for scene safety when the event involves a child. Be aware of hazards that can incapacitate you as a rescuer.

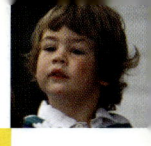

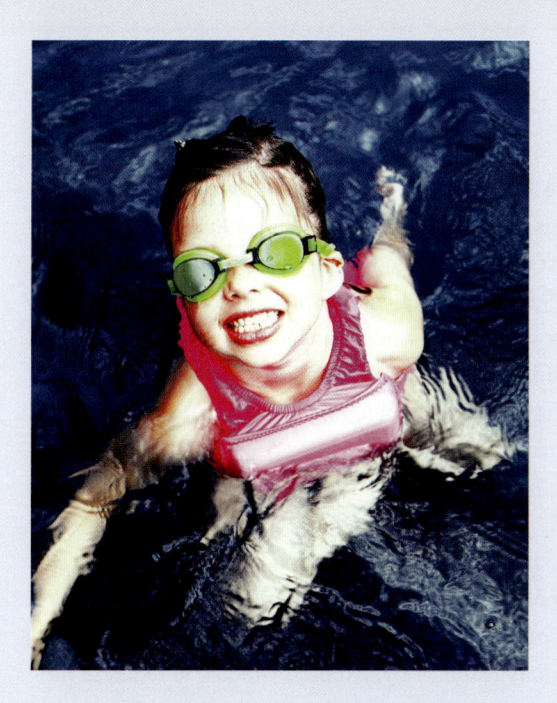

Another potential hazard is malfunctioning electrical equipment (lights, heaters) in home swimming pools. Electricity transmitted through the water may not only have caused the victim to drown, but also may be a potential hazard to the rescuer.

Initial Assessment

General Impression and Level of Consciousness
Determine a general impression as you approach the patient. Does the child appear unresponsive? Is the child restless or combative? Are there obvious wounds or injuries? What is the appearance of the child's skin (pale, cyanotic, and so on)?

Airway and Cervical Spine
Cervical spinal cord injury with paralysis or a head injury with loss of consciousness may prevent even the expert swimmer from staying above the water. Common causes of aquatic head and neck injuries include head-first dives into shallow water, surfing, water skiing accidents, and boating mishaps.

Always consider the potential for spinal cord injury. If there is a history of trauma, evidence of trauma (cuts or bruising on the head, face, or neck), or no history is available, assume there is a spine injury and take manual control of the cervical spine. You may start mouth-to-mask (with barrier device) ventilation on the apneic submersion victim while still in the water. Once the child is out of the water, begin aggressive resuscitation efforts. If the child is apneic or having inadequate respirations, open the airway using the modified jaw-thrust maneuver and attempt to ventilate with a bag-valve mask. If ventilation is difficult or impossible, suspect an airway obstruction.

Never perform a blind finger sweep on a child. Use the maneuvers suggested for the removal of a foreign body in an infant or child. Remove the object only if it is visualized, and ventilate the child between attempts at foreign body removal. Have suction ready, as these maneuvers may precipitate reflux of water from the lungs or stomach.

> **PEARLS**
>
> Consider that children with submersion injury may have cervical spine and head injuries.

Pediatric Submersion Injuries

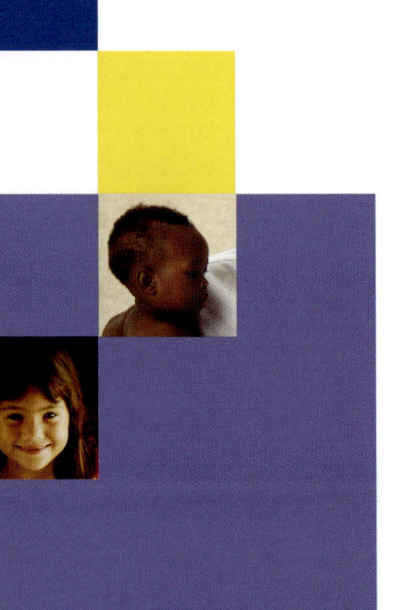

Breathing

If the child is being ventilated, always use 100 percent oxygen. Do not waste valuable time trying to "drain" water from the lungs by using various maneuvers that may cause aspiration. In freshwater submersion, most of the aspirated water will probably have been absorbed through the lungs into the circulation. In a saltwater submersion, there may be water in the lungs; however, time is better spent on airway management and ventilation than on trying to "drain" the lungs. The child who is awake and able to protect his own airway should be placed on 100 percent oxygen by nonrebreather mask. Carefully monitor these children for signs of respiratory distress and failure.

Circulation

If a pulse is not present, begin CPR immediately. Take the pulse for 1 full minute. Many cold-water submersion victims are extremely bradycardic. If a pulse is present, determine the rate and check for the capillary refill. Compressions may still be needed. The submersion injury's effects on the respiratory system may result in hypoxemia, which can increase the risk of arrhythmias, including ventricular tachycardia, ventricular fibrillation, and asystole. The presence of metabolic acidosis may further lower the threshold for developing arrhythmias. Stop all active sources of bleeding.

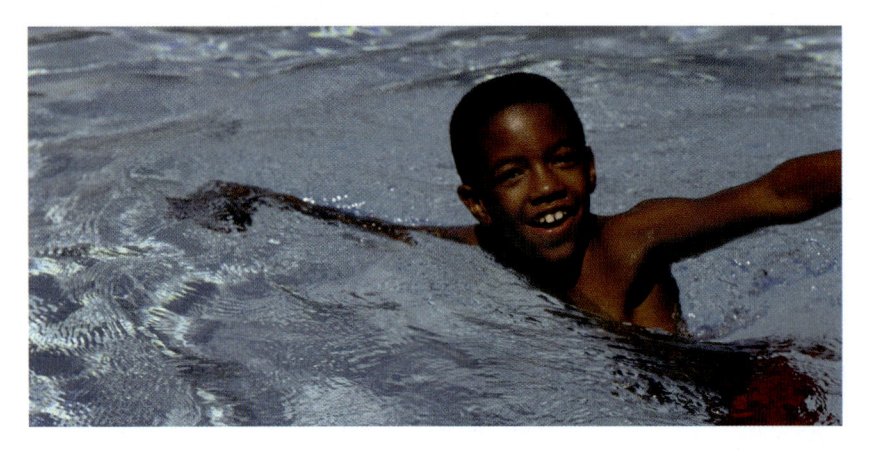

Rapid Trauma Survey

In addition to the rapid head-to-toe assessment, perform a brief neurologic assessment. Although the lungs are affected first, the brain is most susceptible to permanent damage from cerebral hypoxia. Direct all resuscitation efforts at getting oxygen to the brain. Beware of the fact that a head injury, alcohol or drugs, seizures, or hypoglycemia can result in an altered mental status and may complicate drowning.

Critical Interventions and Transport Decisions

Rapidly package and transport any child with an unstable airway, respiratory insufficiency, shock, or altered mental status. Attempt to resuscitate any child who has been submerged for 1 hour or less, particularly if the water is cold. Children who have fallen through ice may become hypothermic very quickly, and this hypothermia may offer some protection against anoxic brain injury. There are a number of case reports of children surviving cold-water drowning, even after prolonged submersion times. Children in cardiac arrest following cold-water submersion require transport to a hospital capable of instituting advanced rapid rewarming techniques, including cardiopulmonary bypass.

Pediatric Trauma Life Support

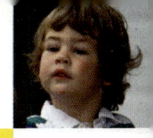

Airway

The most important actions in resuscitating critical submersion victims are managing the airway and ventilation with 100 percent oxygen. Perform endotracheal intubation on any child who is apneic, unconscious, with a GCS less than 8, or inadequately ventilating. The most experienced person present should perform such intubation while maintaining cervical spinal motion restriction. If you can effectively oxygenate and ventilate the child with a bag-valve mask and the transport time is short, you may delay intubation for the receiving facility. Carefully monitor the child for emesis and have suction readily available. If the child's airway is open, keep him on 100 percent oxygen during transport. If the child is intubated, rapidly confirm endotracheal tube placement with an $EtCO_2$ monitor or device.

Apply appropriate spinal motion restriction as soon as it is feasible. During the log roll of the child onto the backboard, assess the child's back, being careful to avoid moving the cervical spine.

Breathing

If the child is intubated, make sure the endotracheal tube is correctly positioned and there are equal bilateral breath sounds. Secondary confirmation of endotracheal tube placement, with an $Et\ CO_2$ device, is mandatory. If the child is not intubated, carefully monitor the respiratory status during transport. If the child is hypothermic, then you may use warmed and humidified oxygen. If a pulse oximeter is available, use it to maintain the oxygen saturation above 95 percent. The pulse oximeter may not provide an accurate reading in a child who is hypothermic and hypotensive. You may attempt various sites in order to improve the device's accuracy.

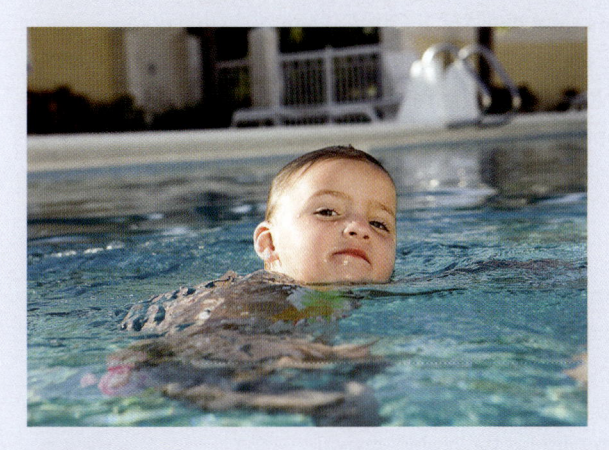

Circulation

Attach the cardiac monitor to the child. Cardiac arrhythmias are common in submersion victims because of the combination of hypoxia, acidosis, and hypothermia. Cardiac arrhythmias are treated according to the ACLS/PALS guidelines, with one important exception. If the child is severely hypothermic (less than 86° F [30° C]), the heart may not respond to cardiac medications. Therefore, in the presence of severe hypothermia, only give one round of ACLS/PALS drugs prior to the time the child is warmed to 92° F (33.9° C). Obtain IV access en route to the hospital (this may include an IO line). Run IV fluids at a keep-open rate unless the child shows signs of shock. Keep fluid boluses to 20 mL/kg to avoid aggravating head and pulmonary injuries from excessive fluids.

Pediatric Submersion Injuries

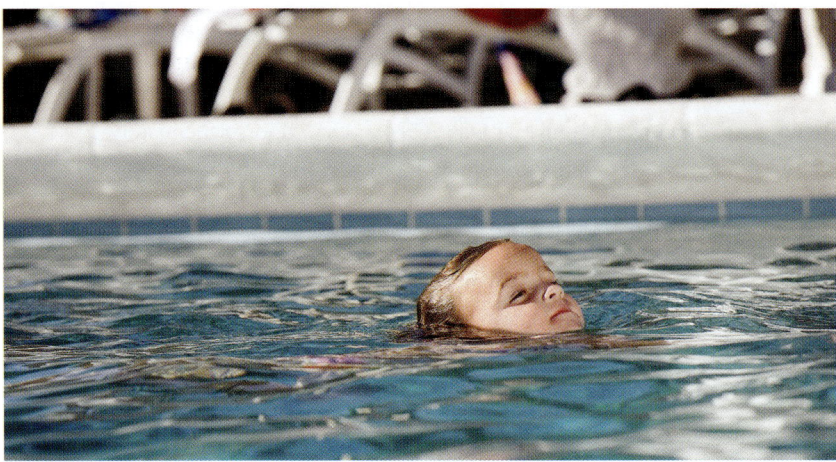

Thermoregulation

Hypothermia is a common finding in submersion victims, particularly children, whose body surface (heat exchange) area to body mass (heat generating) ratio is greater than that of adults. Because the body loses heat much faster when immersed in water than in air of comparable temperature, hypothermia develops quickly. Immersion hypothermia occurs in both summer and winter.

In general, do not treat hypothermia in the field. However, it is possible to prevent further heat loss and worsening hypothermia in a child by removing wet clothes, drying the child, and wrapping him in blankets.

If available, use warmed IV fluids; warmed, humidified oxygen; and portable gel warmers. Manage severe hypothermia (less than 86° F [30° C]) aggressively, as some children who have fallen through ice and who have been submerged for prolonged periods have survived neurologically intact. Rapidly package and transport these children to a hospital capable of providing cardiopulmonary bypass.

ITLS Secondary Survey

While en route to the hospital, perform the ITLS Secondary Survey, if time allows. Pay special attention to the neurologic examination. Note the level of consciousness, pupillary reaction, and motor and sensory response.

Transport the child quickly to the nearest appropriate facility, calling ahead to allow the emergency department time to prepare for the child's arrival.

SPECIAL CONSIDERATIONS

Certain events may initiate a submersion injury, such as cervical spine injury, head injury, use of alcohol or drugs, seizures, hypoglycemia, and child abuse. Seizures, even while the child is in shallow water, may result in aspiration and subsequent drowning. Children with a seizure disorder have a four-fold increase in drowning risk. Hypoglycemia with loss of consciousness while in the water may lead to a drowning event. Although diabetic children are usually carefully controlled, extra exercise or poor eating can lead to hypoglycemia. Suspect child abuse when submersion events occur under questionable circumstances, such as in bathtubs, buckets, or toilets.

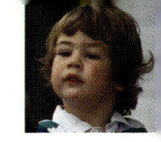

The prehospital provider is in a unique position to gather important historical information and observe the incident scene. Careful observation and documentation will provide important information to the emergency physician and appropriate authorities.

PROGNOSIS

In general, studies indicate that a majority of children who survive submersion incidents or children who need brief CPR will have a good outcome. The major determinant of a good outcome is the success of resuscitation at the site of submersion injuries. It has been shown that individuals who are conscious on arrival to the hospital after being successfully resuscitated have an excellent chance of surviving intact. Most studies support that the longer the duration of submersion, the poorer the outcome. Also, cold-water submersion is associated with better outcomes compared with warm-water submersion injuries.

Warm-Water Drowning

Victims with submersion times of less than 5 minutes who develop a return of spontaneous circulation within 10 minutes of ACLS/PALS resuscitation will likely have a good outcome. Factors thought to adversely affect outcome include prolonged submersion, delay in initiating CPR, severe acidosis, asystole on arrival at a medical facility, fixed and dilated pupils, and unresponsiveness (GCS less than 5).

Cold-Water Drowning

Falls through ice or submersion in water less than 40° F (4.4° C) offer the best chance for full neurologic recovery. Children are likely to be caught unaware and offer no struggle, and this may result in their brains being protected as their body temperature drops rapidly. Hypothermia may result from one of two situations. The first is a "true" cold-water drowning in which the child falls through ice. Because severe hypothermia greatly reduces cerebral oxygen requirements, the brain may be able to withstand anoxia for a longer period. These children have been reported to survive neurologically intact even after being under the water for an hour. Cold-water drowning requires aggressive resuscitation.

The second situation that may result in severe hypothermia is brain death. As the brain dies, the ability to control body temperature is lost and the patient becomes progressively cold. Never make this diagnosis in the field. Transport all such patients to an appropriate medial facility with rewarming capacity.

PREVENTION

Drowning outranks motor vehicle collisions and pedestrian trauma as the single leading cause of injury and death in children less than five years old. Recent legislation and public information campaigns targeted to the use of child seats and restraints are largely responsible for this disparity. Attention now needs to focus on preventing drowning because nearly all drowning deaths are preventable. The American Academy of

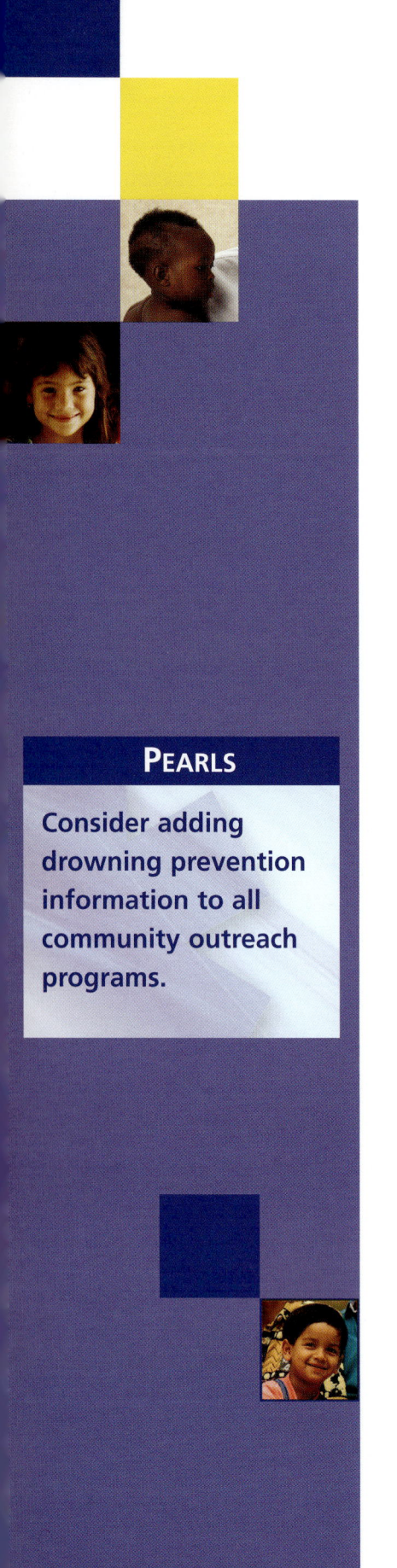

Pediatrics Committee on Injury and Poison Prevention has developed a list of 23 recommendations to decrease the incidence of submersion injuries. Toddlers may even drown in five-gallon buckets or toilets; prevention strategies that minimize a toddler's exposure to areas of standing water are critical. Most submersion injuries that result in death occur in private pools, either at the child's own home or at a neighbor's home. It has long been believed that parental supervision is the key to drowning prevention. Even so, as history has proven, it takes only a momentary lapse in supervision to result in catastrophe for a child. Other protective mechanisms must be present to "save" the child during lapses of parental supervision.

Pool Enclosures, Covers, and Alarms

Complete pool fencing has emerged as a promising prevention strategy. More stringent laws governing total pool enclosure are needed in most states. This means installing a fence no less than four feet high on all sides of a pool. A house cannot be considered the fourth side of the pool enclosure because children would then have direct access to the pool. The fence must also have a self-closing, self-latching gate. Pool covers are designed only to retain heat in pools and hot tubs and to keep debris out. Young children may climb onto the covers, slip beneath them, and drown. More rigid pool covers have been advocated, but because their application can be cumbersome, few are in use in the United States today.

The Consumer Product Safety Commission recently evaluated pool alarm systems. No satisfactory system exists, and further study is needed.

Public Information Campaigns

Because prompt resuscitation is vital to survival, pool owners should be mandated to learn CPR. All too often, bystanders pull children from the water and wait for emergency medical service personnel to arrive and initiate CPR. Prehospital and other health care providers can teach parents to empty their buckets after chores, to never allow children to bathe alone without adult supervision, and to enroll their children in swimming classes at an early age.

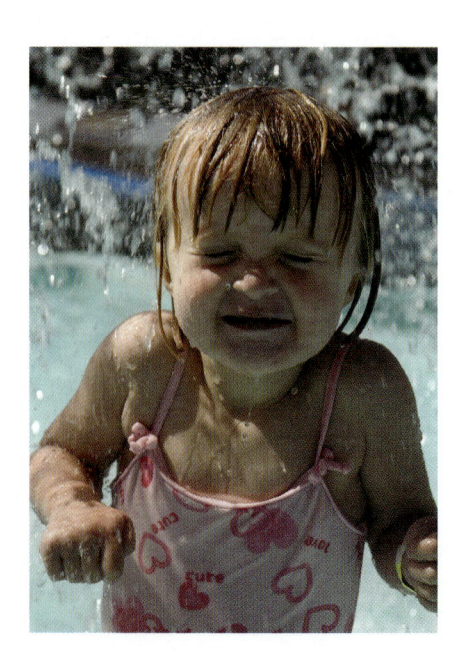

PEARLS

Consider adding drowning prevention information to all community outreach programs.

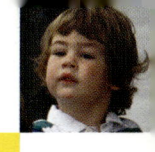

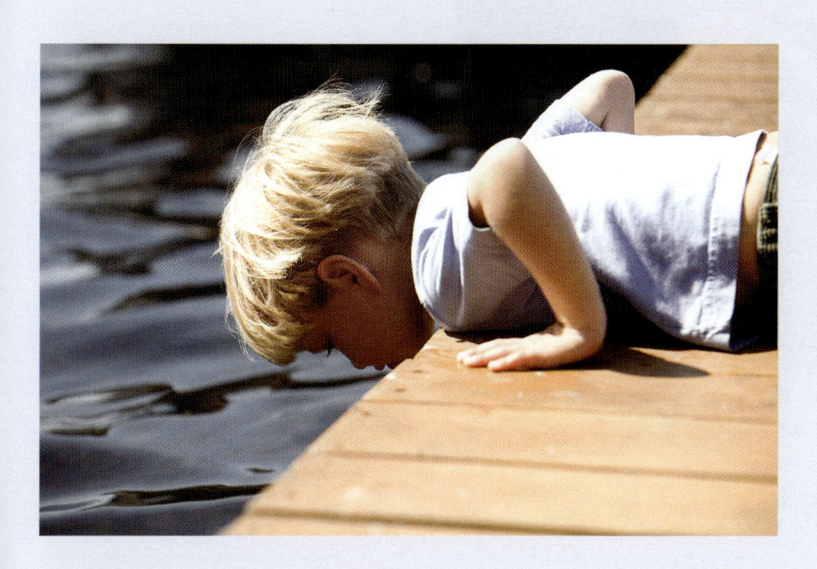

Case Study *continued*

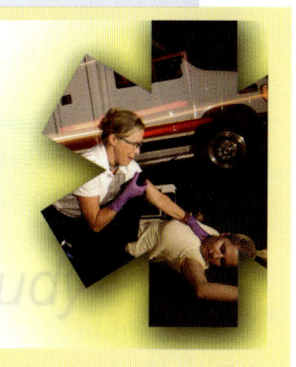

After a Scene Size-Up, John begins the ITLS Primary Survey and finds that the child has a manually opened airway but is apneic. Susan starts bag-valve-mask ventilations with 100 percent oxygen. The child does have a femoral pulse of 90 beats per minute. John then performs a Rapid Trauma Survey and finds no obvious injuries to the child. However, a brief neurological exam reveals that the child's pupils are 5 mm and nonreactive. The child's Glascow Coma Score (GCS) is 6 (E=1, V=1, M=4). With Bob's assistance, John applies a spinal motion restriction device to the child and rapidly transports the patient to a nearby pediatric emergency department. An IV line is placed during transport.

The trauma team is waiting on arrival. In view of the markedly decreased level of consciousness and the possible ventilatory support, the child was intubated and ventilated taking full spinal precautions. Subsequent imaging of the head and spine revealed the presence of cerebral edema and a stable cervical spine fracture.

The child was admitted to the pediatric intensive care unit and after a long hospital stay, discharged to an extended care facility for rehabilitation.

Pediatric Submersion Injuries

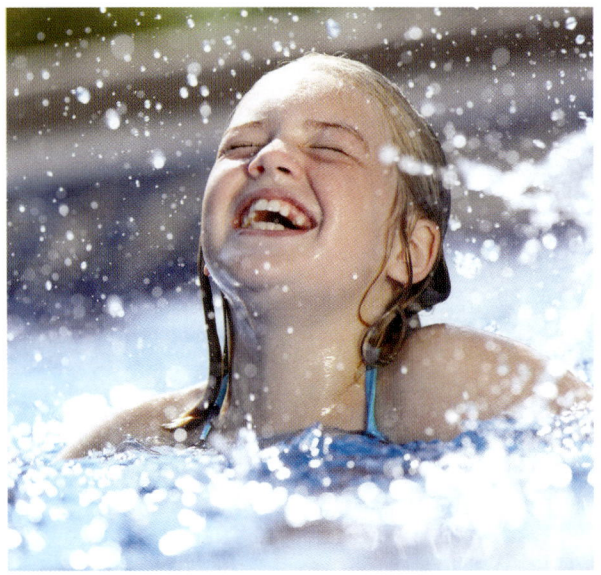

Case Study wrap-up

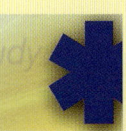

Drowning is the second leading cause of accidental deaths in children ages 14 and under. The case study illustrates the importance of preventative measures and the importance of anticipating additional injuries in addition to the effects of submersion itself. The team followed the ITLS patient assessment procedures and provided timely, optimal care for this child, which led to her survival.

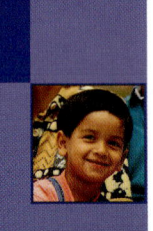

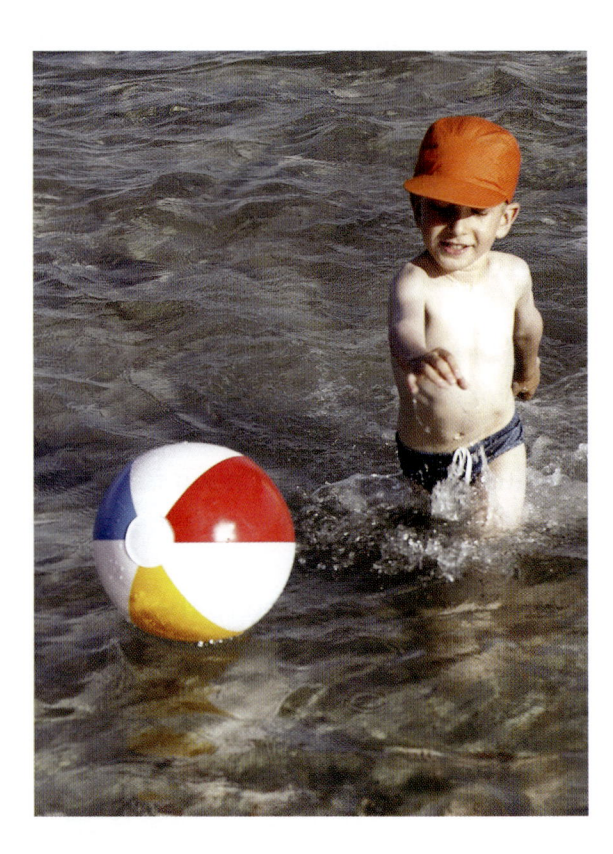

SUMMARY

1. Childhood drowning is largely preventable with common sense, education and barrier devices such as fencing around swimming pools.
2. Rapid completion of the ITLS Primary Survey along with early, aggressive CPR as needed, rapid airway management; and transport to a pediatric center offer the best hope for drowning survival.
3. While children submerged in cold water (< 40° F [4.4° C]) have a better chance for survival than those submerged in warm water, prevention remains the ultimate intervention.

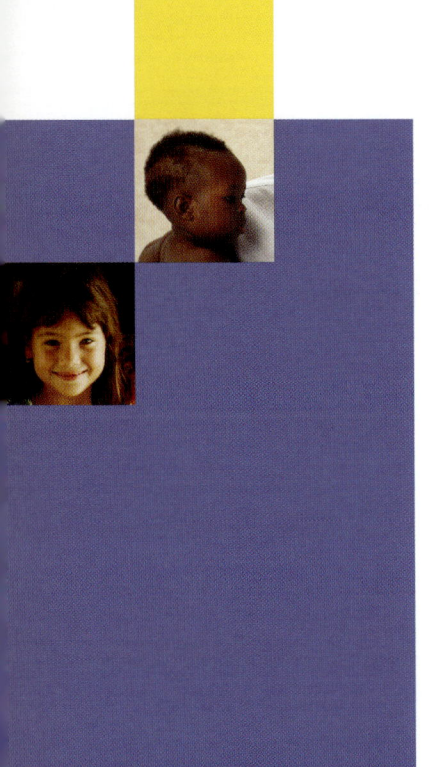

Recommended Reading

Campbell, John Emory, ed. "Drowning, Barotrauma, and Decompression Injury." In *International Trauma Life Support for Prehospital Care Providers*, 6th ed., 384–90. Upper Saddle River, N.J.: Pearson/Prentice Hall, 2008.

Causey, Alan L., John A. Tilelle, and Mark E. Swanson. "Predicting Discharge in Uncomplicated Near-drowning." *American Journal of Emergency Medicine* 18 (2000): 9–11.

Graf, William D., Peter Cummings, Linda Quan, et al. "Predicting Outcome in Pediatric Submersion Victims." *Annals of Emergency Medicine* 26 (1995): 312–19.

Huang, Vivian, Frances Shofe, Dennis R. Durbin, et al. "Prevalence of Traumatic Injuries in Drowning and Near Drowning in Children and Adolescents." *Archives of Pediatrics and Adolescent Medicine* 157 (2003): 50–3.

Quan, Linda and Peter Cummings. "Characteristics of Drowning by Different Age Groups." *Injury Prevention* 9 (2003): 163–68.

Salomez, Frederick and Jean-Louis Vincent. "Drowning: A Review of Epidemiology, Pathophysiology, Treatment and Prevention." *Resuscitation* 63 (2004): 261–68.

Van Beeck, Edward F., Christine M. Branche, David Szpilman, et al. "A New Definition of Drowning: Toward Documentation and Prevention of a Global Public Health Problem." *Bulletin of the World Health Organization* 83 (2005): 853–56.

16

CHAPTER 16
Pediatric Traumatic Cardiopulmonary Arrest

Patricia M. Hicks, MS, NREMT-P
Steven J. Shaner, EMT-P
George Waterman, MD

Objectives
Upon completion of this chapter, you should be able to:

1. Discuss the causes of traumatic cardiopulmonary arrest.
2. Compare outcomes from pediatric and adult traumatic cardiopulmonary arrests.
3. Discuss critical interventions in the management of the pediatric traumatic cardiopulmonary arrest.

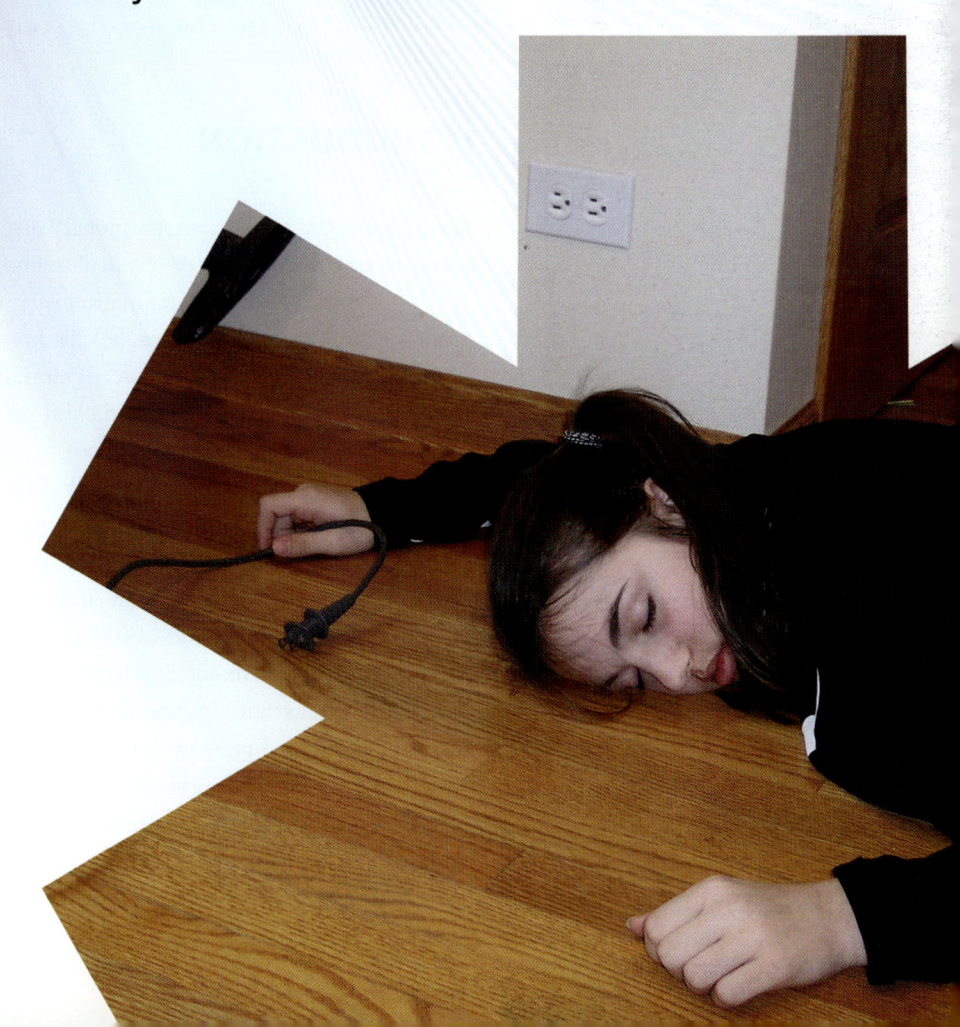

Case Study

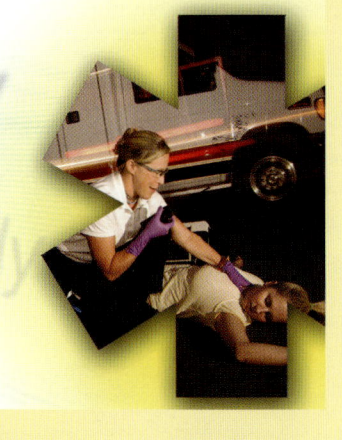

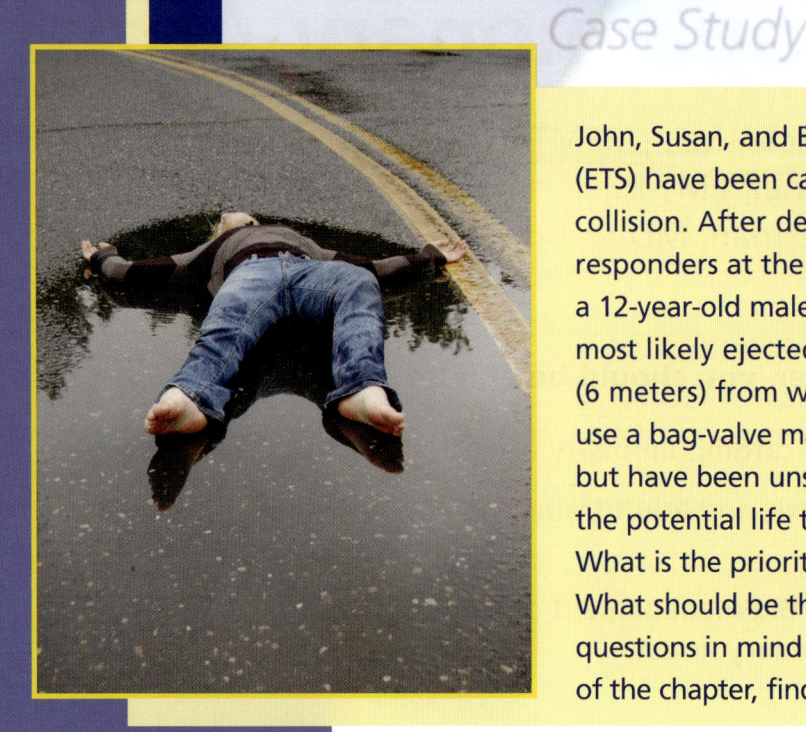

John, Susan, and Bob of the Emergency Transport System (ETS) have been called to the scene of a train vs. automobile collision. After determining the scene was safe, first responders at the scene tell the team that the patient, a 12-year-old male riding in the rear seat of the car, was most likely ejected and was found approximately 20 feet (6 meters) from where the car stopped. They have tried to use a bag-valve mask to ventilate the unresponsive child but have been unsuccessful due to facial trauma. What are the potential life threats that may present with this child? What is the priority of the prehospital team at this time? What should be their immediate actions? Keep these questions in mind as you read the chapter. Then, at the end of the chapter, find out how the rescuers completed this call.

INTRODUCTION

The pediatric traumatic cardiopulmonary arrest is defined as cardiorespiratory arrest occurring as a direct result of physical trauma to one or more body systems. According to the U.S. National Pediatric Trauma Registry, one-half to two-thirds of all pediatric trauma deaths occur before the child reaches the hospital. Traumatic cardiopulmonary arrest in the adult population has a near 99 percent mortality rate. While there is less information on traumatic cardiopulmonary arrest in children, pediatric traumatic cardiopulmonary arrest may have a lower mortality rate. A look at 584 traumatized children who received CPR in the prehospital setting showed that 450 of the patients died; however, 134 survived to discharge from the hospital. While morbidity data was not available, these figures may suggest that, with proper intervention, pediatric traumatic cardiopulmonary arrest patients have a slightly better outcome than adult traumatic cardiopulmonary arrest patients.

In another study, a cohort of 957 pediatric trauma patients who received CPR in the prehospital setting were noted to have an overall survival rate of 23.5 percent. This study also examined mortality in subgroups. The study showed that, once the child arrived at the hospital, if the blood pressure was still less than 60 mmHg systolic or if the child was comatose, the chance of survival was dismal.

As in medical arrests, the primary cause of traumatic cardiopulmonary arrest is usually due to airway or respiratory compromise. If hypoxia is ignored or not treated immediately and effectively in the pediatric trauma patient, it will lead to respiratory arrest and, ultimately, cardiopulmonary arrest. You must therefore maintain the airway and deliver oxygen promptly to prevent hypoxemia.

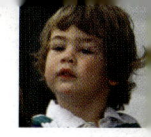

Circulatory compromise may also lead to arrest. A prolonged insult to the vascular system may cause the vital organs to die as a result of impaired perfusion and oxygenation. Early recognition and prompt intervention may control the body's response to shock and prohibit needless morbidity or mortality.

PATIENT ASSESSMENT

Assessing the child in traumatic cardiopulmonary arrest is the same as in any other situation and should be performed in the following order:

1. ITLS Primary Survey
    A. Scene Size-Up
    B. Initial Assessment
    C. Rapid Trauma Survey or Focused Exam
    D. Critical Interventions and Transport Decisions
    E. Contact medical direction as needed.
2. ITLS Secondary Survey and/or Ongoing Exam

Table 16.1: Causes of Traumatic Cardiopulmonary Arrest

1. **Airway Problems**
    a. Foreign body
    b. Tongue prolapse
    c. Swelling

2. **Breathing Problems**
    a. Pulmonary contusion
    b. Sucking chest wound
    c. Flail chest
    d. High spinal-cord injury
    e. Carbon monoxide inhalation
    f. Smoke inhalation
    g. Aspiration
    h. Near-drowning
    i. Central nervous system depression from drugs/alcohol
    j. Apnea secondary to electric shock or lightning strike

3. **Circulatory Problems**
    a. Hemorrhagic shock (empty heart syndrome)
    b. Tension pneumothorax
    c. Pericardial tamponade
    d. Myocardial contusion
    e. Acute myocardial infarction
    f. Cardiac arrest secondary to electric shock

Pediatric Traumatic Cardiopulmonary Arrest

ITLS Primary Survey

Scene Size-Up
The mechanism of injury may provide valuable information regarding the cause of the arrest. Rapidly investigate the scene for clues that may suggest how the actual injury occurred. Knowing the cause of the arrest will help determine the appropriate intervention for managing the arrest. Table 16.1 shows the causes of traumatic cardiopulmonary arrest.

Initial Assessment
General Impression
Identifying traumatic cardiopulmonary arrest usually occurs rapidly. The mechanism of injury and position of the patient may provide clues to the cause for arrest.

Airway and Cervical Spine
An uncorrected airway obstruction may lead to a respiratory arrest followed by a cardiorespiratory arrest. In a child already in arrest, open the obstructed airway to provide any opportunity for resuscitation. You can usually relieve an obstruction by the tongue or a foreign body with basic airway maneuvers. You may also need to suction blood and mucus from the oropharynx to maintain a patent airway. Immediately initiate bag-valve-mask ventilation. Intubation is necessary for patients who cannot be successfully ventilated with a bag-valve mask. Maintain manual spinal motion restriction during all assessments and interventions to prevent further injury. Correct airway compromise before continuing the assessment.

> **PEARLS**
>
> Always consider hypoxia, regardless of the cause, when dealing with the traumatic cardiopulmonary arrest.

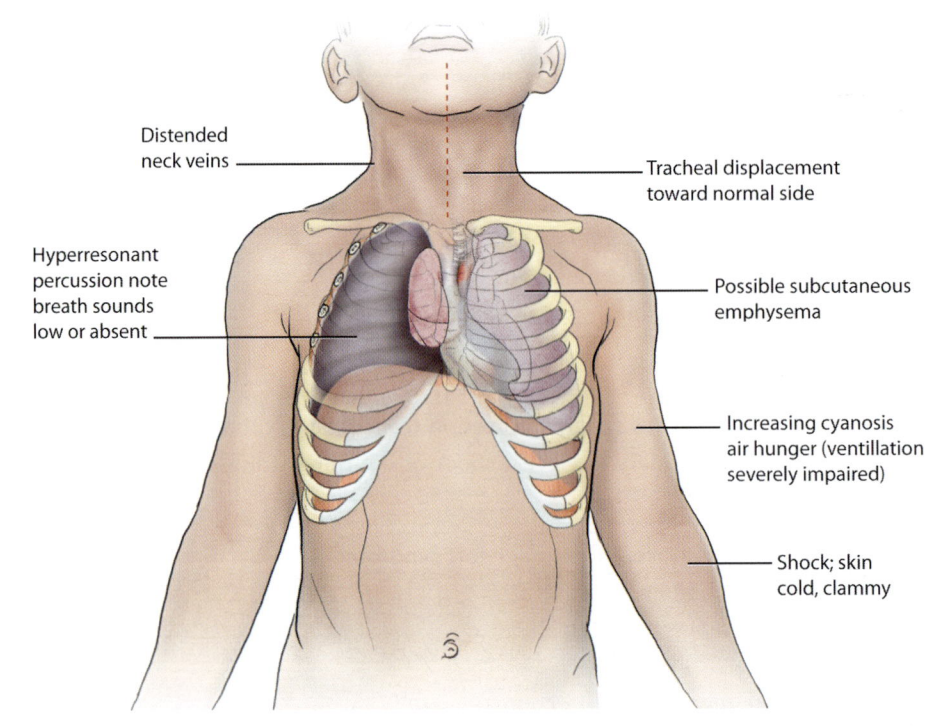

Figure 16.1 *Tension pneumothorax is one cause of traumatic cardiopulmonary arrest that can be corrected in the prehospital setting.*

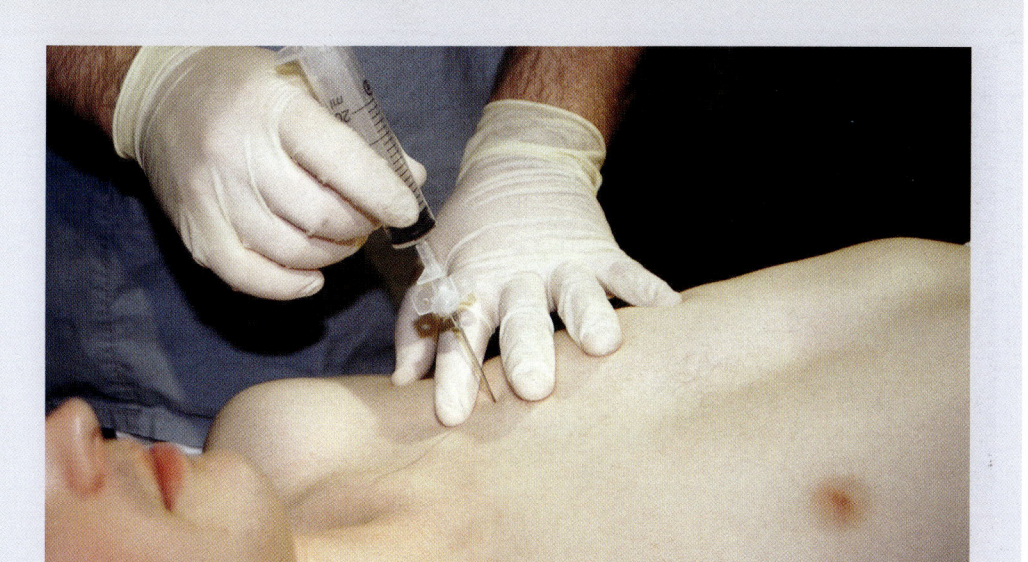

Figure 16.2 *Needle decompression to correct a tension pneumothorax is usually life-saving if performed before the patient goes into cardiopulmonary arrest.*

Breathing

Always consider hypoxia, regardless of the cause, when dealing with the traumatic cardiopulmonary arrest. One cause of arrest, while not common, is tension pneumothorax, a life-threatening situation that can be corrected in the prehospital setting (Fig. 16.1). Rapid needle decompression will usually be life-saving if performed before the patient has deteriorated to the point of cardiac arrest (Fig. 16.2). Administration of 100 percent oxygen and airway management is also essential. Upper cervical cord injuries may also result in respiratory paralysis and even arrest; therefore, you must maintain spinal motion restriction.

Circulation

Hemorrhagic shock may also cause arrest (empty heart syndrome). Initiate CPR if the pulse rate or blood flow is not adequate to perfuse the brain. Control all acute external hemorrhage. If you cannot control bleeding by pressure, tourniquet, or hemostatic agents, immediately transport the pediatric patient to the closest hospital with a staffed emergency department. Consider massive intra-abdominal bleeding or pericardial tamponade as potential etiologies of shock, and aggressively identify and manage them. Cardiac arrest from an electrical shock produces ventricular fibrillation or secondary hypoxic arrest from respiratory paralysis; you may successfully reverse this type of cardiopulmonary arrest with pediatric ACLS/PALS protocols.

Rapid Trauma Survey

The Rapid Trauma Survey should include brief exam of the head, neck, abdomen, pelvis, and extremities. In this case, the sole purpose of the Rapid Trauma Survey is to look for immediate life threats. After initiating CPR, you can complete the Rapid Trauma Survey. Control all active bleeding. Auscultate the lungs to rule out the possibility of tension pneumothorax as a cause of arrest.

> **PEARLS**
>
> **A structured, consistent approach is important and may alleviate the stress experienced by responders, particularly in traumas involving pediatric patients.**

Pediatric Traumatic Cardiopulmonary Arrest

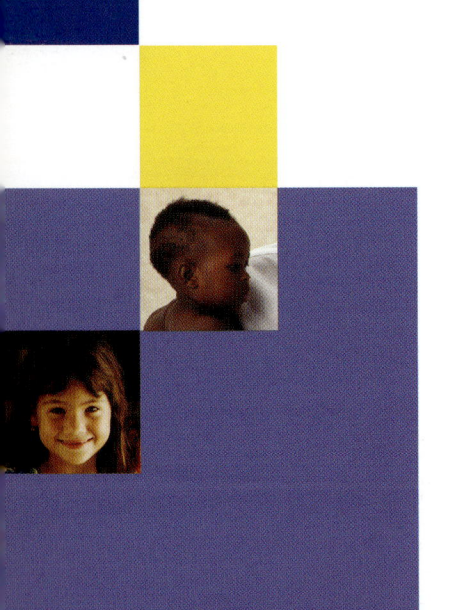

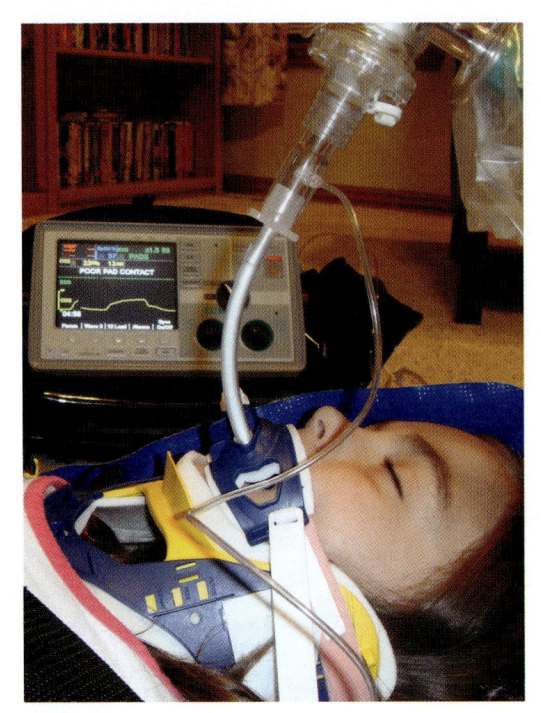

Figure 16.3 *Capnography should be used to confirm the placement of the endotracheal tube if it is available.*

Critical Interventions and Transport Decisions

The traumatic cardiopulmonary arrest is always a situation in which you must make a time-versus-benefit decision. The decision to transport to the closest appropriate facility by ground or by air may be a difficult one. Your medical direction physician can help you make this decision. Traumatic cardiopulmonary arrest is always a load-and-go situation.

Aim your approach to managing the traumatic cardiopulmonary arrest at treating the cause of arrest. Establish complete spinal motion restriction interventions before transport.

Airway and Breathing

Initially, treat airway compromise and hypoxemia. Initiate basic airway management, suctioning, and bag-valve-mask ventilation. If basic airway management is not effective and the patient needs more definitive airway management, perform endotracheal intubation. If basic airway maintenance is effective, intubation may be accomplished after arrival at the hospital. Confirm the position of the endotracheal tube by auscultation and at least two other methods, such as end-tidal CO_2 monitoring and pulse oximetry (Fig. 16.3). If tension pneumothorax is suspected, perform chest decompression as discussed in Chapter 6.

Circulation

Initiate temporizing therapy such as intravenous or intraosseous fluid resuscitation and give as boluses of 20 mL/kg en route to the hospital. Refer to Chapters 7 and 8.

Follow pediatric ACLS/PALS protocols in cases of cardiopulmonary arrest that do not respond to aggressive airway management and fluid resuscitation. Current American Heart Association (AHA) guidelines call for a compression-to-ventilation ratio of 30:2 (single rescuer) for all ages. However, if an advanced airway is in place, coordination of compressions and ventilations is not necessary. The use of cardiac medications such as epinephrine and defibrillation for ventricular fibrillation may be appropriate if airway management and fluid resuscitation have been unsuccessful.

Pediatric Trauma Life Support

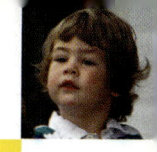

ITLS Secondary Survey and Ongoing Exam

In a traumatic cardiopulmonary arrest situation, there may not be sufficient time to perform an ITLS Secondary Survey. If you cannot determine the cause of the arrest, the ITLS Secondary Survey may reveal subtle clues as to the etiology of the arrest. In these pediatric patients, perform the ITLS Ongoing Exam every 5 minutes. This will enable you to identify changes in the child's condition and help you determine further interventions.

Case Study continued

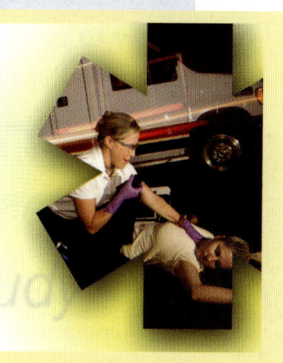

The prehospital team begins the assessment by ensuring the scene is safe. Bob, acting as the Team Leader, maintains the cervical spine manually and opens the airway via modified jaw thrust. The child has an obvious facial injury and is difficult to ventilate by bag-valve mask due to poor face seal. The child has no respiratory effort at this time. The apical heart rate is now < 40 beats per minute (bpm). Bob initiates CPR and intubates the child. Susan helps to control bleeding, and the child is placed in a pediatric spinal motion restriction device and transported by helicopter to a pediatric tertiary care center. Since IV access was not obtained in two attempts or within 30 seconds, Bob establishes an intraosseous line and administers a fluid bolus en route. Upon arrival at the emergency department, the child is reassessed and found to have an airway in place, being ventilated at 30 liters per minute. The radial pulse is now 120 bpm. The child is admitted to the ICU and dies two days later. The family donates the child's viable organs. An organ procurement team is able to use the heart, liver, and pancreas and other organs that eventually saved or improved the lives of four other children.

Case Study wrap-up

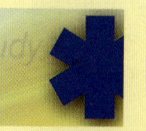

The child who is in traumatic cardiopulmonary arrest may present as one of the most challenging and stressful situations a prehospital provider encounters. This case study illustrates how the ITLS patient assessment procedure can be applied to a traumatic cardiopulmonary arrest situation.

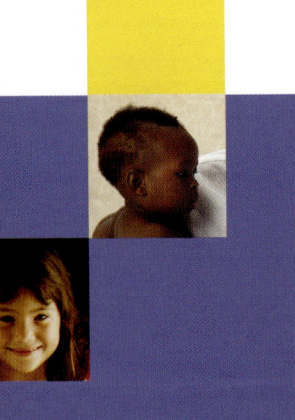

A rapid, well-organized assessment is key to recognizing possible causes of traumatic cardiopulmonary arrest. A structured, consistent approach will also help to alleviate the natural stress experienced by responders, particularly in traumas involving pediatric patients. Interventions can then be used to stop or reverse a potentially fatal situation. Bob and the team provided optimum care for the boy, avoiding a prehospital death. The survival for two days in hospital provided the opportunity for the parents and family to consider and agree to organ donation which saved or improved the lives of other four children.

SUMMARY

1. The early recognition and management of hypoxia, respiratory failure, and circulatory compromise is key to preventing or reversing traumatic cardiopulmonary arrest.
2. The best treatment for traumatic cardiopulmonary arrest is to respond to potential causes before the arrest occurs.
3. Providers who implement the ITLS Primary Assessment and repeat the ITLS Ongoing Exam in an efficient and rapid manner increase the chances for survival of pediatric patients who would otherwise die from their injuries.

Recommended Reading

American Heart Association. "2005 American Heart Association Guidelines for Cardiopulmonary Resuscitation and Emergency Cardiovascular Care: Pediatric Advanced Life Support." *Circulation* 112 (2005): IV167–87.

American Heart Association. "2005 American Heart Association Guidelines for Cardiopulmonary Resuscitation and Emergency Cardiovascular Care: Pediatric Basic Life Support." *Circulation* 112 (2005): IV156–66.

Campbell, John Emory, ed. "The Trauma Cardiopulmonary Arrest." In *International Trauma Life Support for Prehospital Providers*, 6th ed., 306–14. Upper Saddle River, N.J.: Pearson/Prentice Hall, 2008.

American Heart Association. *Advanced Cardiovascular Life Support Provider Manual*. Dallas: Author, 2007.

Ralston, Mark, Mary Fran Hazinski, Arno L. Zaritsky, Stephen M. Schexnayder, and Monica E. Kleinman, eds. Pediatric *Advanced Life Support Provider Manual*. Dallas: American Heart Association, 2007.

Li, Guohua, Nelson Tang, Carla DiScala, Zachary Meisel, Nadine Levick, and Gabor Kelen. "Cardiopulmonary Resuscitation in Pediatric Trauma Patients: Survival and Functional Outcome." *Journal of Trauma* 47 (1999): 1-7.

Perron, Andrew D., Ronald Sing, et al. Research Forum Abstracts. "Predicting Survival in Pediatric Trauma Patients Receiving CPR in the Prehospital Setting." *Annals of Emergency Medicine* 30 (1997): 381.

17

CHAPTER 17
Child Abuse

Jeanette Foster, MSW, LISW-S

Objectives
Upon completion of this chapter, you should be able to:

1. Discuss the role and responsibility of prehospital providers who encounter potential child abuse.

2. Describe the "red flags" that may suggest non-accidental injury.

3. Describe characteristic marks that may indicate physical abuse.

4. Discuss strategies for dealing with family members.

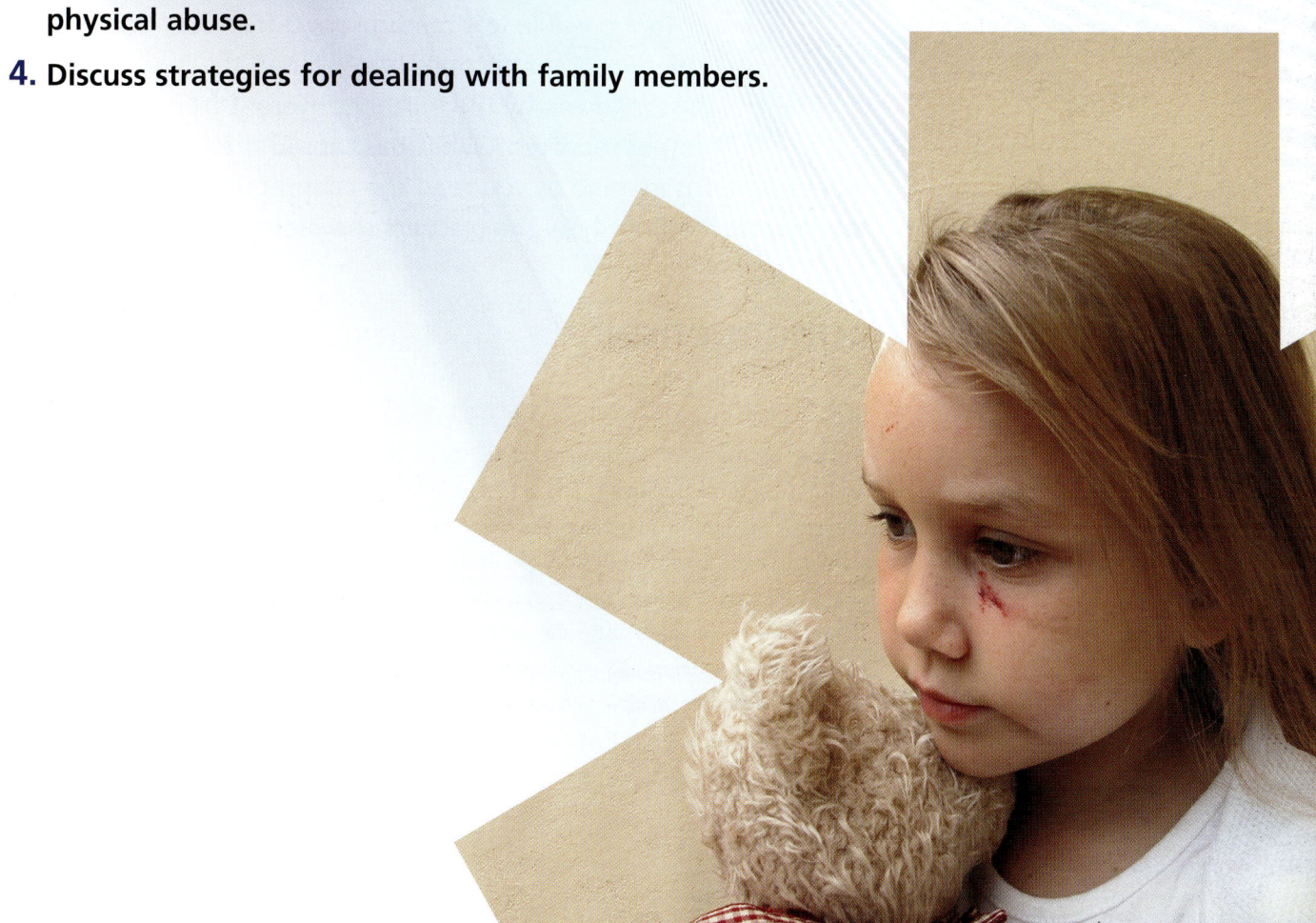

Case Study

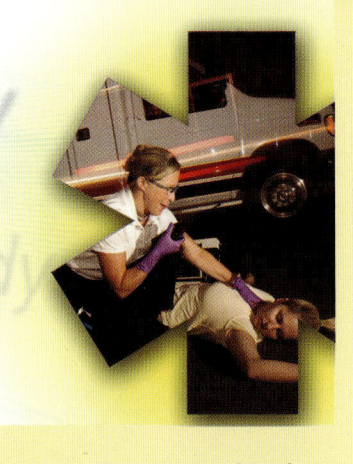

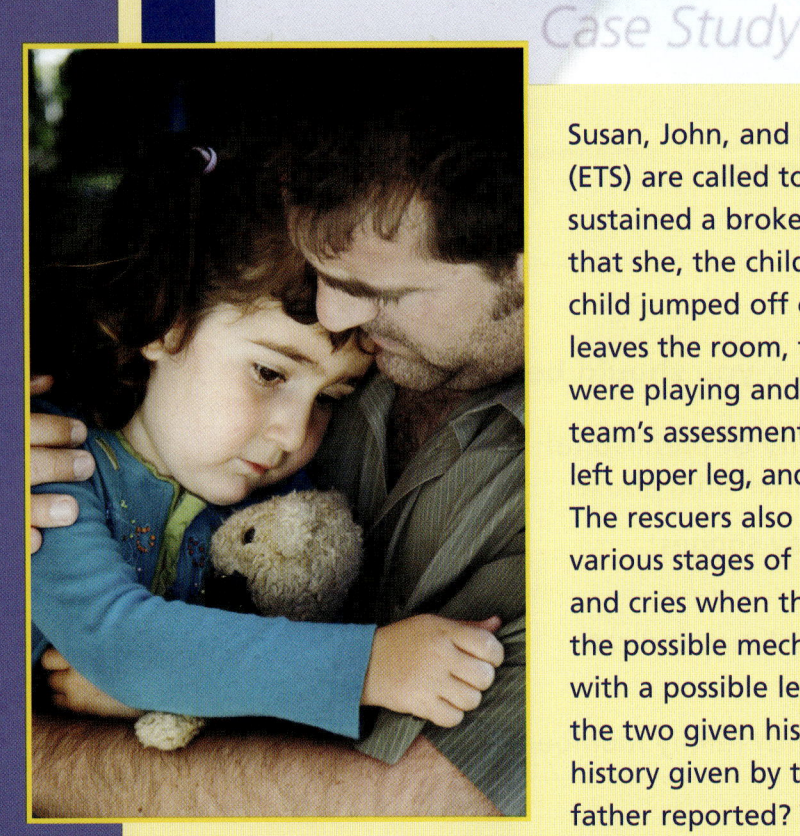

Susan, John, and Bob of the Emergency Transport Service (ETS) are called to a home where a 2-year-old child has sustained a broken leg. As they arrive, the mother says that she, the child, and the father were playing and the child jumped off of the couch, injuring her leg. As she leaves the room, the father says only he and the child were playing and that the child fell down the steps. The team's assessment of the child reveals a deformity of the left upper leg, and a mid-shaft femur fracture is suspected. The rescuers also notice several bruises over the body in various stages of healing. The child clings to the father and cries when the mother reenters the room. What are the possible mechanisms of injury in this 2-year-old child with a possible left femoral shaft fracture? Can either of the two given histories have caused the injury? Why is the history given by the mother different from what the father reported? What has caused the bruises? Keep these questions in mind as you read the chapter. Then, at the end of the chapter, find out how the rescuers completed this call.

PEARLS

It is vital for prehospital providers to be aware of indicators of abuse, recognize high-risk situations, obtain pertinent information, and convey this critical information to the appropriate authorities.

INTRODUCTION

In the United States, child abuse (the non-accidental injury of a child) is no longer just a problem occasionally encountered in the field. Nearly 1,500 children died in 2004 as a result of child maltreatment. The actual number of child deaths as a result of abuse and neglect is thought to be greater. There are three million reports of suspected child abuse and neglect made to Child Protective Services each year.

As these encounters have increased in frequency, perpetrators have become more sophisticated in manipulating abuse injuries and histories to avoid detection. It is vital for prehospital providers to be aware of indicators of abuse, recognize high-risk situations, obtain pertinent information, and convey this critical information to the appropriate authorities.

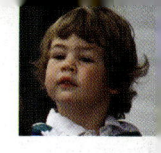

At the scene, you, the prehospital provider, have advantages in your role as gatherer of information. You are given initial explanations of an injury, often before a consensus has been reached. You are able to observe the environment in which the alleged accident occurred. You may be able to identify and describe the mechanism of injury. You are also in the company of family, friends, and others who may or may not come to the emergency department; all of these people may express their perspective on the event and individuals involved. These advantages place you in a unique position to detect or suspect non-accidental injury to a child.

Initially, it is important to listen to all histories. Do not assume that the family was "so upset they couldn't think straight." Although that may be true to some extent, you must document different explanations for an injury. The greater the discrepancy between the stories, the more concerned you should be. Histories that seem rehearsed, similarly worded, and without detail may also be cause for concern.

It is prudent to recognize the discrepancies between two stories as a potential problem. It is not uncommon for family members to try to protect each other, even when only one is guilty of abuse. In addition to noting the discrepancies between stories and documenting them, you should assess the likelihood of the explanations. Fractured femurs from falls are uncommon in two-year-old children. Note the location of the steps and whether they are carpeted or not. If the parent describes a scalding tub burn, notice the tub, its height, the height of the faucets, the type and location of faucets, and so on. Is the child's developmental ability consistent with the story? A nine-month-old child is not generally considered able to turn on a faucet; close the drain, allowing water to pool; and climb into a tub. Take advantage of your ability to assess the area of the alleged accident, and take notes.

SUSPECTING CHILD ABUSE

Remember that child abuse can happen in any family. Some families may have more chronic patterns of abuse; some may generally function well but under acute stress experience a breakdown in normal coping abilities and abuse the child. Remember to pay attention in homes that seem "safe" or "nice," because on those occasions you may make errors by attributing inconsistencies to stress or by believing "far out" stories. Children are hurt and killed in all kinds of homes. However, there are some indicators associated with high-risk households, including neglect (lack of heat, food, clothes, supervision, cleanliness, or delay in seeking care) and the presence of drugs, alcohol, or unsecured weapons. Document your observations of these conditions with facts. The presence of large groups of observers at a scene also increases the likelihood that you will be told something that a well-meaning family member may not communicate to the hospital. Pay attention to these histories, get names when you can, and document them.

Ideally, you should obtain private and individual histories, but sometimes you do not have this luxury because of the critical medical needs of the child or the environment. In general, you should obtain histories from those present while the child is being treated. The ride to the emergency department may be a good time to ask a parent or the child (if the child seems willing to talk) about the history of the injury.

PEARLS

The prehospital provider has advantages as a gatherer of information. Consider "SPICER":

Suspect: consider abuse.

Protect the child and your team.

Inspect the child for injury.

Collect evidence, especially information.

Expect the unexpected — believe the child who discloses.

Respect the child and family with non-judgmental care.

PEARLS

Child abuse can happen in *any* family and in *any* setting.

Child Abuse

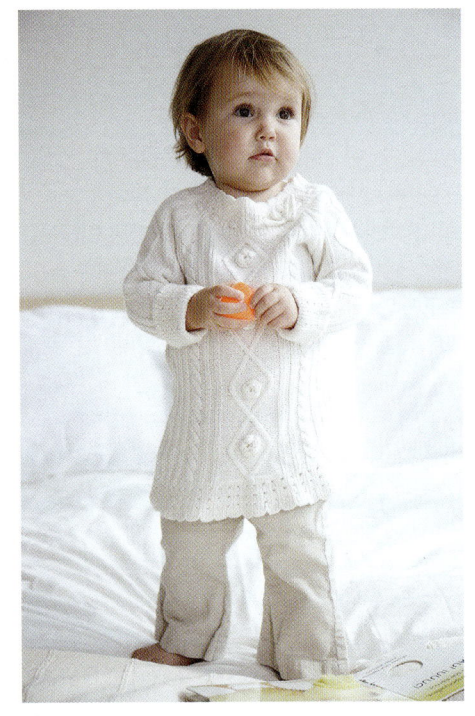

Figure 17.1 *A child who demonstrates fear of a particular person is a red flag for potential child abuse.*

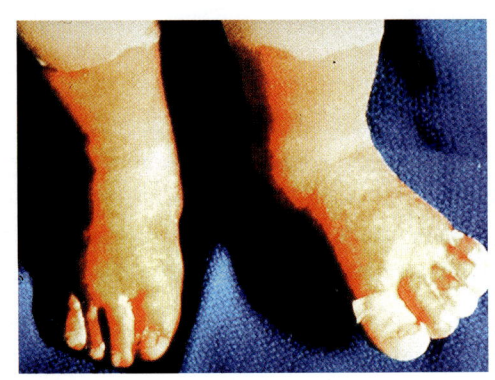

Figure 17.2 *The burn pattern as shown is common in child abuse cases, resulting from submerging the feet in boiling water.*

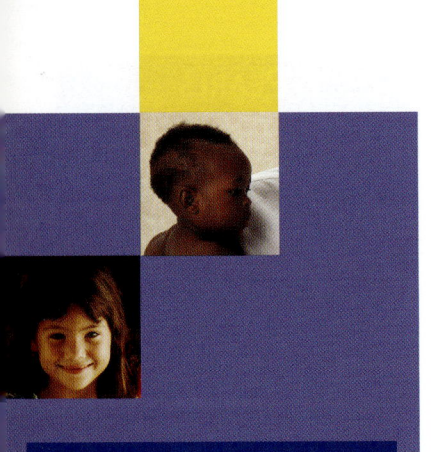

Pearls

"Red flags" that may suggest intentional injury include: injuries with inconsistent histories; changing histories; witnesses who report abuse or suspicion of domestic violence; inappropriate affect of historians; or a child who demonstrates excessive fear or withdrawal from a particular person(s) or who discloses abuse.

Red flags that may suggest non-accidental injury include: injuries with inconsistent histories; changing histories to find the "right" explanation; witnesses who report abuse or suspicion of domestic violence; inappropriate affect of historians; and a child who demonstrates excessive fear or withdrawal from a particular person(s) (Fig. 17.1). Other indicators of acute stress include wreckage (after a domestic violence episode); financial problems expressed by the family; marital problems expressed by the family; family members with chronic medical problems, drug/alcohol abuse, or isolation; and a child who reports being abused.

Physical findings that may indicate possible physical abuse include:

1. Unexplained injuries
2. Marks with the appearance of such man-made objects as belts, belt buckles, cords, and spatulas
3. Cigarette burns
4. Pinch marks
5. Adult-sized bite marks
6. Immersion burns, particularly "glove" or "sock" patterns (Fig. 17.2)
7. Rope burns
8. Burns in the shape of heated forks, spoons, irons, and so on, on unlikely body surfaces (back of the hand, back, leg, or face)
9. Unexplained mouth or dental injuries, fractures (especially in infants)
10. Bulging fontanel in infants
11. Unexplained abdominal or head trauma

Head injuries and abdominal injuries as the result of abuse are the first and second most common causes of death, respectively, in infants and toddlers.

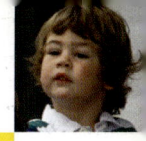

CARE AND SAFETY ISSUES

In situations where abuse is suspected, the family members present will likely show some signs of anxiety as they attempt to avoid detection. There is tremendous family pressure not to disclose information and to minimize the damage done.

The decision to transport the child can be difficult. While some children will automatically be taken to the emergency department for assessment and treatment of their injuries, others may not require further medical evaluation. When abuse is suspected, consider transporting the patient. The trip to the emergency department may be a better means of assessing the history, injury, and family reaction. The child's safety is of paramount importance!

If parents resist having the child taken to the hospital, stress the need for emergency department assessment. In situations of suspected abuse, some families may refuse treatment or transportation. Immediately follow local procedures in such instances. This may include contacting the EMS supervisor in addition to reports to Child Protective Services and law enforcement. Should law enforcement personnel agree with the assessment of emergency medical personnel, they can make the child be transported to the emergency department for evaluation.

Again, it is imperative in suspected abuse cases to minimize additional trauma to the child. One of the easiest ways to manage this is to calmly assess the situation and transport the child whenever possible to the emergency department for assessment and case management. Do not confront family members with discrepancies at the scene; just listen, remember, and document (Fig. 17.3). If the child is in a dangerous situation and parents are demanding that you leave, leave and *immediately* contact law enforcement for assistance. When responding to a situation with serious injury or death of a child, it is important to be sensitive to legitimate emotional needs of the family while preserving the scene for investigators. Immediately contact appropriate backup and follow local protocols.

> **PEARLS**
>
> **Do not confront family members with discrepancies; listen and document. If the child is in a dangerous situation and parents or caregivers are demanding that you leave, leave and *immediately* contact law enforcement for assistance.**

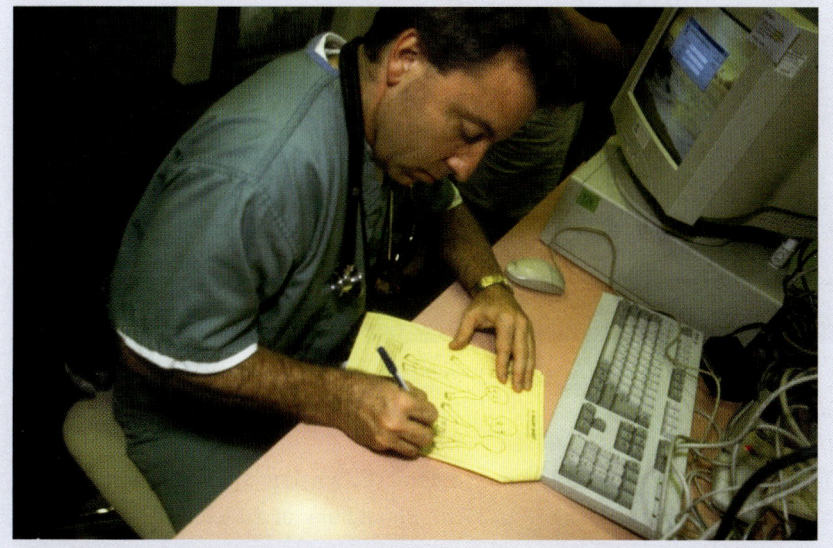

Figure 17.3 *Prehospital providers should always document their findings and suspicions of abuse.*

Child Abuse

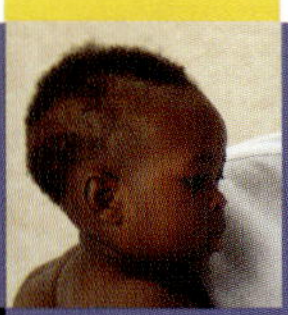

PREHOSPITAL PROVIDER CONSIDERATIONS

Families may be anxious, afraid, remorseful, and defensive following the non-accidental injury of a child. It is perfectly normal for the prehospital provider to feel a wide range of emotions, including anger toward the family. Allow yourself to have opinions and feelings, but remain objective in your tasks of information gathering, assessment, and treatment. Not only will your calmness prevent further emotional escalation in the family and further trauma to the child, but family members may actually tell you something. A person feeling guilty may share some of the guilt with a non-threatening prehospital care provider. Gather information calmly and relay it to the emergency department. In the United States, as a Mandated Reporter, you are responsible to directly report your suspicions to Child Protective Services or law enforcement even if you give information to another medical provider such as a hospital. Know your local laws concerning your responsibility for reporting suspected child abuse.

FAMILY MEMBERS' EMOTIONS

Although there are a number of different presenting characteristics for family members of an abused child, the primary emotion is generally fear (Fig. 17.4). The consequences of being discovered may include jail, disruption of family, income loss, jeopardized marriages, further domestic violence, and rejection by family and friends. For many, there is also the fear of not being discovered and knowing the abuse will continue and worsen. When people are afraid, their normal coping patterns do not work as well. They are more apt to become violent, fight, flee, or lose control. Your primary task is to remain calm and in control. The quickest way to diffuse an individual who is on the verge of losing control is to be calm and stable.

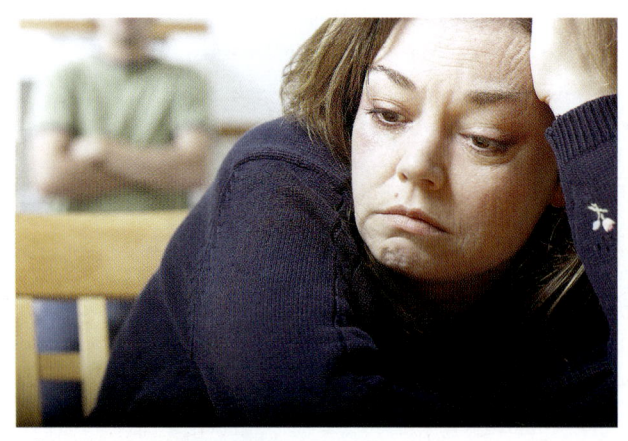

Figure 17.4 *The primary emotion that family members of abused children feel is fear.*

Other family reactions may include increased domestic tension, arguing, pacing, drinking alcohol, using drugs, or fleeing (Fig. 17.5). Should any of these or other reactions interfere with the treatment of the child or become a personal threat, contact supervisors and/or law enforcement agencies as well as your medical director. A way to diffuse family members' reactions is to assure them of your concern for the family. You might say, "I am concerned about all of you, but I need to focus on the child right now." This will place the

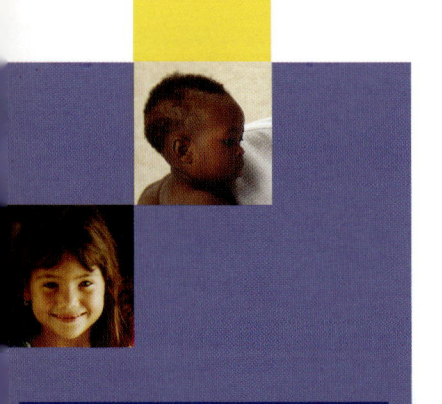

PEARLS

Know your local laws concerning your responsibility for reporting suspected child abuse. In addition to reporting to the emergency department staff, direct reporting to Child Protective Services ensures follow-up with the family and enhances the child's protection.

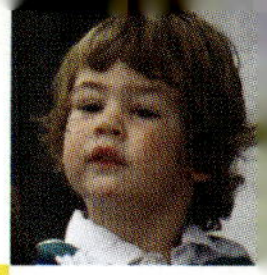

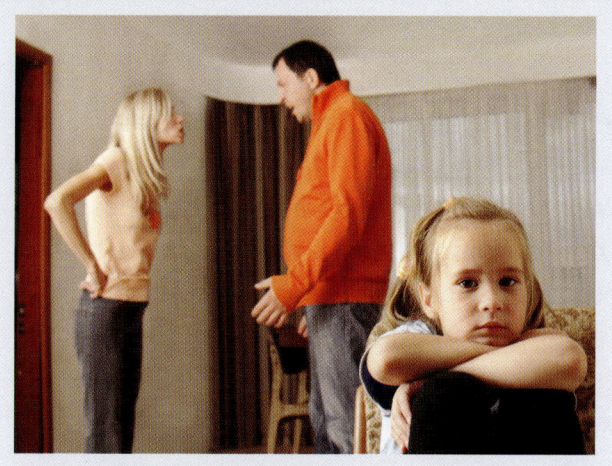

Figure 17.5 *Increased tension and arguing are other common reactions to child abuse within a family.*

family in a position of being supportive of you. Allow families to ask questions, and give them concrete answers. People under stress hear and remember less than ten percent of what they are told; with that in mind, keep it simple. Your volume, tone, and rate of speech convey a greater message than your words. Continually reassure family members you are caring for their child and that the child will be transported to the emergency department for a comprehensive evaluation.

ARRIVAL TO THE EMERGENCY DEPARTMENT

On arrival to the emergency department, it is essential to share all the gathered information with the appropriate individuals. If the child is transported to an emergency department, convey the information to the attending physician, charge nurse, or social worker. In addition to reporting to the emergency department staff, direct reporting to Child Protective Services or law enforcement ensures follow-up with the family and enhances the child's protection. If the child is not transported to the emergency department, but there are suspicions about the incident, report your concerns to the appropriate child protection and law enforcement agencies as soon as possible. Timeframes for reporting are also mandated and generally provide for a 24-hour time period.

Case Study *continued*

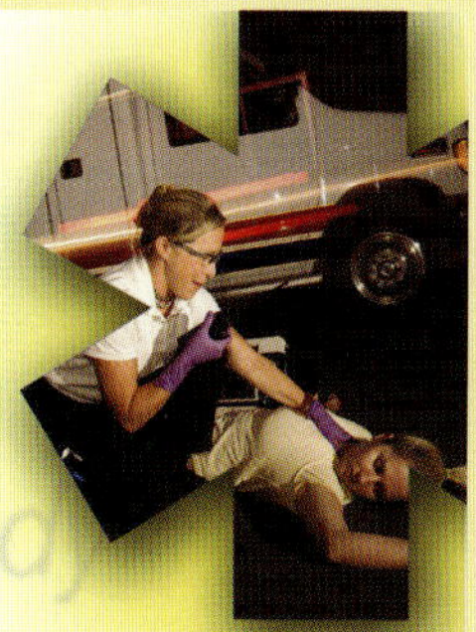

Susan and John pad and splint the injured extremity, and the father accompanies the child to the emergency department. En route, the crew gains additional history on the previous injuries sustained and clarifies the circumstances and information provided by the father

Child Abuse

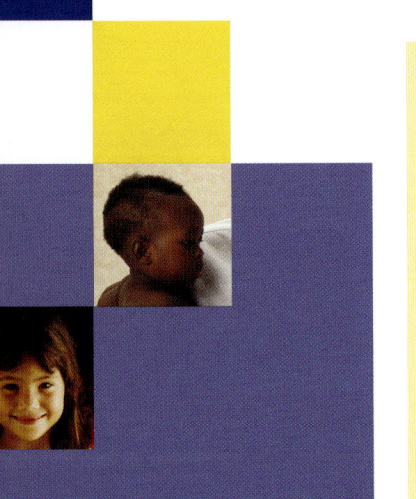

related to the current injury. The child remains calm, crying occasionally from the uneven road surface.

Upon arrival at the hospital, the child's care is transferred to hospital staff, and the crew advises the receiving nurse of the variance in the information provided by the father and mother as to the cause of the injury. The crew completes all required patient care documentation and submits a report to the social worker in the emergency department, knowing the appropriate service will investigate the cause of the injury and circumstances in the home.

The child is assessed by the trauma team and admitted under the joint care of the orthopedic and pediatric teams. Care and safety issues were all addressed before the child is discharged from hospital.

Case Study *wrap-up*

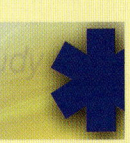

In the United States, child abuse is no longer just a problem occasionally encountered in the field. Children are hurt and killed in all kinds of homes. Remember that child abuse can happen in *any* family. John, Susan and Bob cared for the child well, listened and collected as much information as possible and reported their findings to the hospital staff. This enabled the social worker and the physicians to provide comprehensive care for the child who was a victim of child abuse.

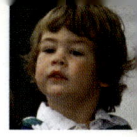

SUMMARY

1. The only real losers in unreported child abuse are: the child who is repetitively abused and perhaps killed, and the family who goes without intervention. You may be the child's last chance.
2. Many obstacles may deter an individual from reporting as required by law. Concerns about retaliation, paperwork, personal beliefs, going to court, or conflicts with law or protective services personnel are just a few.
3. Provide all information gathered at the scene to the emergency department staff and document the information objectively in the run report. Know your local laws, and what you are to report, how, and to whom.
4. Do not confront the family at the scene.
5. Mandated Reporters are required to report suspected abuse and neglect according to regional/state laws. This generally requires that the report be made *directly* to the Child Protective Service or law enforcement agencies. It is critical that Mandated Reporters understand they do not need to *prove* abuse or neglect. They are to report suspicions or concerns of child abuse or neglect.

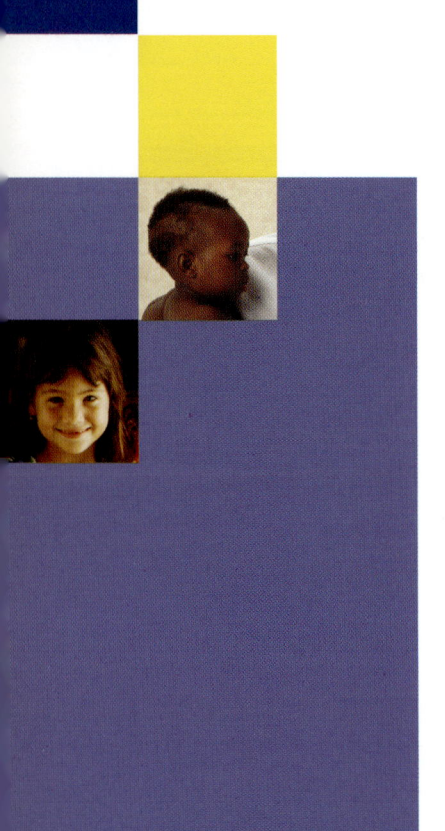

Recommended Reading

Compassionate Friends USA. For *First Responders: Dealing with the Sudden Death of a Child*. Oak Brook, I.L.: Author, 2007.

Hodge, Dee III and Stephen Ludwig. "Child Homicide: Emergency Department Recognition." *Pediatric Emergency Care* 1 (1985): 1.

Hohenhaus, Susan M. EMSC – *C.A.R.E. Child Abuse Recognition Education*. Raleigh, N.C.: North Carolina Office of Emergency Medical Services, 2007.

Krugman, Richard. "Child Abuse and Neglect: Critical First Steps in Response to a National Emergency." *American Journal of Diseases of Children* (1991): 145.

Markinson, David, et al. "A National Assessment of Knowledge, Attitudes, and Confidence of Prehospital Providers in the Assessment and Management of Child Maltreatment." Pediatrics 119 (January 2007): 3103–8.

U.S. Department of Health and Human Services, Children's Bureau. Child Maltreatment 2004. Washington, D.C.: U.S. Government Printing Office, 2004.

Weintraub, Barbara, et al. "Child Maltreatment Awareness for Prehospital Providers." *International Journal of Trauma Nursing* 8 (July-September 2002): 81–83.

18

CHAPTER 18
Death of a Child

Nancy B. Nelson, MSW, LISW
Jeanette Foster, MSW, LISW-S

Objectives
Upon completion of this chapter, you should be able to:

1. Describe the common grief reactions exhibited by family and friends.

2. Discuss recommendations for notifying and assisting the family of a child who dies.

3. Acknowledge the impact that a child's death can have upon you.

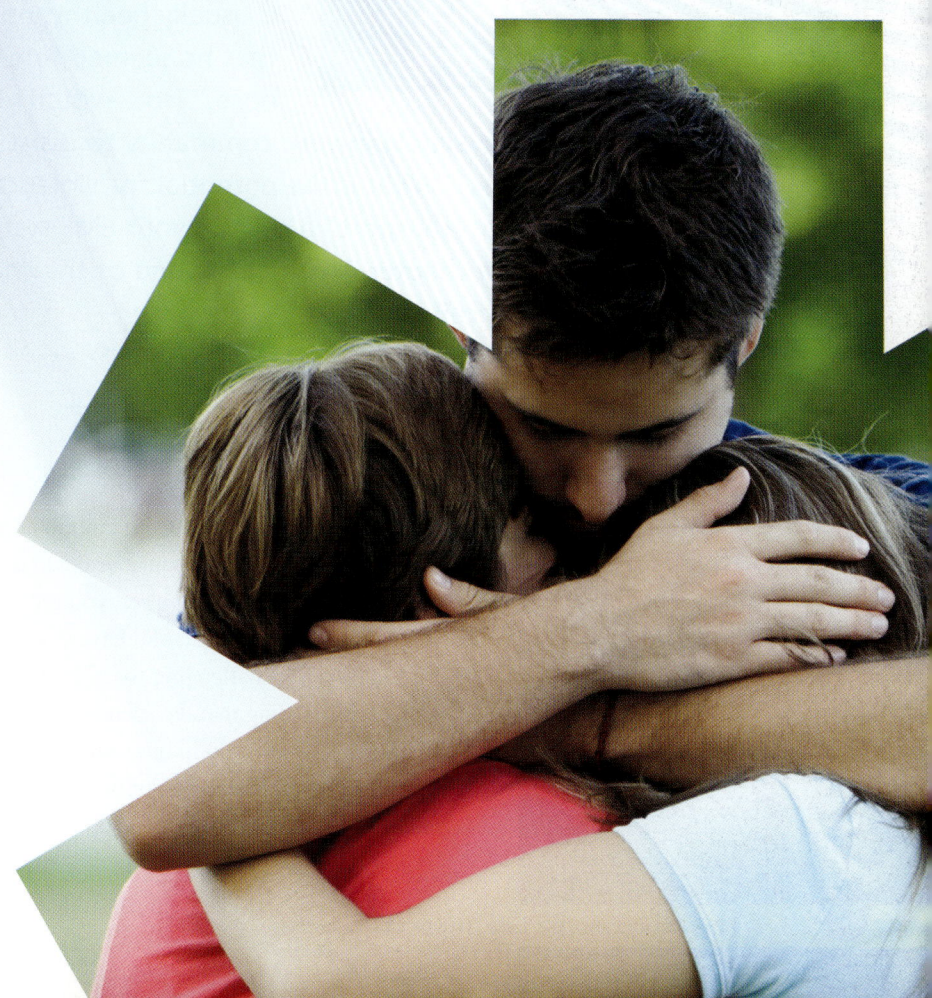

Case Study

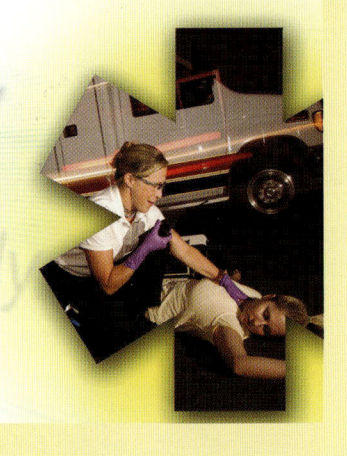

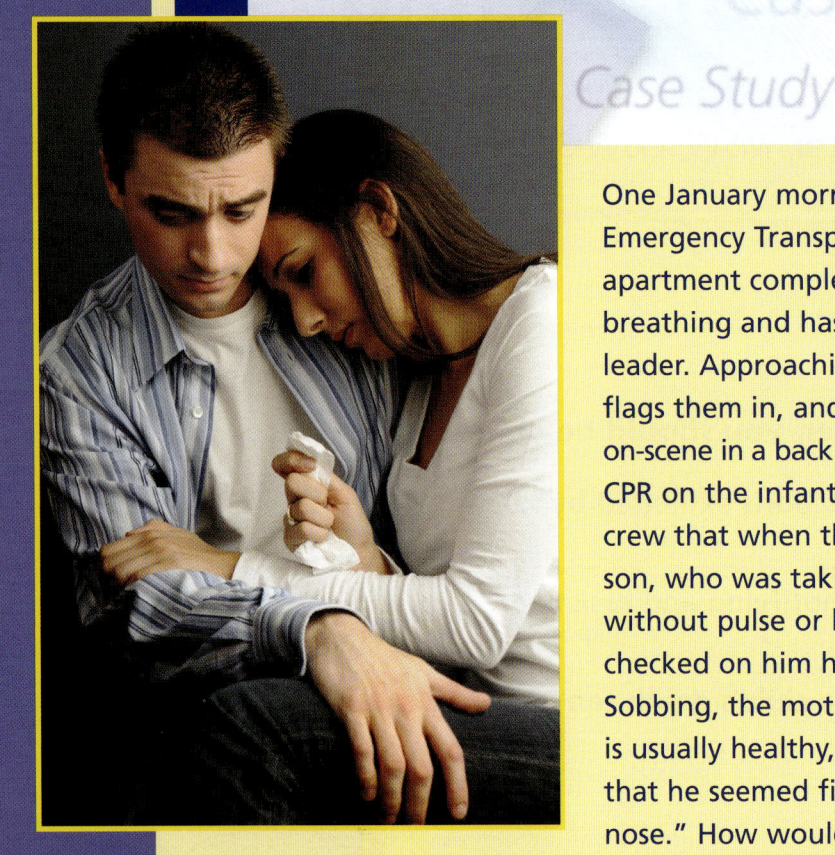

One January morning, John, Susan, and Bob of the Emergency Transport System (ETS) are called to an apartment complex for a 6-month-old boy who is not breathing and has no pulse. Susan will act as the team leader. Approaching the address given, a family member flags them in, and the scene appears safe. As they arrive on-scene in a back bedroom, they find a woman performing CPR on the infant. Another woman tearfully tells the crew that when the boy's mother went to check on her son, who was taking a "very long nap," she found him without pulse or breathing. The last time someone had checked on him had been about 90 minutes before. Sobbing, the mother is able to tell the crew that her son is usually healthy, on no medications, has no allergies and that he seemed fine that morning except for a "runny nose." How would you approach this situation? What resources are available in your community to assist the family members through the grieving process? What is the potential for violence on this call? And why? Are you allowed to "not transport" a child in your EMS system? Keep these questions in mind as you read the chapter. Then, at the end of the chapter, find out how the rescuers completed this call.

INTRODUCTION

There is perhaps no crisis more emotionally challenging and stressful for the prehospital provider than the critical injury or death of a child. Not only are you challenged by arduous medical tasks, but often you are also confronted with overwhelming demands from parents and families who have been thrust into an unexpected and catastrophic event. It is additionally challenging for prehospital providers to balance the needs of the surviving family while seeing that the scene of death is preserved intact for proper authorities.

The death of a child in our society is often regarded as the "ultimate tragedy." Children are not supposed to die, certainly not before their parents. The death of one's child is potentially the most profound and devastating experience of one's life. Although the nature

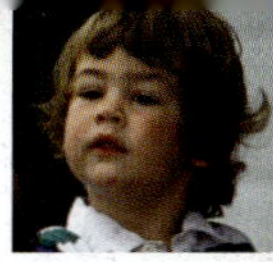

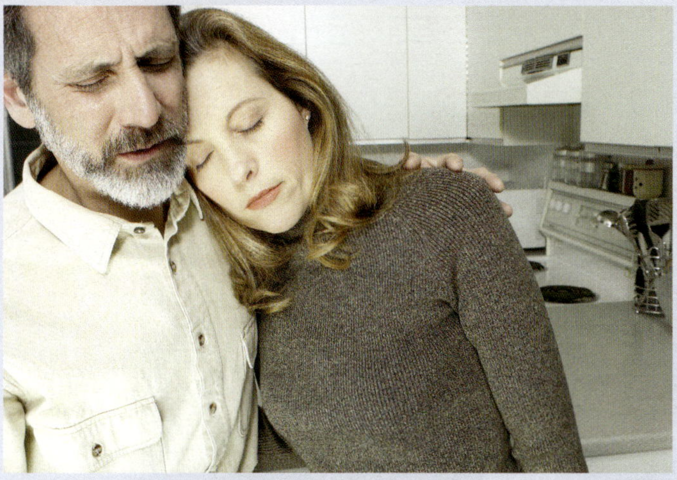

Figure 18.1 *Shock is the first stage in the initial process of grief.*

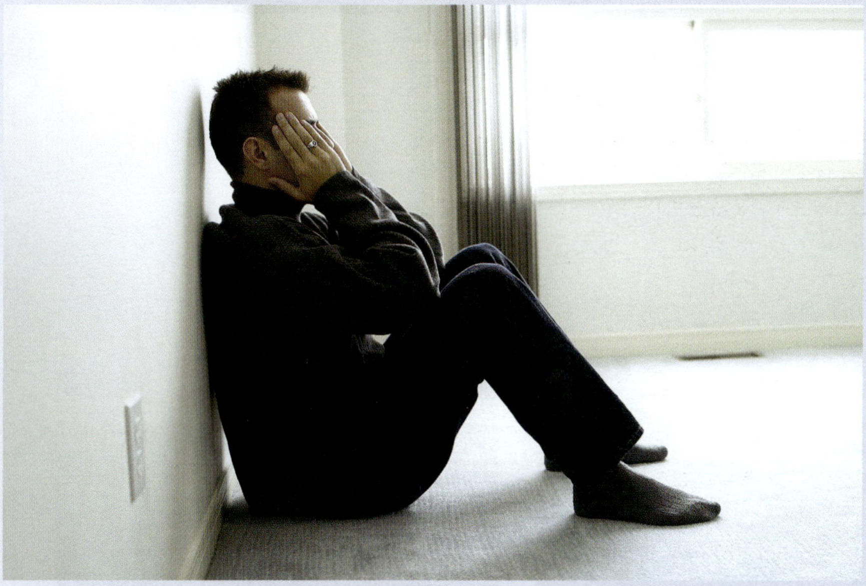

Figure 18.2 *Family members in shock may demonstrate numbness, internal conflict, denial or guilt as part of the first stage of grief.*

Pearls

There is no "right" way for families to grieve. During the initial stages of grief, parents, family members, and close friends of critically injured and dying children may display many different behaviors such as hysterical crying, flatness of affect, anger, or hostile reactions that may appear to be directed toward you and other prehospital providers.

and specific circumstances surrounding a child's death can be very different, parental reactions are overwhelmingly similar. Even where differences do occur, most can be considered acceptable and expected within a wide continuum of reactions.

The following stages are the three common responses in the initial process of grief. These are the stages that the prehospital provider most likely will encounter with the child's family. The first stage is shock, during which the family may demonstrate denial, numbness, internal conflict, or guilt (Figs. 18.1, 18.2). During the second stage, the family experiences an affective or emotional reaction—the internal experience or outward expression of anger, sadness, fear, or anxiety (Fig. 18.3). The third stage, alpha mourning, is the beginning process of mourning, which involves the perception, expression, and acknowledgement of catastrophic loss (Fig. 18.4).

Through these initial stages, parents, family members, and close friends of critically injured and dying children may display the following behaviors: tearfulness, hysterical crying, flatness of affect, and labile behavior that vacillates between different and extreme displays of emotion; angry or hostile reactions that may appear to be directed toward you and other prehospital providers; and feelings of guilt, hopelessness, and loss of control over oneself and the situation (Figs. 18.5, 18.6, 18.7).

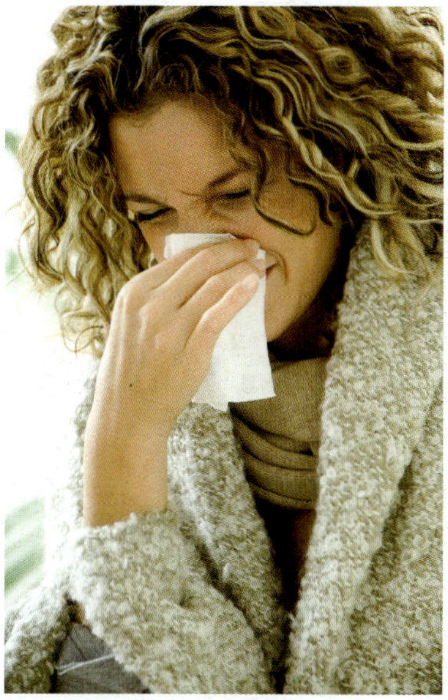

Figure 18.3 *The second stage of grief is characterized by an emotional reaction, such as an expression of sadness.*

Death of a Child

223

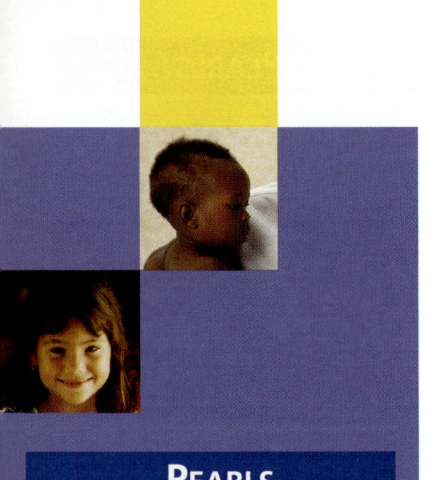

PEARLS

A change in mental status such as agitation or restlessness may signal the early signs of shock; consider rapid "load-and-go" transport.

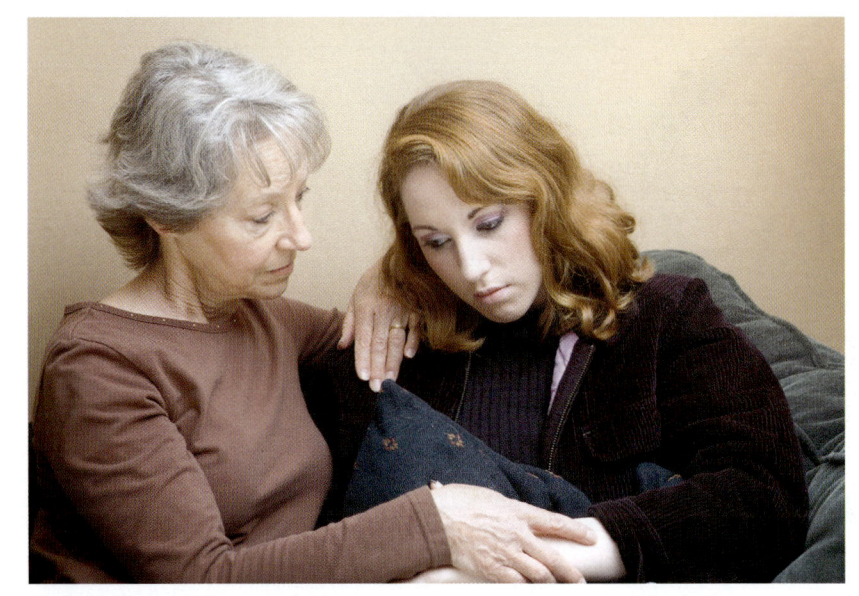

Figure 18.4 *Acknowledgement of catastrophic loss is part of the third stage of grief, sometimes called alpha mourning.*

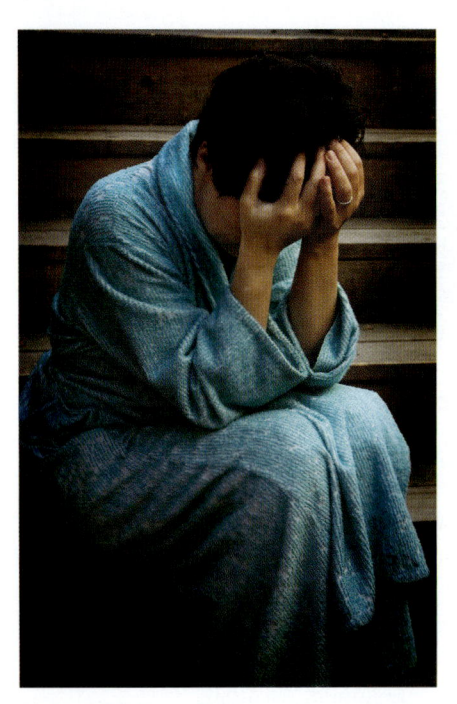

Figure 18.5 *Tearfulness is a common grief reaction during the initial stages.*

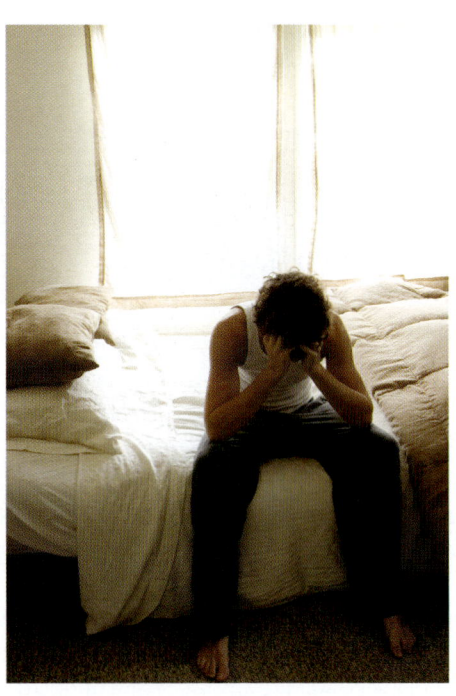

Figure 18.6 *Grieving family members may express guilt or hopelessness.*

GRIEF REACTIONS

Grief reactions may also produce somatic symptoms in acutely grieving parents and can complicate your role as caregiver to the child. The parent who exhibits any of the following symptoms may require emergency medical evaluation as well as support: rapid, tense speech; shortness of breath; chest pain; numbness in the throat; sensitivity to loud noises; tension headaches; muscle spasms; nausea; loss of strength or faintness; restlessness or agitation; hyperactivity; hypertension; and confusion or impaired concentration (Fig. 18.8).

Sudden death generates a different kind of grief, "a harsher variety" than in the case of death after a long illness. Accidental deaths and other kinds of sudden loss are more difficult because there is no opportunity to prepare for the loss. Intensified guilt and

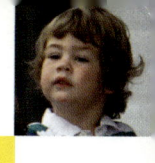

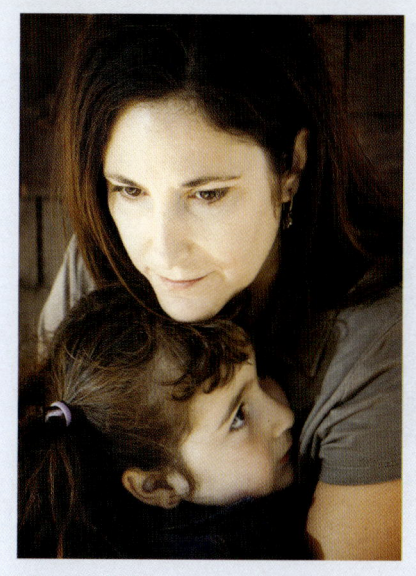

Figure 18.7 *Flatness of affect is another common grief reaction.*

self-blame are common feelings for parents whose children are injured in accidents that they feel they could have, or should have, prevented.

When confronting these intense reactions in others, it is important to identify your own feelings. You may identify with particular people or situations. For example, a five-year-old child who dies may be particularly upsetting for you if you have children of the same age. Your immediate reaction may be to distance yourself from the grieving family, as the intensity of their emotion is overwhelming. You may fear being blamed because you could not save the child, or you may fear not knowing the answers or what to say to the family. It is important to acknowledge your own feelings of powerlessness and helplessness.

Many institutions currently allow parents to be with their child during painful procedures or resuscitation attempts. Research directed at families who have experienced the death of a child has found that the family benefits from being close to the child and comforting the child when they are near death. A written policy may assist in guiding prehospital care providers with such situations. When writing the policy, remember that most families participating in the research study did not critique the resuscitation, but instead found the experience of watching the resuscitation reassuring that everything possible had been done for their child. This helped with closure following the child's death. The amount of family involvement should be individually determined, and should not interfere with the delivery of medical care.

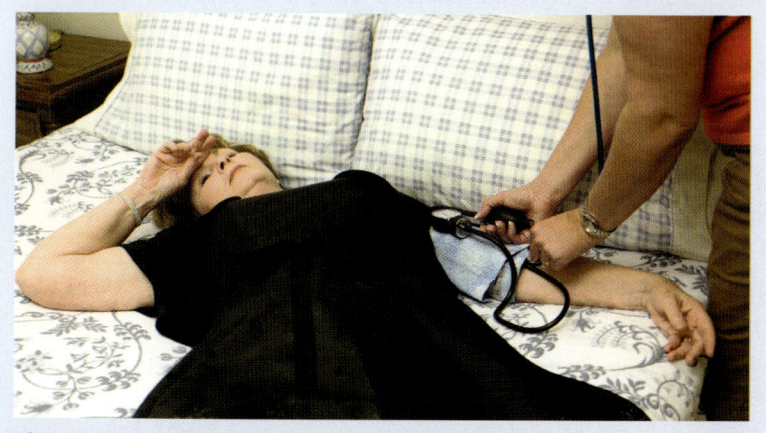

Figure 18.8 *Grief reactions in acutely grieving parents or caregivers may include somatic symptoms, such as faintness or hypertension, that require emergency medical evaluation.*

Pearls

The amount of family involvement and presence during the resuscitation of a child should be addressed by written policies, be individually determined, and should not interfere with the delivery of medical care.

Death of a Child

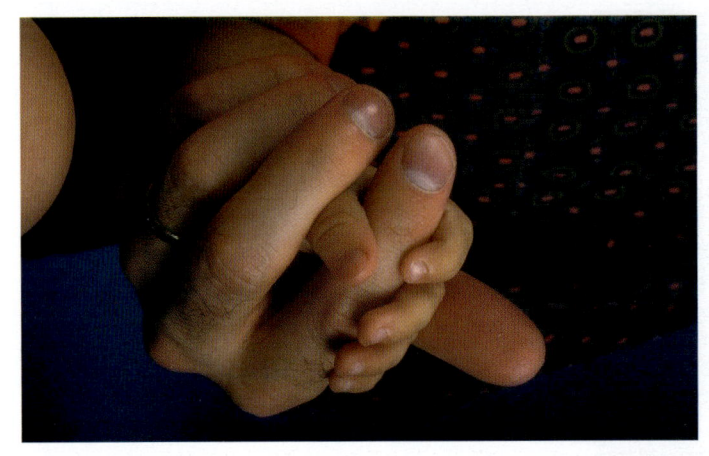

Figure 18.9 *Touch or contact with grieving families offers support and comfort.*

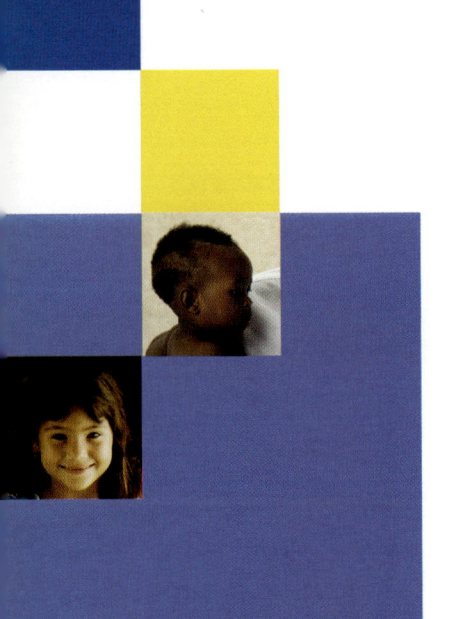

PEARLS

Those who care for children who die after receiving prehospital care are also at risk for emotional distress. Access and referral to appropriate mental health services should be available to provide immediate counseling for the prehospital providers involved.

CRITICAL INCIDENT STRESS DEBRIEFING (CISD)

The death of a child is a very stressful event, not only for the family, but also for the providers who may have feelings of helplessness or guilt that they could not save the child. Critical incident stress debriefing may be very beneficial for all health care providers involved in a pediatric trauma case that results in a death, severe disability, or disfigurement.

RECOMMENDATIONS FOR HOW TO HELP

Compassionate Friends is an organization offering support for bereaved parents and families. The following suggestions have been adapted from their literature:

1. Don't try to find magic words that take away the pain; there aren't any. A hug, a touch, and a simple "I'm so sorry" offer real comfort and support (Fig. 18.9). Be comfortable with silence.
2. Don't be afraid to cry. Sometimes tears express what words cannot.
3. Avoid saying things like "I know how you feel" unless you also have lost a child and have experienced the same depth of loss.
4. Don't try to find something positive in the child's death such as "at least you have other children" or "God must think you are very special to handle this." There are no words that make it all right that their child has died.
5. Avoid judgments of any kind. Saying "you should ..." or "you shouldn't …" is not helpful.
6. Be patient. Remember that different people respond differently to pain. Some scream; others withdraw and are unable or unwilling to talk. Others strike out angrily.
7. Be willing to ask about the child. Even though you may have never known the child, many parents will cherish the opportunity to tell you through their tears how special their child was. This can also be helpful to you as you resolve your own feelings about the death.
8. If possible, give some special attention to surviving children who may be present. They are hurt, confused, and often ignored. Many older children will suppress their painful feelings to avoid adding to their parents' pain. Talk to them and acknowledge their loss.

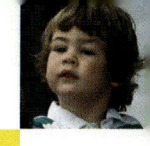

9. Be aware that a child's death can raise serious questions about God's role and the parent's religious beliefs. Ask the family if they have a pastor or minister whom they would like you to contact. Do not presume others' religious beliefs are like your own.
10. Listen, listen, and listen!

Compassionate Friends makes some additional recommendations for prehospital providers who are in the position of notifying parents of the sudden death of their child.

First, never release identifying information to the news media prior to family notification. It is catastrophic for a family member to hear of a child's death by TV or radio.

Second, never notify the family of the death of their child by telephone. Ideally, at least two prehospital providers should make the notification. One should be a provider of information, and the other should be available to observe the reaction of the family. This team should break the news in steps, as follows:

1. Confirm the identity of family members.
2. Tell them there has been an emergency.
3. Tell them that the situation was so serious that a death occurred. Promptly give information about the incident, such as a car accident, fall, and so on.
4. Use the child's name if possible and provide specific, clear information tactfully and honestly.

After notification, do not leave family members alone. Offer to contact neighbors, friends, clergy, and others who can be present to provide support and assistance (Fig. 18.10). In situations in which a dying child is transported to the hospital, the family is often waiting for what seems like a very long time for information. Although the clinical responsibilities may seem overwhelming, make some contact with the child's family.

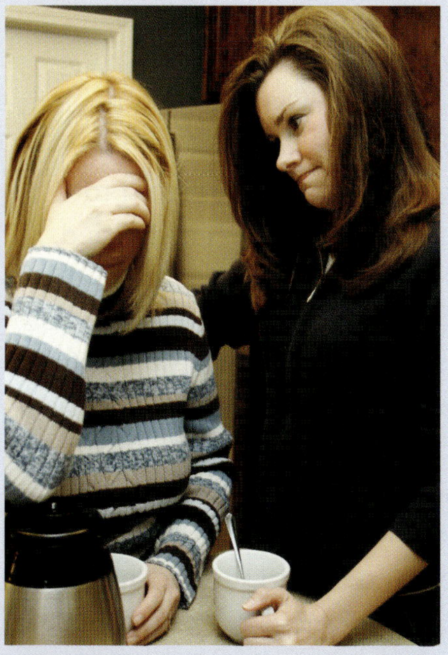

Figure 18.10 *Contact neighbors, friends, clergy or others to provide support to the family that has just been notified of the death of their child.*

> **PEARLS**
>
> **Ideally, two prehospital providers should notify the family of the death of their child. One should give information, and the other should observe the reaction of the family.**

Death of a Child

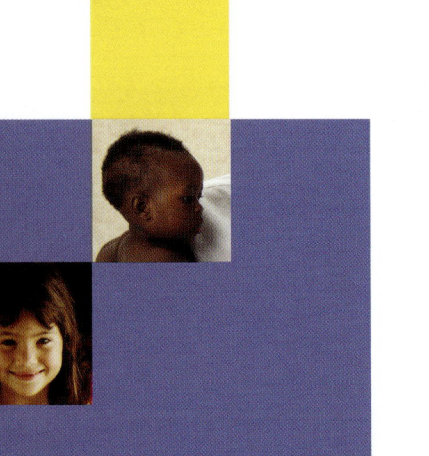

If the child is not doing well, prepare the family gently for bad news. Repeated visits with updated information, even if it is bad, can reduce the trauma to the family. Make sure appropriate hospital staff, social workers and/or the chaplain are aware of the family's situation. These individuals may provide the family with support and convey their important needs and wishes to you. If possible, after the child has died and the family is departing, give the family a name and phone number to contact with their unanswered questions.

Remember, the death of a child is potentially one of life's cruelest and most devastating blows. Responders have the challenge to provide care not only to the child, but to the child's loved ones. Your patience, honesty, and the capacity to listen to the most painful and overwhelming feelings the family is experiencing enable parents to begin to grieve and allow their emotional wounds to begin the long process of healing.

Case Study *continued*

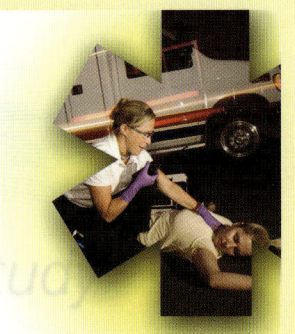

As Susan, Bob and John approach the child, they note that he is very pale. Susan's Initial Assessment reveals that he has no vital signs. John and Bob take over BLS from the neighbor doing CPR, noting the high quality of her performance. Susan also notes that there is a purplish color to the infant's back and posterior lower extremities. Susan attaches the cardiac monitor and simultaneously tries to ascertain any additional history or helpful information. She finds that the cardiac rhythm without CPR is asystole. Further assessment reveals that there are no signs of trauma and no obvious choking hazards in the vicinity. BLS is continued and as per local protocol, Susan notifies medical direction. Medical direction instructs the team to discontinue CPR and stand by for law enforcement arrival. CPR is stopped, and the team sits quietly with the family and neighbors, awaiting law enforcement and the father's arrival. Bob tells the neighbor who performed CPR what an excellent job she had done in trying to resuscitate the child and commends the other neighbor and the mother for being able to provide them with vital information.

The father arrives and is overcome with grief and anger. Susan, John, and Bob stood by and listened as the parents went through several acute grief responses. The team was aware of community resources to support parents in the grieving process, and they were able to facilitate moving the parents into this process.

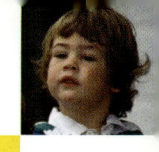

Case Study wrap-up

The death of an infant or child is one of the most difficult experiences a prehospital provider can encounter. Often, prehospital providers are the first to arrive at the scene, and at the same time as making difficult judgments about resuscitation, must deal with the devastating initial shock of caregivers. Understanding the grief process for family members and friends as well as our own vulnerabilities are important factors when dealing with the tragic death of a child. The possibility of violence is very real as parents may lash out as part of their grief response.

SUMMARY

1. The death of a child is an emotionally challenging experience.
2. Acute grief reactions include tearfulness, hysterical crying, a flat affect, anger, hostility, and extreme displays of emotion.
3. Your patience and capacity to listen to the most painful and overwhelming feelings enables parents to begin the long process of grieving and healing.

Recommended Reading

Advanced Life Support Group. "When a Child Dies." In *Pre-Hospital Paediatric Life Support: The Practical Approach*, 2nd ed. London: Blackwell BMJ Books, 2005.

American Academy of Pediatrics, Committee on Pediatric Emergency Medicine, and the American College of Emergency Physicians, Pediatric Emergency Medicine Committee. "Death of a Child in the Emergency Department: Joint Statement by the American Academy of Pediatrics and American College of Emergency Medicine." *Pediatrics* 110 (2002): 839–40.

Compassionate Friends USA. *How Can I Help When a Child Dies?* Oak Brook, I.L.: Author, 1987.

Compassionate Friends USA. *For First Responders Dealing with the Sudden Death of a Child.* Oak Brook, I.L.: Author, 1988.

Holland, Lin and Lee Ellen Rogich. "Dealing with Grief in the Emergency Room." *Health and Social Work* 5 (1980): 12–7.

International Society for Traumatic Stress Studies. Trauma Loss and Traumatic Grief, Revised. Amsterdam, Netherlands: Author, 2005. http://www.estss.org/resources/sudden_traumatic_loss.cfm (accessed December 1, 2007).

Knapp, Ronald J. *Beyond Endurance: When a Child Dies*, 77. New York: Schocken Books, 1986.

Paul, Barbara J. "Reactions to Sudden or Traumatic Loss." *AARP* (2007): 19–95. http://www.aarp.org/families/grief_loss/a2004-11-15-reations.html (accessed December 1, 2007).

Truog, Robert D., et al. "Sudden Traumatic Death in Children: We Did Everything, but Your Child Didn't Survive." *Journal of the American Medical Association* 295 (June 14, 2006): 2646–54.

CHAPTER 19
Trauma In the Newborn

Joanne E. Lapetina, MD, MS, FAAP, FACEP

Objectives
Upon completion of this chapter, you should be able to:

1. Discuss the best supportive care for the unborn fetus exposed to trauma.
2. Describe positioning of the pregnant patient over 20 weeks' gestation.
3. Describe appropriate interventions when meconium staining is present.
4. Discuss resuscitation guidelines and interventions.
5. Explain why minimal blood loss can be critical.

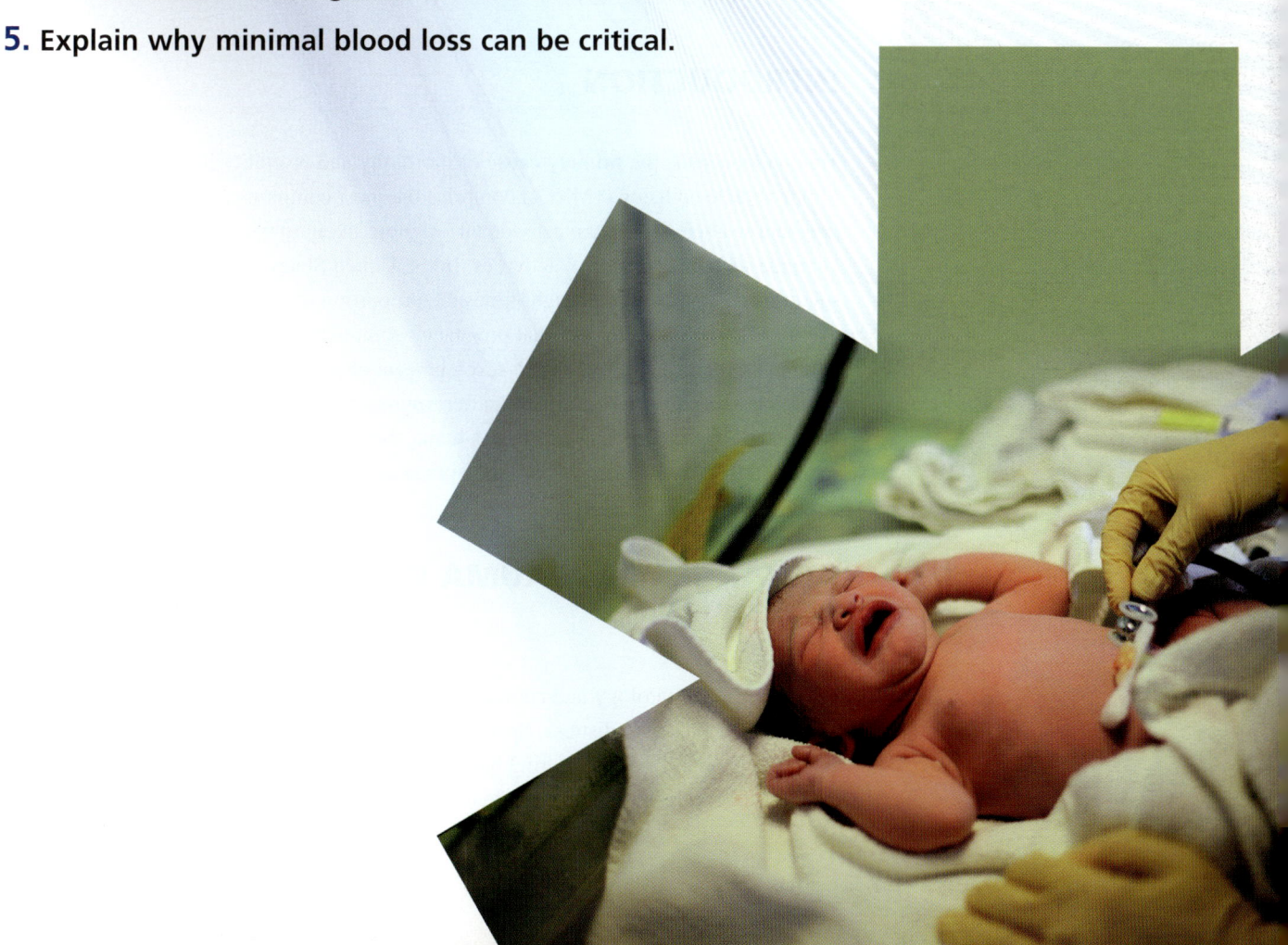

Case Study

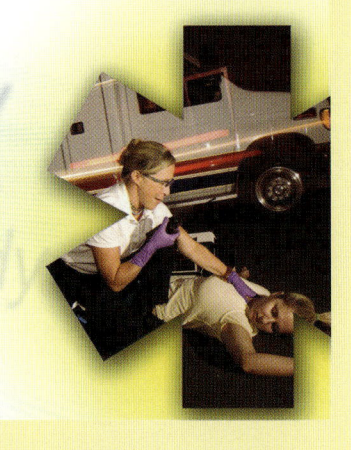

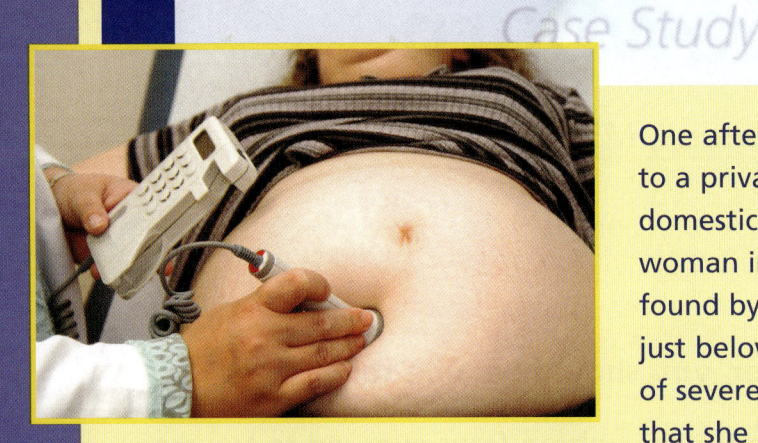

One afternoon, John, Susan, and Bob are called to a private home by the police after a 911 domestic violence call. They are informed that a woman in her 20s, who is visibly pregnant, was found by the police with a knife in her abdomen, just below the umbilicus. The woman complains of severe abdominal pain. Police assure the team that she is the only person in the house. What injuries should the team anticipate? Is the unborn fetus in danger? Who is the priority patient? What interventions should the team perform on each patient? What are the immediate risks? Keep these questions in mind as you read the chapter. Then, at the end of the chapter, find out how the rescuers completed the call.

INTRODUCTION

Trauma represents the primary cause of morbidity and mortality in the pregnant woman. Motor vehicle collisions (MVCs) comprise the most common cause of major trauma in pregnant women, as today most women are more likely to work outside the home and continue with pre-pregnancy activities. In the United States, MVCs, domestic violence, and suicides account for almost eight times the proportion of deaths in females of reproductive age than those related to maternal pregnancy complications. Trauma is actually quite common in pregnancy, with six to seven percent of pregnant women requiring emergency department or obstetrical evaluation after traumatic events (Fig. 19.1). While most maternal and fetal deaths are secondary to blunt trauma, there has been a disturbing rise in penetrating trauma in the United States. Pregnant women are more likely than non-pregnant women to be victims of domestic assault.

ADVANCES IN TRAUMA CARE OF THE NEWLY BORN INFANT

Advances in perinatology and neonatology in the last ten years have greatly increased survival of neonates in distress. Specialized equipment, surfactant therapy for premature infants, and aggressive monitoring have increased survival of infants born as early as 24 to 26 weeks' gestation. Review of more than 100,000 trauma admissions of pregnant women requiring emergency Caesarean section and neonatal resuscitation revealed an infant survival rate of almost 75 percent if the infant was greater than 25 weeks' gestation and had fetal heart tones capable of being read on a Doppler device on arrival at the trauma center (Fig. 19.2). This review also identified a subset of infants who suffered preventable deaths, because while their mothers were found to have mild to moderate injuries, lack of aggressive monitoring missed signs of fetal distress until the infant died. These deaths were almost uniformly caused by abruptio placentae, or separation of the fetus from its blood supply. The most common direct cause of fetal death in the traumatic situation was skull fracture and brain injury as a result of blunt trauma and fracture of the maternal pelvis.

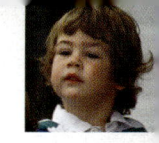

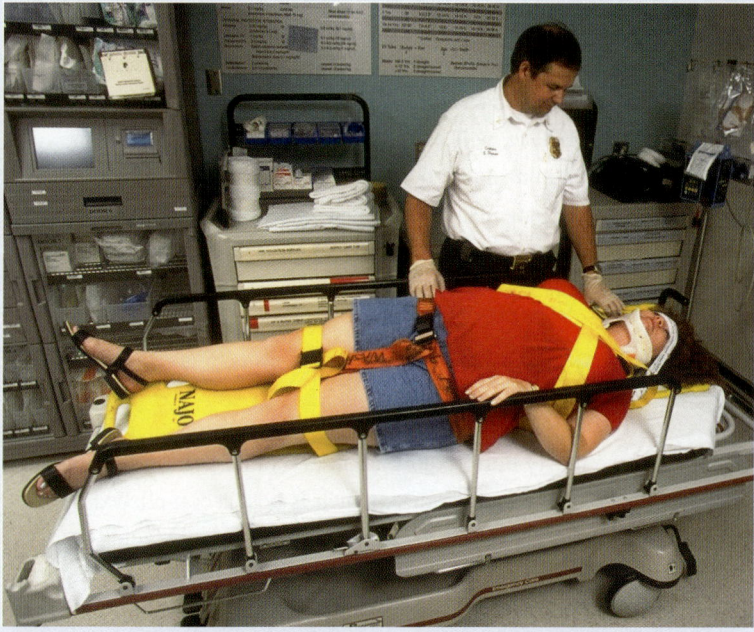

Figure 19.1 *Trauma represents the primary cause of morbidity and mortality in the pregnant woman.*

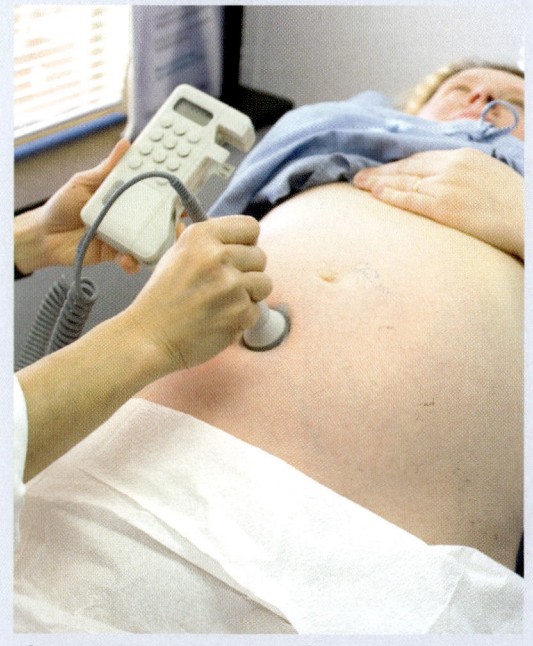

Figure 19.2 *A Doppler device reads fetal heart tones and is useful to evaluate the fetus after a traumatic incident to the pregnant patient.*

PEARLS

Trauma is actually quite common in pregnancy, with 6 to 7 percent of pregnant women requiring emergency department or obstetrical evaluation after traumatic events.

Trauma in the Newborn

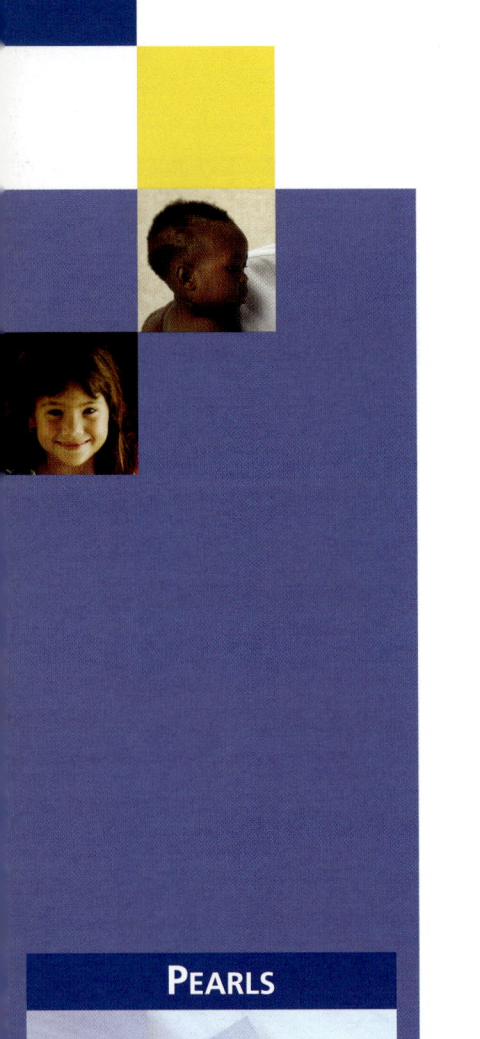

Traumatologists now advocate documentation of fetal heart tones in all traumatized pregnant women during the initial assessment of the patient. As Doppler capability is not generally present in the field and stethoscopes may be unreliable in detecting fetal heart tones, the fetus must be presumed alive in the prehospital situation. The presence of fetal heart tones necessitates immediate obstetrical consultation and continuous fetal monitoring. Any fetal distress detected in a fetus greater than 25 weeks' gestation warrants consideration for immediate delivery. Interestingly, rapid delivery of the fetus has been shown to improve maternal outcome as well.

New concepts in neonatal resuscitation put forth by the International Liaison Committee on Resuscitation (ILCOR) have been adapted by the European Resuscitation Council (ERC) and the American Heart Association (AHA). These recommendations, listed in the following section, compromise the 2005 recommendations that the American Academy of Pediatrics (AAP) and AHA incorporated in the *Neonatal Resuscitation Textbook*. Resuscitation of the *newly born*, a term now utilized to distinguish the neonate less than 28 days of age from the *just born*, will be outlined. It is exceedingly rare to encounter a newly born infant in a trauma situation, and there are no published guidelines for this special population of pediatric patients. Basic resuscitation principles are covered, with an emphasis on changes since the previous recommendations released in 2000, and the basic trauma principles where indicated.

NEONATAL RESUSCITATION

The overwhelming majority of the newly born require no intervention at birth beyond the general principle of maintenance of body temperature, which is best accomplished by drying the infant, performing a simple suction of the mouth and nose, and placing the infant on the mother's chest (Fig. 19.3). Approximately 10 percent of infants will require some resuscitation, mainly establishment of adequate ventilation, and only 2 or 3 in 1,000 infants ever require code medications. The neonatal resuscitation inverted pyramid visually demonstrates that while drying, warming, and suctioning form the base of resuscitation, there is a progression of procedures necessary for the sickest, most depressed hypoxic babies (Fig. 19.4). The inverted pyramid moves from drying, warming and suction to establishing effective ventilation, then performing chest compressions, and finally administering drug therapy if necessary.

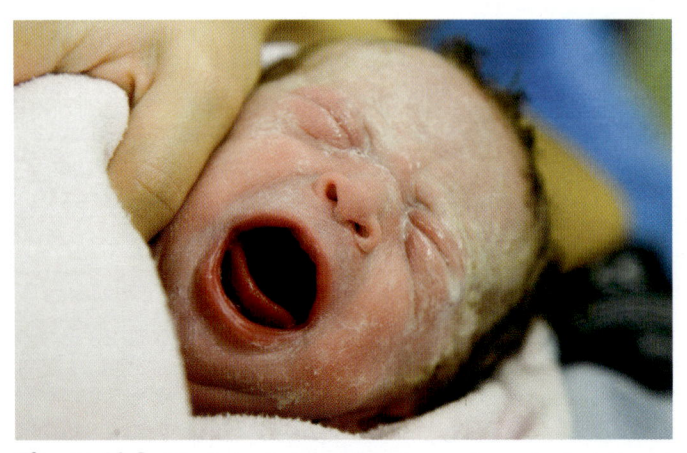

Figure 19.3 *Most newly born infants require only drying and a simple suction of the mouth and nose before placing the infant on the mother's chest.*

> **PEARLS**
>
> The fetus must be presumed alive in the prehospital situation.

Neonatal Resuscitation Inverted Pyramid

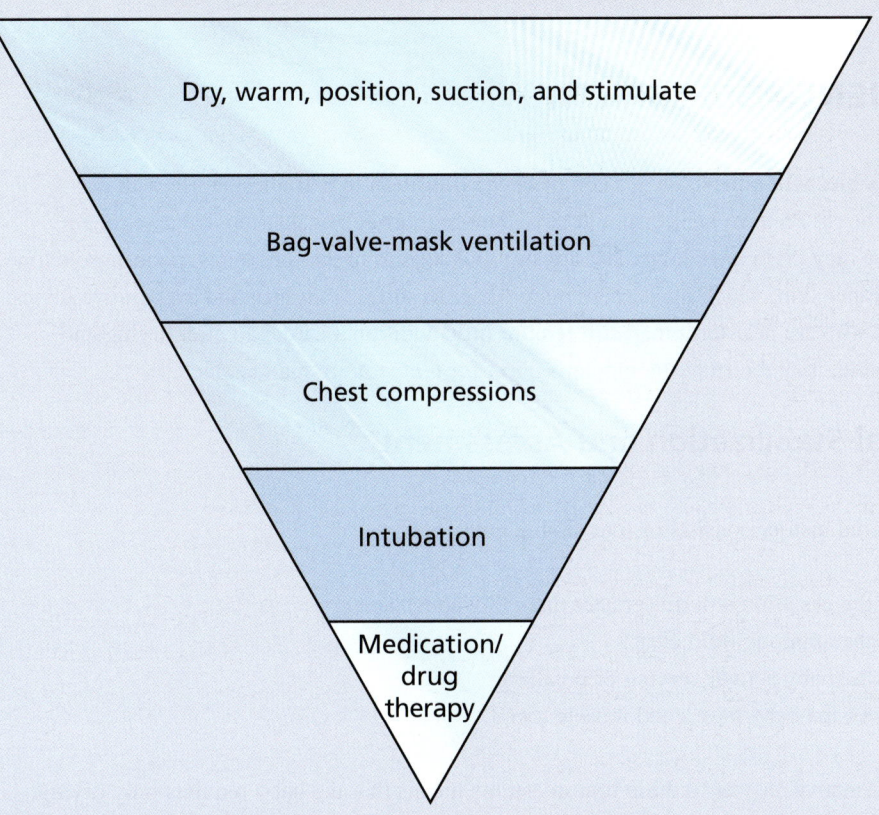

- Dry, warm, position, suction, and stimulate
- Bag-valve-mask ventilation
- Chest compressions
- Intubation
- Medication/drug therapy

Figure 19.4 *The inverted pyramid of neonatal resuscitation shows the progression of procedures that may be necessary to perform on newly born infants. As the inverted pyramid narrows, the frequency of the necessity of the intervention decreases.*

There is currently argument in the literature on whether 100 percent oxygen or room air (21 percent oxygen) should be used for neonatal resuscitation if bag-valve-mask ventilation or endotracheal intubation are used. AHA currently recommends 100 percent oxygen for resuscitation. A survey of delivery room resuscitations in the United States reveals a lack of uniformity in management of evaporative loss of low birth weight babies, oxygen delivery practices and adherence to ILCOR/AHA guidelines. More worrisome is that only 32 percent of programs use CO_2 detectors for confirmation of endotracheal tube placement, despite numerous articles and studies that these monitors confirm placement more quickly and accurately than physical assessment can. CO_2 monitoring of intubated patients is not only necessary but should be a standard for both prehospital and inhospital patients.

Recommendations for initiation of neonatal resuscitation call for a warm, well-lit, draft-free area with a flat resuscitation area under a radiant heater. Other recommendations include at least one well-trained neonatal resuscitation provider, regularly checked and operational resuscitation equipment, and the ability to acquire the additional equipment to resuscitate the preterm infant (< 37 weeks' gestation) in a timely fashion. As the prehospital environment may be poorly lit, cold, and devoid of any form of radiant heating, keep in mind that quick and thorough drying, a flashlight, and placing the infant against warm skin may be all that is required for a successful intervention. The resuscitation process occurs very quickly, and better outcomes will occur with ongoing assessments that occur in 30-second intervals, and forethought that includes environment and needs for specialized equipment (such as contained in a prepacked pediatric kit or Broselow bag).

Pearls

As the prehospital environment may be poorly lit, cold, and devoid of any form of radiant heating, keep in mind that quick and thorough drying, a flashlight, and placing the infant against warm skin may be all that is required for a successful intervention.

PATIENT ASSESSMENT

Term babies will almost always complete the transition to extrauterine life with no intervention. Preterm babies should have a more thorough evaluation and assessment because they often have lungs that are stiff and require higher pressures, poor muscle tone, and thinner skin, which make them more likely to suffer from heat and evaporative losses. Babies who are near term may still require little additional care, and after drying and suctioning, may return to the mother's chest for temperature maintenance.

Initial Stabilization and Assessment

The initial history consists of four simple questions:

1. Is the gestation at term (greater than 37 weeks)?
2. Is the amniotic fluid clear?
3. Is the baby actively crying or breathing?
4. Does the baby have good muscle tone?

An affirmative answer to these four questions means that the baby requires only drying, warming, and suctioning before being placed on mother's chest (Figs. 19.5, 19.6).

When assessing the baby's breathing, it is important to remember that *gasping is the same as apnea*. The newborn should make vigorous efforts to breathe, which drives the intralung fluid across capillary membranes, creating a low pulmonary vascular system where a high-pressure system existed moments before. This allows the alveoli to fill with oxygen for transport to the tissue. Interruptions to this process may culminate in the following clinical findings: poor tone, apnea or tachypnea with continued cyanosis, bradycardia, and weak pulses secondary to end-organ oxygen deprivation (Fig. 19.7). If the baby is not breathing well, *intervene*.

Good tone in the healthy newly born infant is characterized by flexed, active extremities. The depressed infant will have flaccid, straight extremities that do not recoil when pulled or flicked during stimulation.

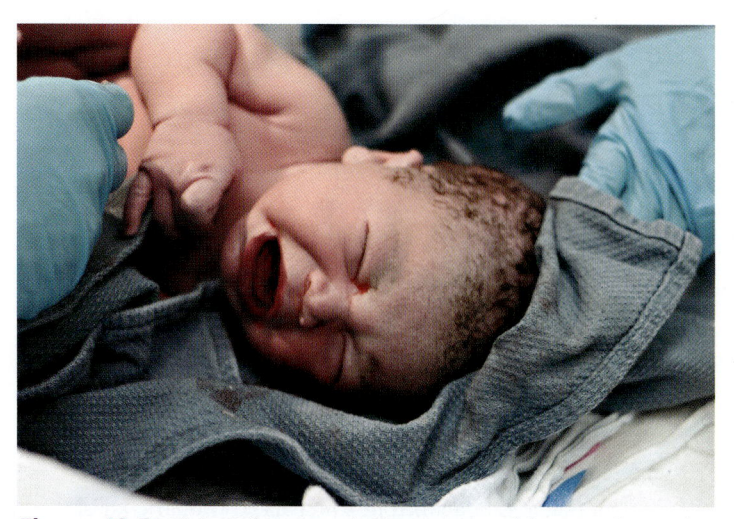

Figure 19.5 *If the infant is actively crying and has good muscle tone, the only interventions usually required are drying, warming, and suctioning.*

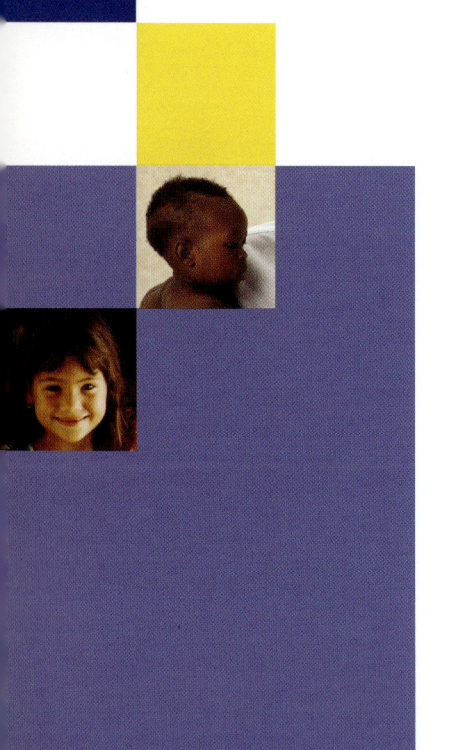

PEARLS

The initial history consists of four simple questions:
1. Is the gestation at term (greater than 37 weeks)?
2. Is the amniotic fluid clear?
3. Is the baby actively crying or breathing?
4. Does the baby have good muscle tone?

Pediatric Trauma Life Support

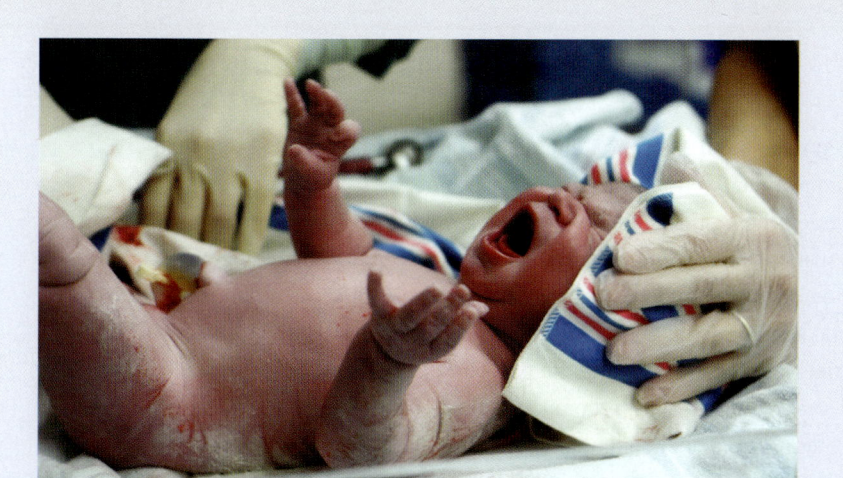

Figure 19.6 *Thoroughly dry the newly born infant and suction the mouth and nose before placing the baby on the mother's chest.*

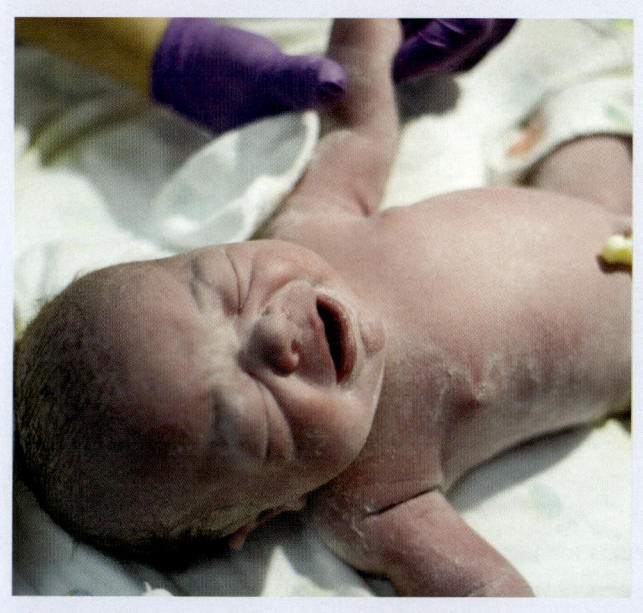

Figure 19.7 *A weak pulse, bradycardia, apnea or tachypnea with continued cyanosis, and poor tone result when a newly born infant is having difficulty breathing.*

Special Situations

Preterm infants pose a particular challenge in that they have large surface area for heat loss, thin skin, and poor fat deposition. Most fat deposition in the fetus occurs after the 36th week of gestation. Neonatology guidelines and the AHA now recommend that infants born at less than 28 weeks' gestation may be placed, below the neck, in a reclosable polyethylene bag, without first drying the skin to reduce heat and resorptive loss. Use a standard 1-gallon, plastic food-storage bag such as the type that can be purchased in a grocery store. This item should become part of the prehospital pediatric kit. Further resuscitation can take place as needed.

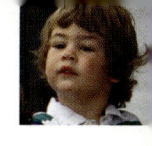

Meconium aspiration can be a deadly disease in neonates, causing a severe aspiration pneumonitis. Efforts in the past to remedy this problem required intrapartum suctioning of the baby before delivery of the shoulders; however, recently completed studies show no benefit to this maneuver, and ILCOR and the AHA no longer recommend this procedure. Therefore, fully deliver the baby before beginning any assessment of the meconium-stained infant. Studies have also shown that babies who have experienced meconium aspiration and are vigorous and have good tone and cry should be treated as other well-appearing, newly born babies. However, you should immediately suction the mouth of babies who do *not* have good tone or cry with a large (12-14 French) suction catheter and then immediately intubate for suctioning of the trachea. Direct connection of the endotracheal tube to the suction catheter is recommended and requires a special adapter. After suctioning, remove the endotracheal tube along with whatever material was suctioned during the procedure. Then proceed with resuscitation as for any other depressed infant. Past recommendations differentiated between thin and thick meconium but there is no evidence that this makes any difference during resuscitation.

APPROACH TO THE NEWLY BORN INFANT WITH AN ABNORMAL INITIAL ASSESSMENT

Newly born infants failing any of the initial stabilization questions or assessment must undergo further resuscitation and stabilization. As with any resuscitation effort, attention to the ABCs is paramount to successful outcome. Prehospital resuscitation of the newly born is accomplished on a firm surface (usually a short backboard). Maintaining the airway in sniffing position (achieved by extending the head while simultaneously flexing the neck) holds the cervical spine in neutral position (Fig. 19.8). While cervical spine injuries may occur during the birth process and are theoretically possible as a consequence of trauma, the occurrence is quite rare. Babies with Down syndrome, however, are at risk for high spinal injury because of anatomic alterations that predispose these patients to atlantoaxial dislocation.

Airway

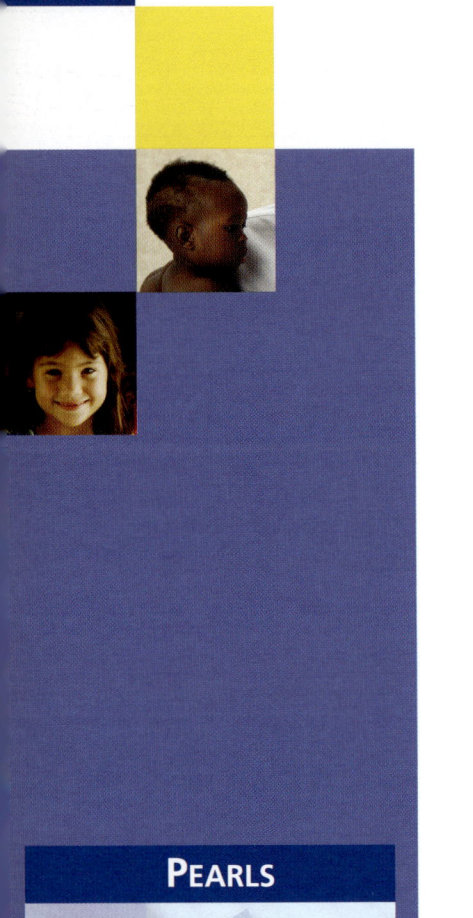

If there is any concern about trauma to the newly born infant, institute spinal motion restriction precautions and use cervical spine stabilization with all airway maneuvers (Fig. 19.9). After drying, warming, and suctioning, use the bulb syringe in the infant's mouth first and then the nose to prevent aspiration of material that may have collected in the mouth prior to or during delivery. Then place the baby in sniffing position with the body horizontal to the flat surface. Placing a small towel roll beneath the infant's shoulders is helpful in maintaining the trachea in neutral position, as the infant's relatively large occiput predisposes the infant to forced airway flexion. Avoid hyperextension from downward forces on the baby's forehead, and flexion from inattention to shoulder elevation, as both

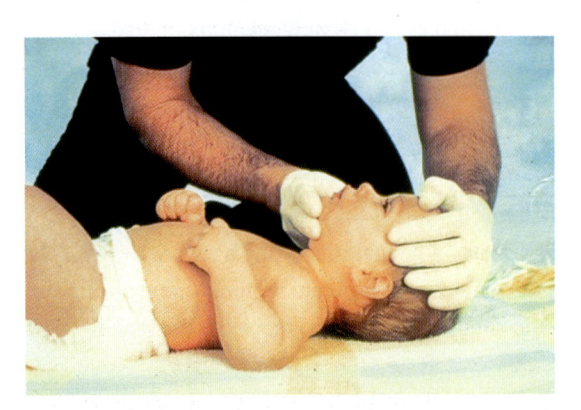

Figure 19.8 *Maintaining the airway of an infant in sniffing position holds the cervical spine in neutral position.*

PEARLS

If there is any concern about trauma to the newly born infant, institute spinal motion restriction precautions and use cervical spine stabilization with all airway maneuvers.

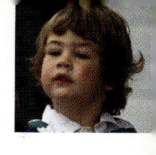

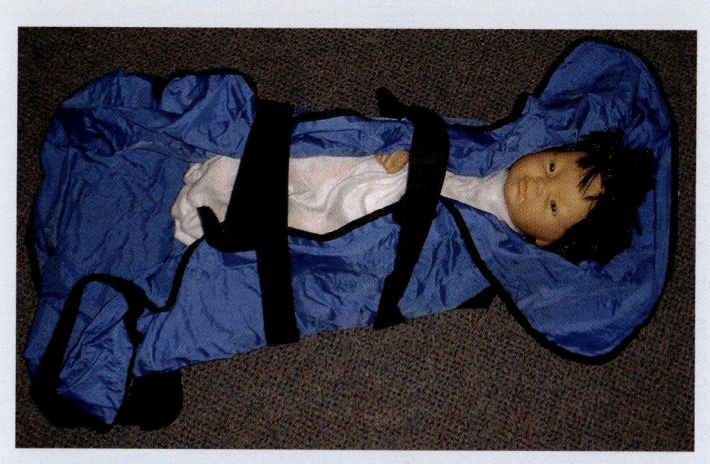

Figure 19.9 *An infant spinal motion restriction device such as a vacuum splint or a papoose may be necessary to minimize motion when performing interventions.*

retard airflow through the trachea. Also avoid Trendelenburg positioning, as it has been associated with intracerebral bleeding in preterm infants. As previously discussed, perform tracheal suctioning on babies with presence of meconium if they do not have good tone or cry. Take care to avoid deep or prolonged suctioning, as this may precipitate an episode of apnea and bradycardia.

Breathing

Newly born infants not responding to simple measures after 30 seconds will require oxygen, ventilation, or both. Babies with good respiratory effort but who remain cyanotic may have a trial of 100 percent oxygen delivered by the blow-by technique. This is accomplished by bag-valve mask or cupping the end of the oxygen tubing over the nose to blow or waft oxygen past the infant's face. As infants are obligate nose breathers, placing oxygen at the nose provides the highest concentration possible. Proficiency with bag-valve-mask ventilation is necessary for successful resuscitation of the newly born infant who requires assistance. Early recognition of the infant requiring ventilatory assistance is the first and foremost skill required. It is vitally important to use an appropriately sized face mask that covers the nose and mouth without encroachment of the eyes or extension beyond the chin (Fig. 19.10). The seal of the mask must not leak. This allows for appropriate pressure to be delivered to open atelectatic airways and provide oxygenation to the alveoli. Most prehospital providers will use a self-inflating bag (Ambu bag) and should use an infant bag that has a volume of 200 to 750 mL. To prevent volutrauma, hold tidal volumes to 5 to 8 mL/kg. In delivering this amount to the patient, watch for the chest to rise just a small amount as an indicator of correct volume delivery. Overzealous bagging, either by rate or high pressure/volume, may precipitate pneumothorax or intracranial hemorrhage.

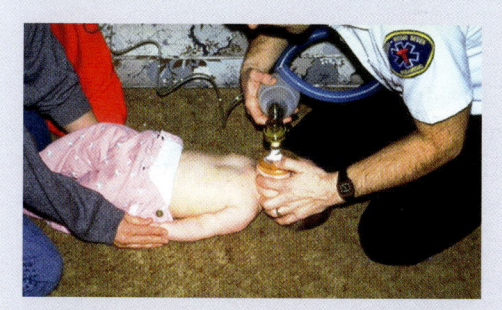

Figure 19.10 *An appropriately sized mask for an infant should cover the mouth and nose without encroaching on the eyes or extending beyond the chin.*

Trauma in the Newborn

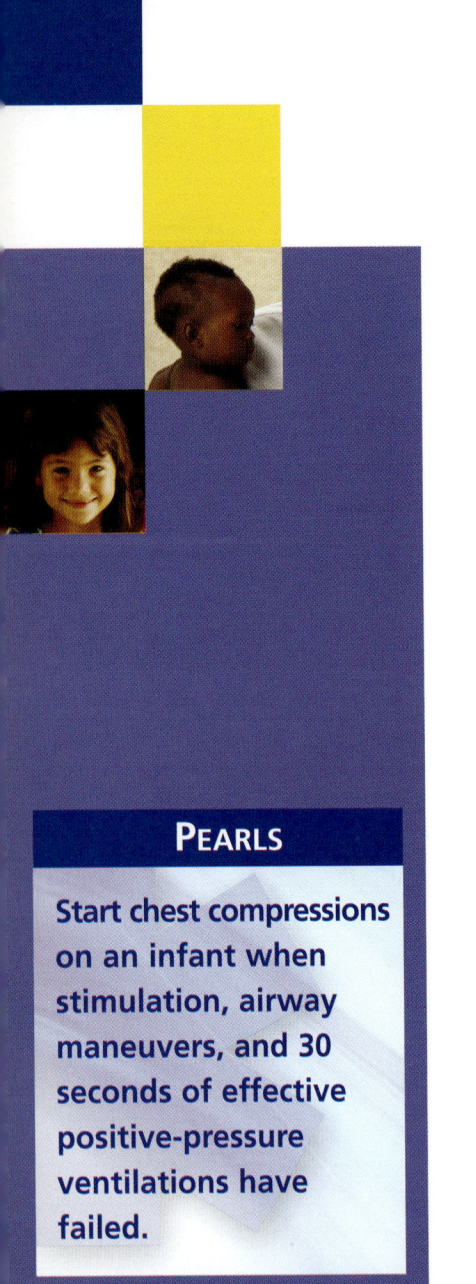

The bag-valve-mask ventilation rate for the persistently cyanotic or apneic infant should be 40 to 60 times per minute with reassessment in 30 seconds. The heart rate, if less than 100 beats per minutes (bpm), should almost immediately rise with intervention. Checking the pulse at the base of the umbilicus is most useful for infants with good heart rates, but those with bradycardia are better evaluated by apical auscultation with a stethoscope. As heart rate rises, color and tone should almost simultaneously improve. Evaluation of lung fields in the newly born is best checked in each axilla to minimize confusion by transmitted sounds across the precordium. If the infant is intubated, this becomes more important in order to recognize and correct right mainstem intubation.

Quickly reassess the airway of infants who do not immediately improve with bag-valve-mask ventilation. Is the airway blocked by secretion or position? Is the seal of the mask inadequate to deliver oxygen to the alveoli? Is the Ambu bag connected to oxygen? Does it have a leak? Does squeezing the bag make the chest rise? If there is no problem with the airway or equipment, you may need to intubate. If the baby has a heart rate less than 60 bpm after 30 seconds of effective bag-valve-mask ventilation, chest compressions are warranted. You may institute intubation either before or after chest compressions. Most will try a trial of chest compressions for 30 seconds prior to intubation so as not to delay resuscitation efforts.

Intubation can be challenging in the newly born term and preterm infant secondary to the sheer size and anterior location of the airway. The posterior pharynx and vocal cords are best seen by sliding a 0 or 1 Miller (straight) blade past the base of the tongue to the vallecula and lifting forward in the direction of the handle. The uncuffed endotracheal tube (ETT), 2.5 for preterm babies and 3.0 for term babies, should be advanced through the cords just to the level of the black vocal cord guide on the tube. Advancing beyond this point may cause right mainstem intubation. Note the marking at the baby's gum and carefully secure the tube at that level. Record the depth of the tube noted via the centimeter markings so that it can be checked and rechecked during resuscitation and transfer. It is critical to check placement of the tube, as esophageal intubation can be lethal if not recognized. Acceptable methods for checking placement of the ETT include auscultation in both axillae and over the stomach, chest rise, prompt resolution of cyanosis and bradycardia, rising pulse oximetry, and CO_2 detection.

CO_2 detectors such as continuous wave-form capnography are quite useful in babies with cardiac activity. Prompt color change of the device signifies tracheal intubation. Many prehospital agencies require CO_2 detection and documentation for every intubation. This is an excellent practice and should be instituted on all patients. CO_2 detectors occasionally fail despite accurate tracheal intubation because of very poor cardiac output and insufficient CO_2 exhalation. In this case, you may need to directly visualize the tube by reinserting the blade.

Circulation

When stimulation, airway maneuvers, and 30 seconds of effective positive-pressure ventilation have failed, start chest compressions. The failure of bag-valve-mask ventilation to restore color and tone means that the infant is likely to have low oxygen levels and significant acidosis. Acidosis reduces enzymatic activity at the cellular level which, in turn, reduces myocardial contractility. Poor pump function does not allow for circulation of oxygenated blood to the end organ tissues. Although not addressed in neonatal resuscitation, you must immediately control hemorrhage in a trauma patient—no matter how small.

PEARLS

Start chest compressions on an infant when stimulation, airway maneuvers, and 30 seconds of effective positive-pressure ventilations have failed.

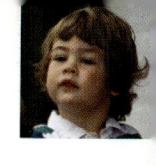

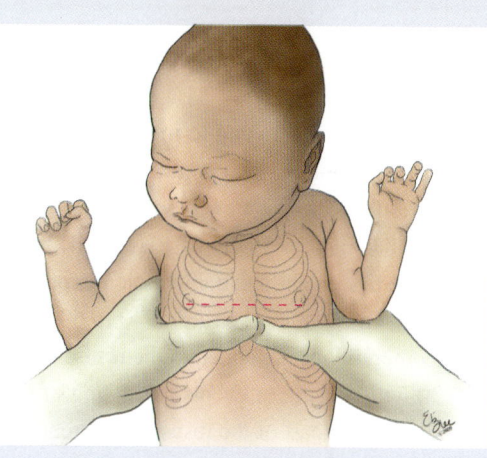

Figure 19.11 *The thumb technique for performing chest compressions is preferred because it is easier to control the depth of compressions.*

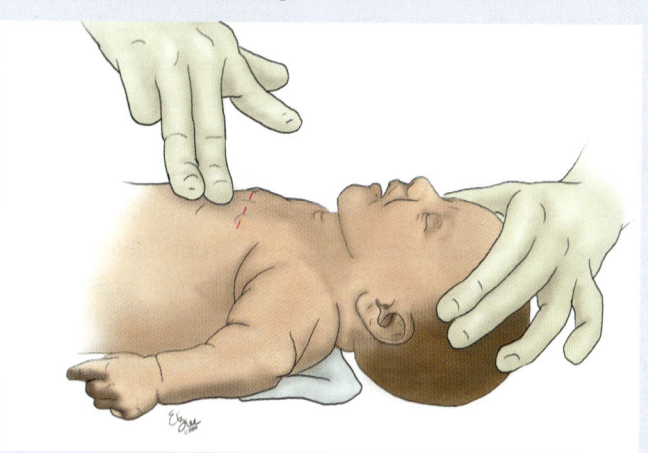

Figure 19.12 *The two-finger technique for chest compressions may be easier on large infants or for providers with small hands.*

If the neonate demonstrates ongoing external bleeding, this must be controlled with direct pressure. Neonates and small infants may bleed to death from lacerations; therefore, immediate direct pressure applied on identified bleeding sites may be life-saving. Other pearls of wisdom not commonly taught to prehospital providers include the importance of leaving at least three inches of umbilical cord next to the infant when cutting the umbilical cord. This facilitates umbilical vessel access by those individuals trained in the placement of such IV lines. Second, the infant should remain at the level of the perineum until the cord is cut to minimize transfusion of blood either toward or away from the attached placenta. Rapid shifts of blood in either direction via gravity may precipitate stroke in neonates, particularly premature infants.

There are two techniques for chest compressions in the newly born infant. The first and more effective for increasing systolic and coronary perfusion pressure is the thumb technique. The thumb technique is where the hands encircle the chest and the thumb pads press vertically on the lower third of the sternum in the center while the fingers support the spine (Fig. 19.11). This technique is preferred because it is easier to control the depth of compressions, which should be one-third of the anterior-posterior (AP) chest diameter, and is less tiring. It does restrict access to the umbilicus for IV medication administration if it should be required.

The second technique for chest compression is the two-finger technique. The two-finger technique may be easier on large infants or for providers with small hands. Use the second hand to support the back and the index and middle fingers to depress the lower third of the sternum one-third of the AP diameter of the chest (Fig. 19.12). With either technique, keep the fingers or thumbs in contact with the sternum to avoid shifts in placement of the compression and to maximize the compression time. There is some evidence that slightly shorter chest compression-to-relaxation time ratios are associated with better blood flow in the newly born infant.

Chest compressions performed incorrectly can damage lungs, rib cartilages, the heart, or intra-abdominal organs. Provide careful attention to placement and compression depth to reduce this risk. While bag-valve-mask ventilation alone occurs at a rate of 40 to 60 bpm, the amount of ventilations is reduced to 30 when compressions are added to the resuscitation. The ratio of compressions to ventilations is 90:30 with a cycle of events consisting of three compressions followed by a positive-pressure breath. This part of the resuscitation requires at least two providers. Continue chest compressions for 30 seconds followed by a reassessment of the pulse. A quick check at the base of the cord will be positive if the heart rate is greater than 60 bpm. If the heart rate is greater than 60 bpm, the compressions can stop with a shift to ventilation at 40 to 60 bpm. Continuing chest compressions when the heart rate is greater than 60 bpm may reduce the effectiveness of the positive-pressure ventilation.

Reevaluate the process if the heart rate remains below 60 bpm after chest compressions. Meanwhile, continue CPR. Is the airway patent? If intubated, is the tube correctly placed or dislodged? Does the chest rise? Is the oxygen tank hooked up and set to deliver 100 percent oxygen? Is it empty? Are chest compressions being performed correctly? Is there a problem with the mask or Ambu bag? Is there a pneumothorax? If no correctable problem is found, drug therapy is indicated with continuation of CPR and reevaluation at 30-second intervals.

Pneumothorax is not an uncommon occurrence after positive-pressure ventilation; evacuate the pneumothorax if it compromises ventilation and perfusion. Recognition of pneumothorax in absence of an X-ray is best accomplished by noting differential breath sounds in the axillae associated with poor cardiopulmonary status. The recommended method for decompression in the newly born infant is placement of an 18-20 gauge IV catheter via the midaxillary approach in the fourth intercostal space. Once placed, withdraw the needle, leaving the catheter. A traumatized neonate could also have a hemothorax, which would be better evacuated initially with a larger IV catheter prior to transport for definitive chest tube placement. Assume the neonate with penetrating trauma to the chest wall to have a hemopneumothorax, which would require decompression in the event of cardiopulmonary compromise. Infanticide is the most common cause of traumatic death in the neonate but is rarely discovered at a point where medical intervention is of benefit. Rates of penetrating trauma to the pregnant uterus during domestic abuse are rising but these infants are not typically born prior to arrival at the emergency department.

Drug Therapy

While D stands for disability in prehospital algorithms, it signifies drug therapy in the neonatal resuscitation inverted pyramid (Fig. 19.13). Only a tiny fraction of infants will require IV placement and drug therapy for transition to extrauterine life. Neonatal training courses teach umbilical vein cannulation for drug administration but this is not a standard for prehospital training protocols. Intraosseous (IO) infusion lines may be used in this population and are more familiar to prehospital providers. Ensure that IO needles are available in all prepared pediatric equipment packs. The usual sites, anterior proximal tibia and distal femur, are still recommended with attention to avoiding the joint space. In very small infants, you may substitute a 20-gauge needle for the IO needle. These infants have small bones and fracture may occur from overzealous placement.

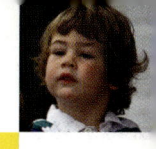

Epinephrine is the mainstay of drug therapy in this pediatric patient population at a concentration of 1:10,000. The dosing is 0.01 to 0.03 mg/kg via the IV route. Higher doses are not recommended and have been associated with hypertensive emergency, intracranial hemorrhage, and worsening cardiac function secondary to increased systemic resistance. Furthermore, endotracheal dosing of epinephrine has been shown to be largely ineffective; however, you may try doses of 0.1 mg/kg of the 1:10,000 preparation while securing another site of access. Doses may be repeated at 3- to 5-minute intervals, while recognizing that 10 minutes of adequate resuscitation without response is cause for ceasing resuscitation efforts.

You may consider volume expansion if the infant appears to have weak, thready pulses with clammy, pale skin and does not respond to other measures. Isotonic crystalloid solutions are recommended at 10 mL/kg given over 5 to 10 minutes. The commonly used isotonic fluid is normal saline, but other medically approved crystalloids are acceptable. Newly born babies with documented blood loss from placenta previa, abruption, or trauma benefit from O negative blood. There is no current literature on the use of the new synthetic blood products in this pediatric patient population.

Narcan (naloxone) is not recommended for prehospital use for the newly born infant because of the risk of seizure. The danger in use of Narcan in infants of drug-addicted mothers outweighs any benefit over bag-valve-mask ventilation for apnea. Also, though Narcan is given via endotracheal intubation in other age groups, it is only recommended to be administered intravenously or intramuscularly in this age group for select babies whose mothers were given a dose of narcotics prior to delivery in the hospital. Atropine does not have a code indication in the newly born infant.

Neonatal Resuscitation Inverted Pyramid

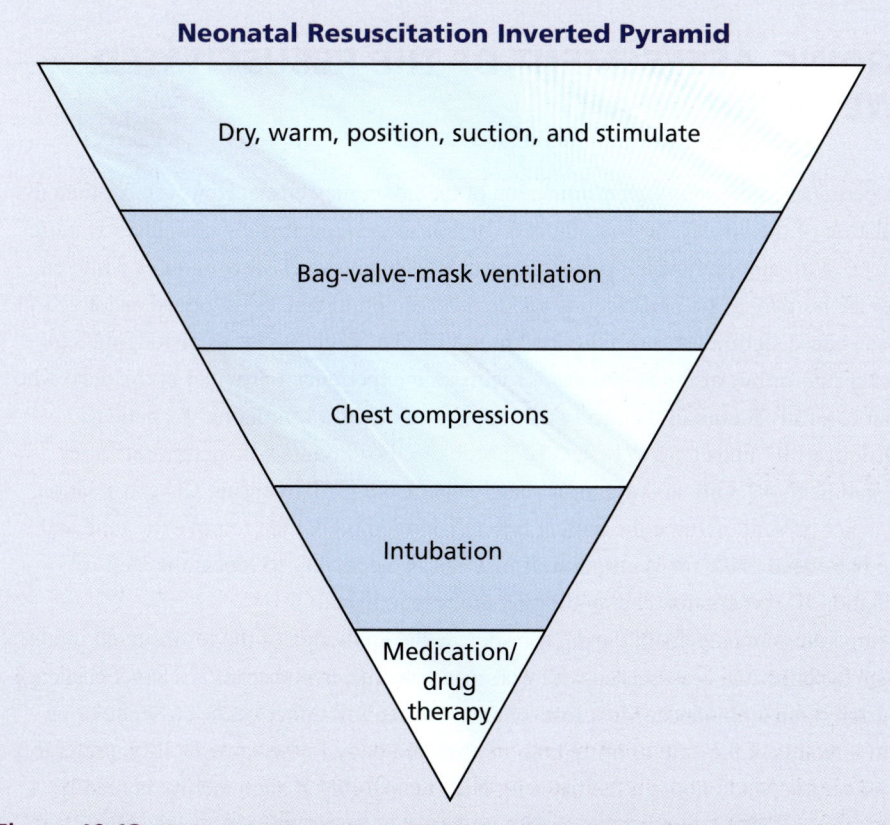

- Dry, warm, position, suction, and stimulate
- Bag-valve-mask ventilation
- Chest compressions
- Intubation
- Medication/drug therapy

Figure 19.13 *Only a small fraction of infants will require IV cannulation and drug therapy, as noted in the neonatal resuscitation inverted pyramid.*

Trauma in the Newborn

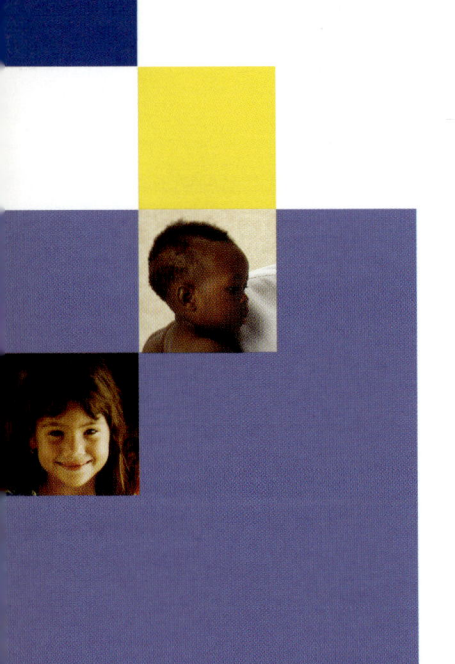

Hypoglycemia, on the other hand, is a common problem in any critically ill neonate or child because of minimal glycogen stores, which are rapidly depleted during stress. The normal blood sugar level for a newly born infant is 40 mg/dL. There is data that hypoglycemia is related to poor outcome but there is no current recommended range to maintain the blood sugar. Those infants with blood glucose levels less than 40 mg/dL should receive 4 mL/kg of 10 percent dextrose IV.

Sodium bicarbonate administration is considered controversial. It is not routinely recommended in the resuscitative phase by the AHA but has indications for judicious use in the post-resuscitative phase at 2 mEq/kg doses (4.2 percent concentration) given no faster than 1 mEq/kg per dose. The European Resuscitation Council recommends administration of sodium bicarbonate if chest compressions are not successful in the resuscitative phase. There may be some benefit in the unwitnessed birth of a prehospital, cold-stressed, depressed infant as this patient would have a greater burden of lactic acidosis.

For infants who respond to drug therapy, once the heart rate rises above 60 bpm, you may cease chest compressions. As the infant's respiratory effort improves, you may wean bag-valve-mask ventilation to 100 percent oxygen delivered by blow-by method. You may undertake post-resuscitative measures such as a glucose check. Infants who do not respond to epinephrine and volume expansion have a poor prognosis but should receive 10 minutes of effective treatment. As these recommendations were written for the in-hospital environment, it may be of value to continue resuscitative efforts all the way to the hospital as long as it does not pose safety concerns to the providers or jeopardize care of other patients in a large multiple casualty event. Parents deal better with the death of their children if they feel everything was done, including resuscitation attempts by the emergency physician and other hospital personnel.

ONGOING ASSESSMENT OF THE RESUSCITATED NEWLY BORN INFANT

If time permits, a more thorough examination of the infant may ensue. However, continuous reevaluation of the airway, airway adjuncts, breath sounds, perfusion, and pulses is more important. With any prehospital patient, repeat assessments every few minutes while en route to the hospital. Care in packaging and transfer are important, as dislodged endotracheal tubes can cause significant morbidity and mortality. The highest risk of dislodging a tube is transfer into or out of the ambulance or with an inexperienced provider at the head who may not carefully maintain the head position and tube while ventilating the patient.

Dislodged IO lines tend to be less of a problem. For infants who deteriorate after initial stabilization, think airway. Immediately check the ETT to ensure CO_2 exhalation. If this is not present, assume the patient has a dislodged tube, then remove the tube and use the bag-valve mask for ventilation. It may not be necessary to repeat the steps of resuscitation if oxygenation and ventilation are reestablished.

Temperature management during transport is the challenge of the resuscitated infant. Although hyperthermia is associated with worsened outcome, hypothermia is a larger challenge in the back of an ambulance. Most resuscitative efforts will either occur on scene or en route to a facility. Take care to bring both mother and baby to the same facility, preferably at the same time, and choose a facility with NICU capability if such facility is readily available. Rapid NICU care is associated with better outcomes for these sick infants.

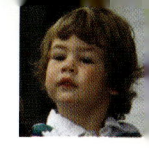

Infants who did not require any resuscitation beyond drying, warming, and suctioning may be transported to hospitals that offer routine obstetrical services and newborn nurseries.

If either mother or baby requires Level I trauma care, immediate transport to a Level I Trauma Center with obstetrical and neonatal resources is indicated. Level I Trauma Centers have access to obstetricians, neonatologists, trauma surgeons, and surgical subspecialists for infants and adults. A timely call to the facility from the field with assessments of both mother and infant will allow time for assembly of the specialized personnel needed for the care of each patient. If the mother is in the same ambulance with the infant, it is appropriate to provide a quick and truthful appraisal of the infant's condition to the mother prior to hospital notification so she asks questions and digests the information before she hears her infant's condition discussed with the receiving facility. If the mother is present, it is important to carefully choose your words in describing the infant's condition without prognosticating outcome in giving the patient report, as your words will be remembered for a lifetime.

Case Study continued

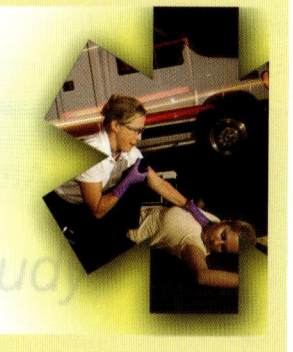

John, Susan and Bob have been called to a scene where a visibly pregnant woman in her 20s has been found with a knife in her abdomen, just below the umbilicus. Police assure the team that she is the only person in the house.

The team, led by John, assesses the situation as load-and-go. Susan immediately provides oxygen while Bob prepares a long board and John performs an ITLS Primary Survey. John notes that the patient is pale, with a thin, rapid pulse. She is breathing quickly and very shallowly. There is very little blood around the knife wound, but her underwear is blood-soaked. The infant is palpable above the umbilicus. The team quickly rolls the patient onto the long board and prepares to take her to the ambulance. Just as they get to ambulance, the patient goes into labor. The team starts two large-bore IVs, and John calls medical direction to report the situation. En route to the hospital, a baby boy is delivered.

Bob and Susan immediately suction the infant, who cries rather weakly, but does pink up. The infant is examined and does not appear to have been stabbed. He is quickly wrapped in warm blankets and given supplemental oxygen. Under instructions from medical direction, the cord is clamped and cut. The mother, although still pale, appears to be in less pain.

Trauma in the Newborn

After they arrive at the hospital, the baby is taken to the NICU, is found to have no injuries, and eventually does well. The mother is rushed to surgery where her lacerated uterus is repaired. She requires several blood transfusions, but she too survives to take her baby boy home.

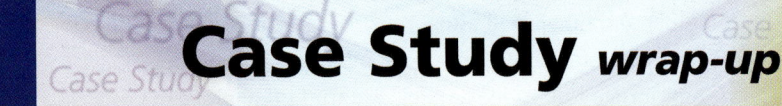

Case Study wrap-up

Assessing and treating a pregnant trauma victim poses additional challenges as the well-being of the unborn child has to be considered as well as the mother's. The best supportive care for the fetus is aggressive optimal management of the mother. Identifying the load-and-go situation from the ITLS patient assessment procedure, prompt oxygenation of the mother, and IV fluid resuscitation en route to hospital resulted in a good outcome for both the mother and newly born baby.

SUMMARY

1. When providing optimal care both for the pregnant mother and the unborn fetus after an injury, it is important to recognize the life threats to the mother and address them promptly in the prehospital phase.
2. As both mother and child will need specialist care, the obstetric and neonatal teams should be alerted en route to hospital.

Recommended Reading

American Heart Association. *Neonatal Resuscitation Textbook*, 5th ed. Dallas: Author, 2006.

American Heart Association. "Neonatal Resuscitation Guidelines." *Circulation* 112 (2005): 185–195.

Colburn, Vicki. "Trauma in Pregnancy." *Journal of Perinatal and Neonatal Nursing* 13 (December 1999): 21–32.

Dean, Michael J., Raymond C. Koehler, Charles L. Schleien, Ivor Berkowitz, John R. Michael, Deborah Atchison, et al. "Age Related Effects of Compression Rate and Duration in Cardiopulmonary Resuscitation." *Journal of Applied Physiology* 168 (1990): 554–60.

Drost, Thomas F., et al. "Major Trauma in Pregnant Women: Maternal/Fetal Outcome." *The Journal of Trauma* 30 (1990): 574–8.

Ralston, Mark, Mary Fran Hazinski, Arno L. Zaritsky, Stephen M. Schexnayder, and Monica E. Kleinman, eds. *Pediatric Advanced Life Support Provider Manual*. Dallas: American Heart Association, 2007.

Kapoor, Sarin H. and Dutta Kapoor. "Neonatal Resuscitation." *Indian Journal of Critical Care Medicine* 11 (2007): 81–9.

Leone, Tina A., Wade Rich, and Neil N. Finer. "A Survey of Delivery Room Resuscitation Practices in the United States." *Pediatrics* 117 (2006): 164–175.

Morris, John D., et al. "Infant Survival after Caesarean Section for Trauma." *Annals of Surgery* 223 (1996): 481–91.

20 CHAPTER 20
Children with Special Health Care Needs

Sherri Kovach, RN, EMT-B
Ann Hoffman, RN, CPN

Objectives
Upon completion of this chapter, you should be able to:

1. Identify the unique aspects of children with special health care needs.

2. Describe the most common complications and emergency management of assistive devices such as tracheostomy tubes, central venous access devices, feeding tubes, and cerebral spinal fluid shunts.

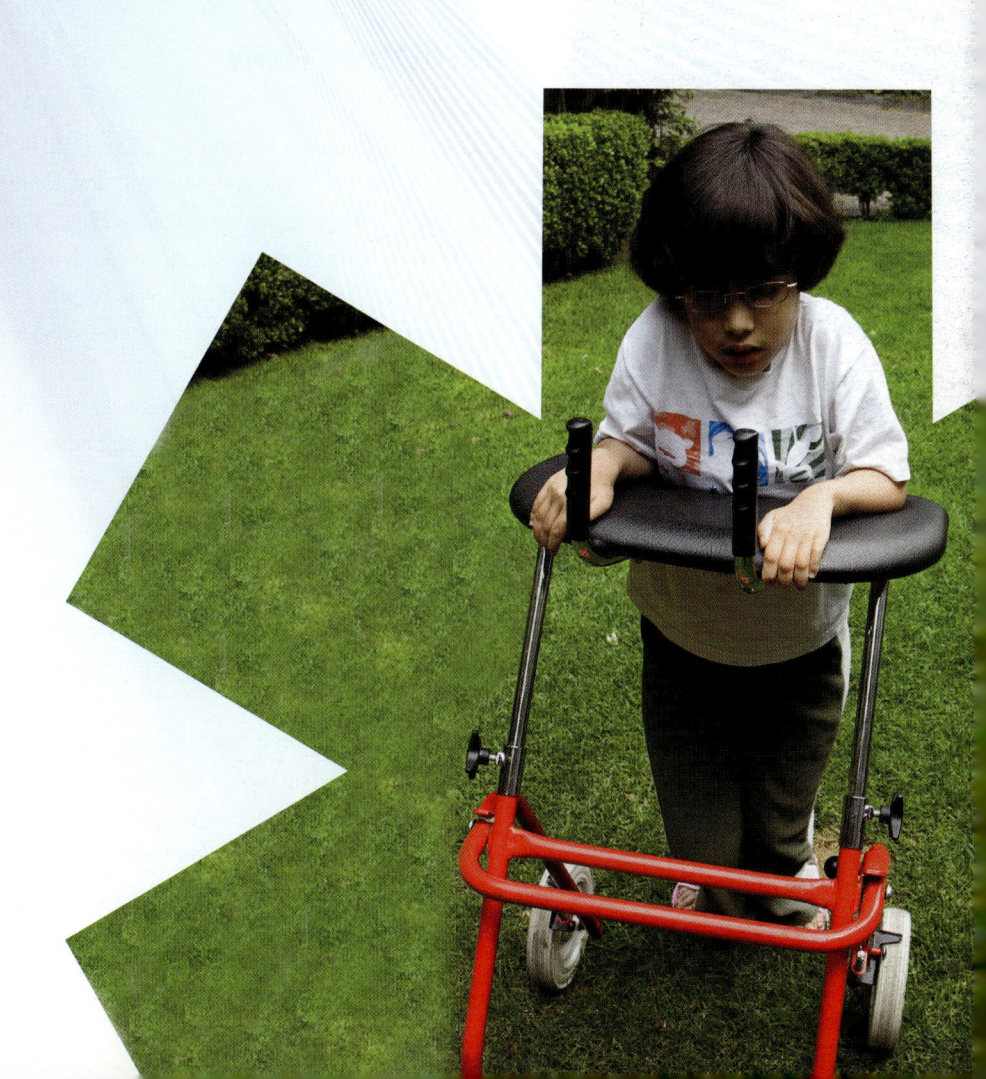

Case Study

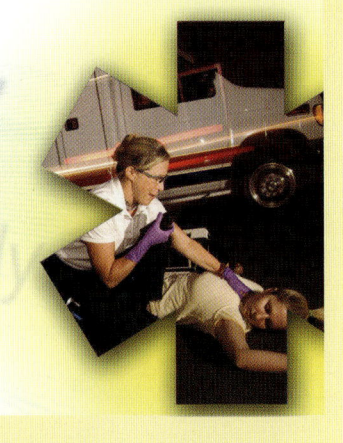

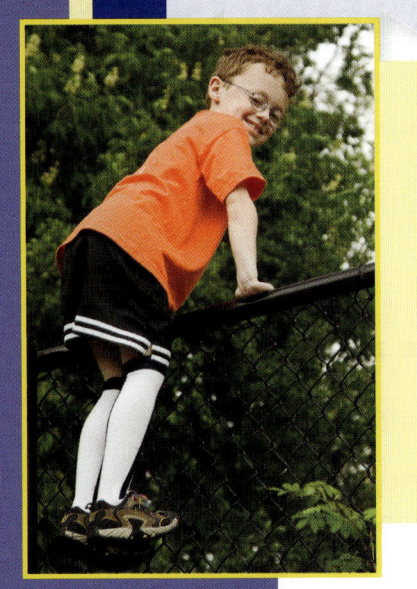

John, Susan, and Bob of the Emergency Transport System (ETS) are dispatched to a school for a 5-year-old child who has fallen and struck his head. This child has a history of ventriculoperitoneal (VP) shunt placement as an infant. The child has become progressively sleepy and has vomited several times. How should the team approach this patient? What specific concerns does this child raise? Keep these questions in mind as you read the chapter. Then, at the end of the chapter, find out how the rescuers completed this call.

INTRODUCTION

Children with special health care needs (CSHCN) are children who have, or are at increased risk for, a chronic physical, developmental, behavioral, or emotional condition, and who also require health-related services that generally go beyond that required by other children. According to an American Academy of Pediatrics Policy on care coordination for CSHCN, "advances in medicine have resulted in increased survival of children with special health care needs who require long-term services from a variety of health care professionals and organizations."

Because of these medical advances, there are a lot of children whose lives depend on highly technical equipment and special advanced care. These may include tracheotomy tubes, mechanical ventilators, central venous access devices, feeding tubes, cerebral spinal fluid (CSF) shunts, oxygen, aerosol nebulizers, apnea monitors, pulse oximeters, colostomy tubes, pacemakers, splints, and crutches or wheelchairs (Figs. 20.1, 20.2, 20.3). These children present with technical problems that prehospital providers are not accustomed to dealing with in the out-of-hospital environment. Also, many of these technology-assisted children (TAC) are living at home; they are no longer institutionalized like they were in the past.

Since these children have increased mobility, they are at risk for being involved in a traumatic event. The basics of pediatric trauma care including assessment, management, and spinal motion restriction are the same in this population of pediatric patients. The following section outlines some common mechanical devices and disease processes that you may encounter and you will need to address in addition to the trauma care.

> **PEARLS**
>
> The basics of pediatric trauma care including assessment, management, and spinal motion restriction are the same for children with special health care needs.

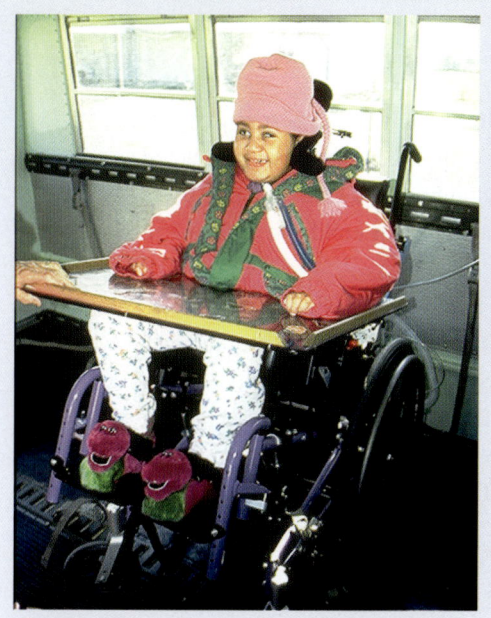

Figure 20.1 *Some technology-assisted children may use a wheelchair to assist their mobility.*

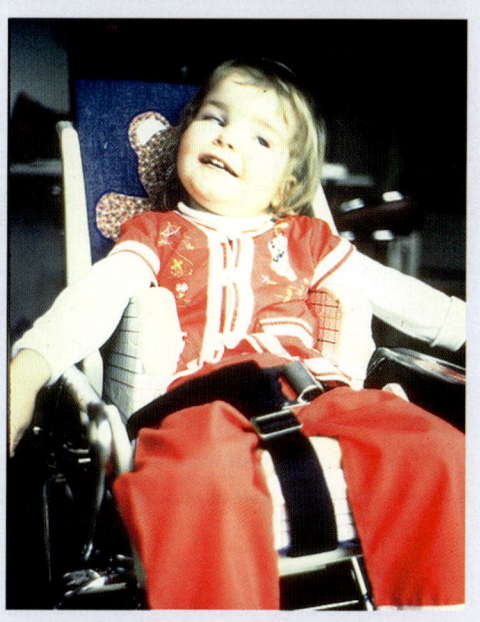

Figure 20.2 *Other children may not have visible equipment to indicate their special health care needs.*

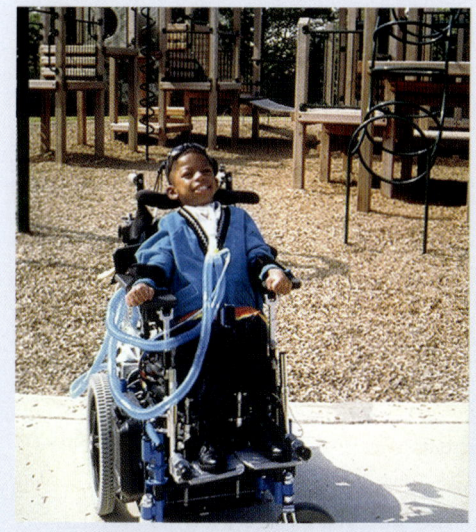

Figure 20.3 *Children requiring oxygen are another special health care need situation providers may encounter in the field.*

EVALUATION

As a prehospital provider, the phrases "children with special health care needs" or "technology-assisted children" are becoming more familiar. If one of these children is involved in a traumatic event, will you be able to provide the appropriate emergency care for his or her chronic medical condition(s)? Will you be able to properly use the life-sustaining equipment and/or troubleshoot problems related to that equipment?

When called to the scene of an injured CSHCN, your initial evaluation should include the Initial and Rapid Trauma Assessments. During your assessment, it is imperative to remember that these children often differ from typical children of the same age in baseline vitals signs, weight, height, and psychosocial development.

The parents or primary caregivers of CSHCN are often the best source of information regarding what is normal for their child. They may have completed specialized training for their child's medical condition, including Basic Life Support (BLS), and are knowledgable in the assessment and management of their child and his or her life-sustaining equipment.

Once you complete ITLS Primary Survey and initiate any appropriate interventions (e.g., oxygen), assess the functional status of the child's specialized equipment. Several of the most common devices used at home for CSHCN are summarized below. These explanations will address basic and advanced level skills for prehospital providers.

The potential complications are listed according to the **DOPE** mnemonic, which reminds providers to look at equipment. **DOPE** stands for the following equipment checks:

Displacement
Obstruction
Pneumothorax, pulmonary thromboembolus, or other complications
Equipment failure

CSHCN Medical Equipment

CSHCN medical equipment may include the following:

Tracheostomy Tube: A breathing tube placed into the trachea through an opening in the neck (stoma) (Figs. 20.4, 20.5).

Uses:
- Bypasses upper airway obstruction
- Provides assisted breathing support via a ventilator
- Removes secretions from the airway when gag/swallow reflexes are ineffective

Types:
- Uncuffed: For infants and young children
- Cuffed: For children > eight years of age
- Fenestrated: Has a hole in the curve of the tube that redirects airflow through the vocal cords to permit talking
- Single lumen or double lumen: Has an inner cannula that can be removed and cleaned

---

PEARLS

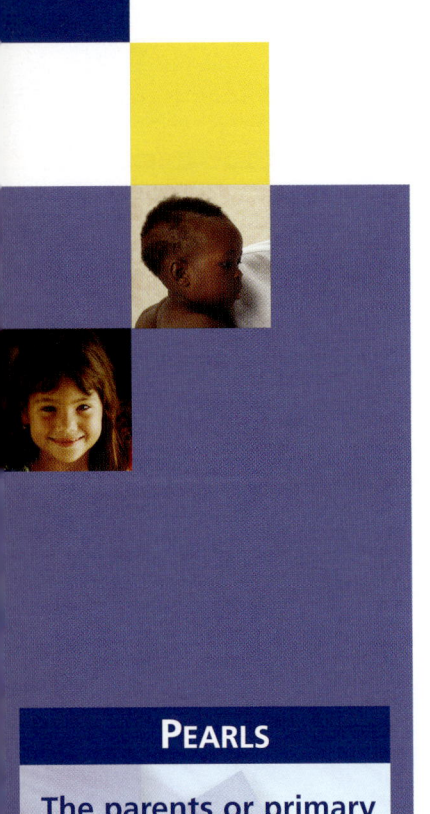

The parents or primary caregivers of children with special health care needs are often the best source of information regarding what is normal for their child.

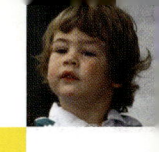

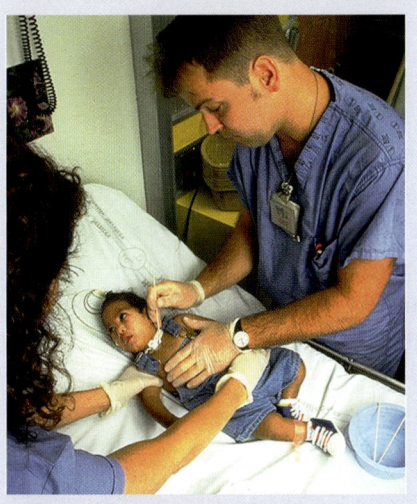

Figure 20.4 *An infant with a tracheostomy tube inserted.*

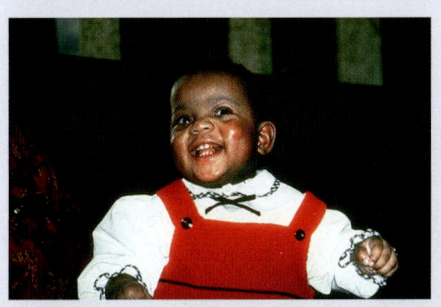

Figure 20.5 *A child with a tracheostomy tube that cannot readily be seen. Be sure to thoroughly check patients for CSHCN equipment.*

Evaluate for DOPE and infection:
  Displaced: Total or partial dislodged tube
  Obstructed: By mucous, blood, or a foreign body
  Pulmonary problems: Aspiration; pneumothorax; pneumonia; bronchospasm
  Equipment: Lack of oxygen; ventilator malfunction; kinked tubing

Treatment:

Basic (BLS)
- If there is no ventilator, administer oxygen via mask or bag-valve mask, or assist ventilation to the tracheostomy tube. Note that children with chronic lung disease may be difficult to ventilate.
- If a ventilator is in use, disconnect and attempt bag-valve-mask ventilation via the tracheostomy tube or an infant mask over the stoma. Call for ALS backup.
- Suction for no more than 10 seconds. For thick secretions, instill 1 mL of saline between suctioning attempts. Insert the suction catheter only 2 to 3 inches (5 to 8 cm).
- If ventilation cannot be achieved, plug the tracheostomy opening and ventilate via the mouth/nose with bag-valve-mask ventilation.

Children with Special Health Care Needs

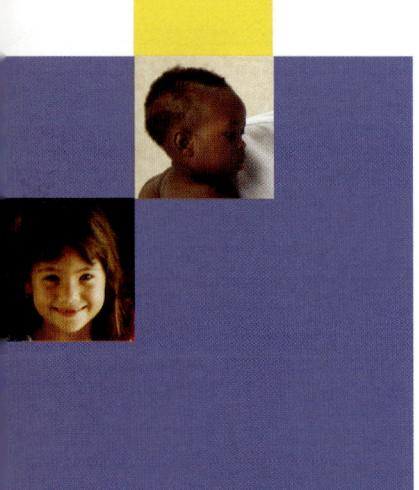

Advanced (ALS)
- If the above treatments fail, deflate the balloon and use a bag-valve mask on the face. If local protocols allow, remove the tracheostomy tube and reinsert a new tracheostomy tube or endotracheal tube of the same size.
- For difficult tracheostomy tube insertion, consider using a suction catheter through the tube. Use a catheter to probe the opening, sliding the tube over the catheter into the stoma, and then remove the catheter.

Central Venous Access Devices (VADs): An intravenous (IV) catheter with the tip in central circulation (superior/inferior vena cava or right atrium) (Fig. 20.6).

Uses:
- Administration of nutrition, medication, and/or blood
- Blood draws

Types:
- **Nontunneled:** Peripherally inserted central catheter (PICC)
- **Tunneled:** Single/multi-lumen catheters (Broviac®, Hickman®)
- **Totally implanted:** Subcutaneous infusion port (SIP), sometimes known as an Impantofix® or Mediport®. These require a specialized Huber needle and sterility to access. Standard hypodermic needles, when inserted into the port, may damage the septum.

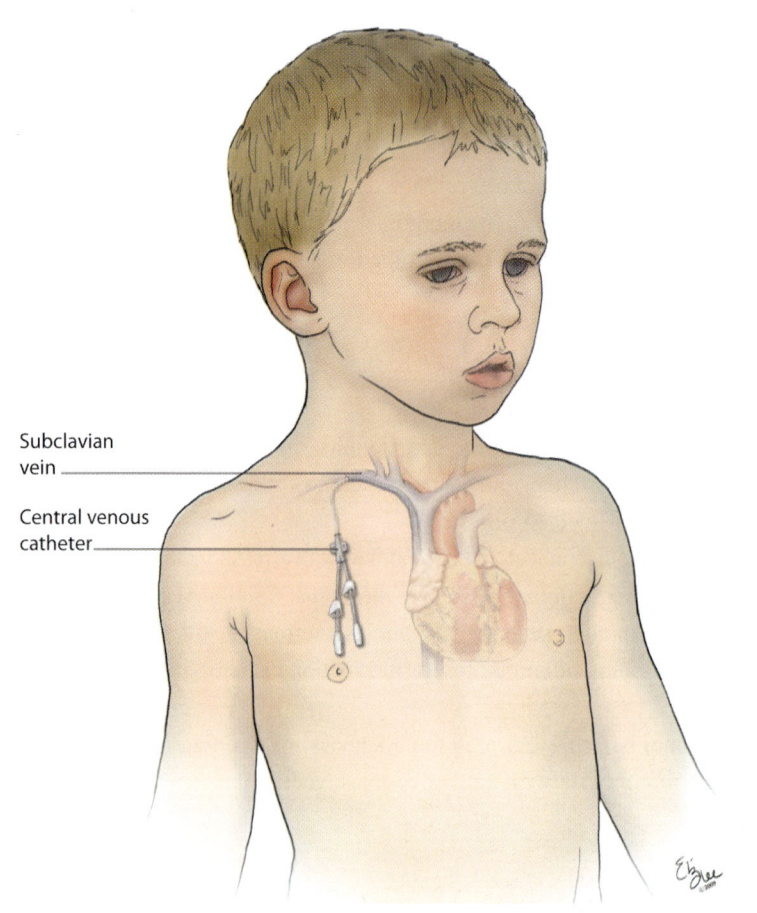

Figure 20.6 *The anatomy and position of a central venous catheter*

Evaluate for DOPE and infection:

Displaced: Partial or total dislodgement from vein

Obstructed: By kinked tubing, or by blood, protein, or crystallized medication

Pulmonary problems: Pneumothorax; pulmonary embolism

Pericardial tamponade: Perforation or migration of the catheter, causing fluid in the pericardial sac

Equipment: Separation or damage to tubing or reservoir

Treatment:

Basic (BLS)
- If bleeding occurs, direct pressure at the site.
- If leaking occurs, clamp the tubing.

Advanced (ALS)
- Aspirate or flush as directed by medical direction or protocol.
- In a stable patient, transport.
- In an unstable patient with functional access, contact medical control regarding use of access.
- In an unstable patient without functional access, administer IV/IO fluids.

Feeding Catheters: A tube providing nutritional supplements to children who cannot take food by mouth (Fig. 20.7)

Uses:
- Total or enhanced feeding and/or medication administration

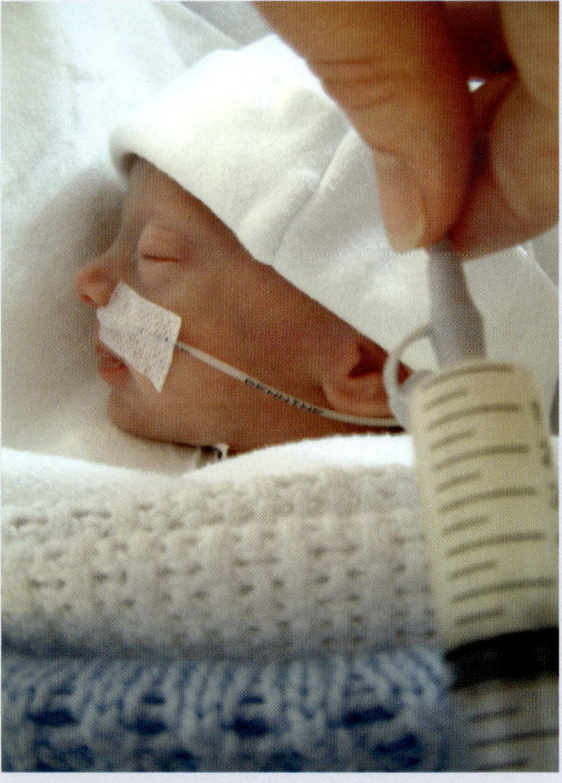

Figure 20.7 *An infant with a nasogastric feeding tube.*

Children with Special Health Care Needs

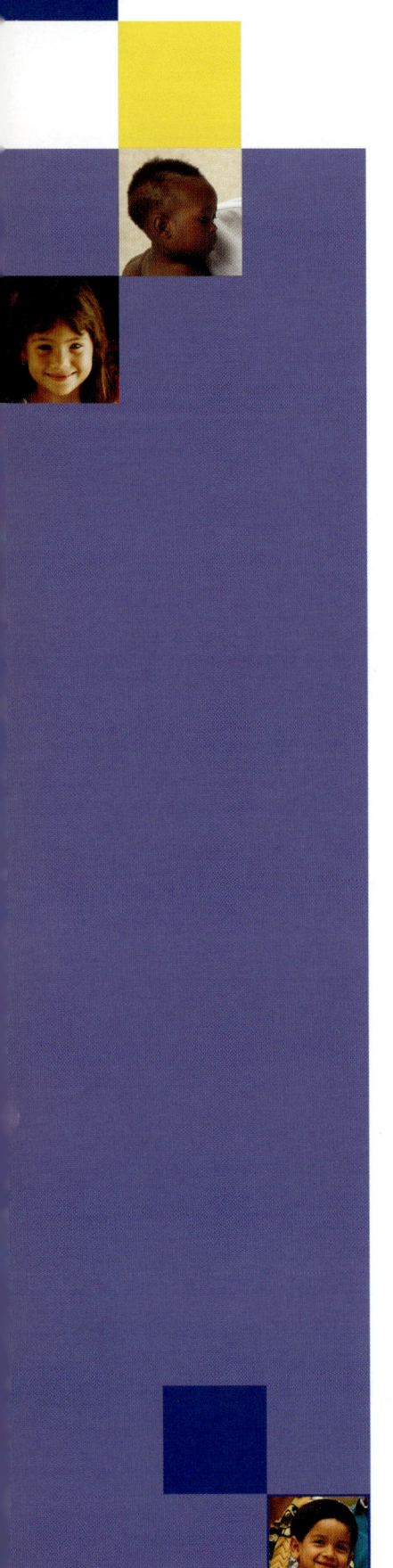

Types:
- **Nasal/oral:** Inserted by physician or parents, for short-term use.
    1. **Nasogastric (NG):** Nose to stomach
    2. **Orogastric (OG):** Mouth to stomach
    3. **Nasojejunal (NJ):** Nose to small intestine (placed by physician)
- **Gastric:** Surgically implanted, for long-term use.
    1. **Catheter type (gastrostomy [G Tube] or jejunostomy [J Tube] tube):** Vent by unclamping the feeding port and attaching a syringe.
    2. **MICKEY button:** Has an antireflux valve. A special adaptor is necessary to vent/decompress the stomach or deliver feedings. Parents will have the adaptor. This may be a G tube, J tube, or both.

Evaluate for DOPE and infection:

Displaced: Partial or total dislodgement of the tube
Obstructed: By blood, abdominal tissue, or crystallized food solution or medication
Peritonitis or **P**erforation: Of the stomach or bowel
Equipment: Kinked tubing; feeding pump failure

Treatment:

Basic (BLS)
- Always stop the feeding and turn off the pump.
- If bleeding occurs, direct pressure at the site. Tape the partially dislodged tube in place.
- If the tube is dislodged, place a dry, sterile dressing over the stoma.
- Transport for evaluation and/or reinsertion of the tube. The stoma can close off within hours. Vent the tube in cases of abdominal distention or vomiting.
- Ask parents for an appropriately sized syringe or tubing adaptor for venting.

Advanced (ALS)
- Aspirate or flush as directed by protocol.
- Administer IV/IO fluids with signs of shock.

Ventriculoperitoneal Shunts: A shunt that travels from the lateral ventricle through the skull to the subcutaneous tissue, runs posteriorly to the ear, and then continues subcutaneously to the abdominal cavity, where the cerebrospinal fluid drains into the peritoneal cavity (Fig. 20.8).

Uses:
- Drains excess cerebral spinal fluid from the brain

Types:
- Polyethylene tubing (catheter) that drains fluid into the abdomen or heart; may or may not have a palpable valve.

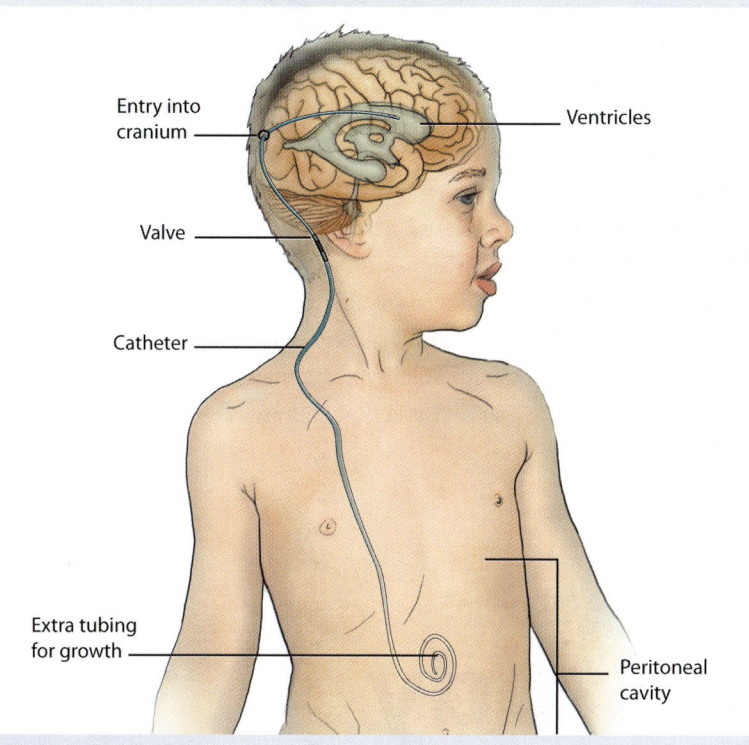

Figure 20.8 *A ventriculoperitoneal shunt drains excess fluid from the brain into the peritoneal cavity of the abdomen.*

Evaluation for DOPE and infection:
    Displaced: Movement of the catheter tip into the abdominal or heart lining
    Obstucted: Narrow tubing may become clotted with blood or protein, or tubing could become kinked causing fluid not to drain properly
    Peritonitis/**P**erforation/**P**seudocyst: Of the stomach or bowel
    Equipment: Damaged, separated, or kinked tubing or valve reservoir

Treatment:

Basic and Advanced (BLS/ALS)
- Administer oxygen as needed.
- Treat as you would any patient with suspected increased intracranial pressure (Table 20.1).
- If neurologic status is altered or there is a change from the baseline: Transport with the head elevated; administer supplemental oxygen; use a cardiac monitor; and reassess frequently and carefully.

Table 20.1: Signs and Symptoms of Increased Intracranial Pressure

- Headache
- Seizures
- Irritability
- Bulging fontanel
- Lethargy

Children with Special Health Care Needs

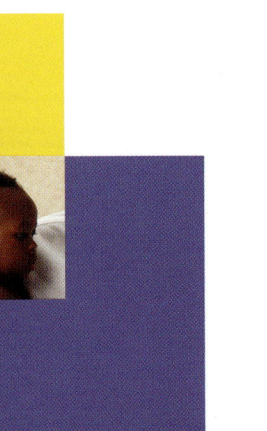

- If altered mental status presents (per the parents' assessment), pupils are equal and reactive, and normal vital signs are present: Transport with the patient's head elevated, administer supplemental oxygenation; do not hyperventilate if bag-valve-mask ventilation is indicated; use a cardiac monitor; and assess closely.
- If altered mental status presents and there are signs of impending herniation (such as unresponsive with unequal pupils, fixed or dilated pupils, or increased BP with decreased HR and irregular respirations [Cushing's triad]): Transport with the patient's head elevated; use bag-valve-mask ventilation with mild hyperventilation; apply a cardiac monitor; and frequently reassess. Note that hyperventilation may cause ischemia because of extreme vasoconstriction.

Case Study continued

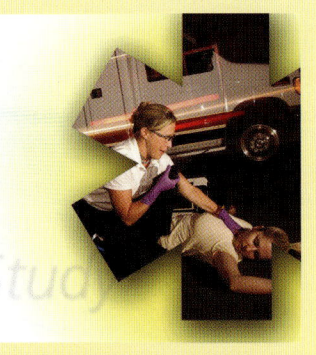

John, Susan, and Bob of the Emergency Transport System (ETS) have been dispatched to a school for a 5-year-old child with a history of ventriculoperitoneal (VP) shunt placement as an infant. The child has reportedly fallen and struck his head. Upon arrival to the scene, the team finds that the child is very sleepy but arousable. The child's airway is open and his breathing is regular. The child's heart rate is 52 bpm and his blood pressure is 120/80. The child is given 100 percent oxygen, and spinal motion restriction is applied. An IV is started and the child is placed on a monitor for transport with the head of the backboard elevated to the nearest trauma center. After a thorough examination at the hospital, the VP shunt is found to be disconnected and the child has developed enlarged ventricles. The child required emergency surgery and ultimately has a complete recovery.

Case Study *wrap-up*

Advances in medicine have resulted in increased survival of children with special health care needs who require long-term services from a variety of health care professionals and organizations. Because of these medical advances, there are a lot of children in our communities whose lives depend on highly technical equipment and special advanced care.

In the case scenario above, the child had a VP shunt in place that became disconnected secondary to minor head trauma. Failure to recognize the possibility of this condition may lead to rapidly increasing intracranial pressure and devastating consequences for the child.

Adhering to the ITLS patient assessment skills combined with evaluation of DOPE and infection will ensure that optimum care has been given to the child.

SUMMARY

1. The Initial and Rapid Assessments should be performed exactly as on any other injured child.
2. Manage immediate life threats identified in the assessment.
3. Oxygen is always administered.
4. CSHCN are highly susceptible to acute medical problems involving their airway, breathing and circulation because of underlying chronic illnesses.
5. Prehospital providers must have a low threshold for transport because significant changes in these children can be subtle.
6. Bring all assistive devices to the hospital with the patient. Be sure you can provide electrical power during transport.
7. Parents and caregivers are important sources of information and should be included in all aspects of their child's care.
8. When transporting these patients, remember they may not be able to lay flat and may need pillows or blankets to assist with positioning of spastic or hypertonic extremities.
9. These patients are prone to skeletal demineralization and are at increased risk for pathologic fractures.
10. Elicit the advice of the parent or caregiver for how to best secure this patient for a safe and comfortable transport.
11. Patients that are dependent upon enteral or IV nutrition may become hypoglycemic when feeds or IV nutrition are turned off during resuscitation or for prolonged transport. Glucose levels need to be monitored closely.

Recommended Reading

Adirim, Terry and Elizabeth Smith. *Special Children's Outreach and Prehospital Education (SCOPE)*. Sudbury, M.A.: Jones & Bartlett, 2006.

American Academy of Pediatrics. "AAP Policy Statement Care Coordination: Integrating Health and Related Systems of Care for Children with Special Health Care Needs." *Pediatrics* 104 (1999): 978–81.

American Academy of Pediatrics. "Children with Special Health Care Needs." In *Pediatric Education for Prehospital Professionals*, 2nd ed., edited by Ronald A. Dieckmann. Sudbury, M.A.: Jones & Bartlett Publishers, 2006.

Emergency Nurses Association. *Core Curriculum for Pediatric Emergency Nursing*, 2nd ed. Sudbury, M.A.: Jones & Bartlett Publishers, 2003.

McPherson, Merle. "A New Definition of Children With Special Health Care Needs." *Pediatrics* 102 (July 1998): 137–9.

Newacheck, Paul W., et al. "An Epidemiologic Profile of Children with Special Health Care Needs." *Pediatrics* 102 (1998): 117.

Reynolds, Sally, Barbara DesGuin, Andrew Uyeda, et al. "Children with Chronic Conditions in a Pediatric Emergency Department." *Pediatric Emergency Care* 12 (June 1996): 166–8.

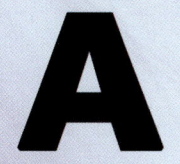

Appendix A
Use of Specialized Pediatric Care Centers

Howard A. Werman, MD, FACEP

Objectives
Upon completion of this chapter, you should be able to:

1. Discuss considerations and guidelines for transportation of children to specialized pediatric care centers.
2. Discuss indicators for high-risk pediatric patients.

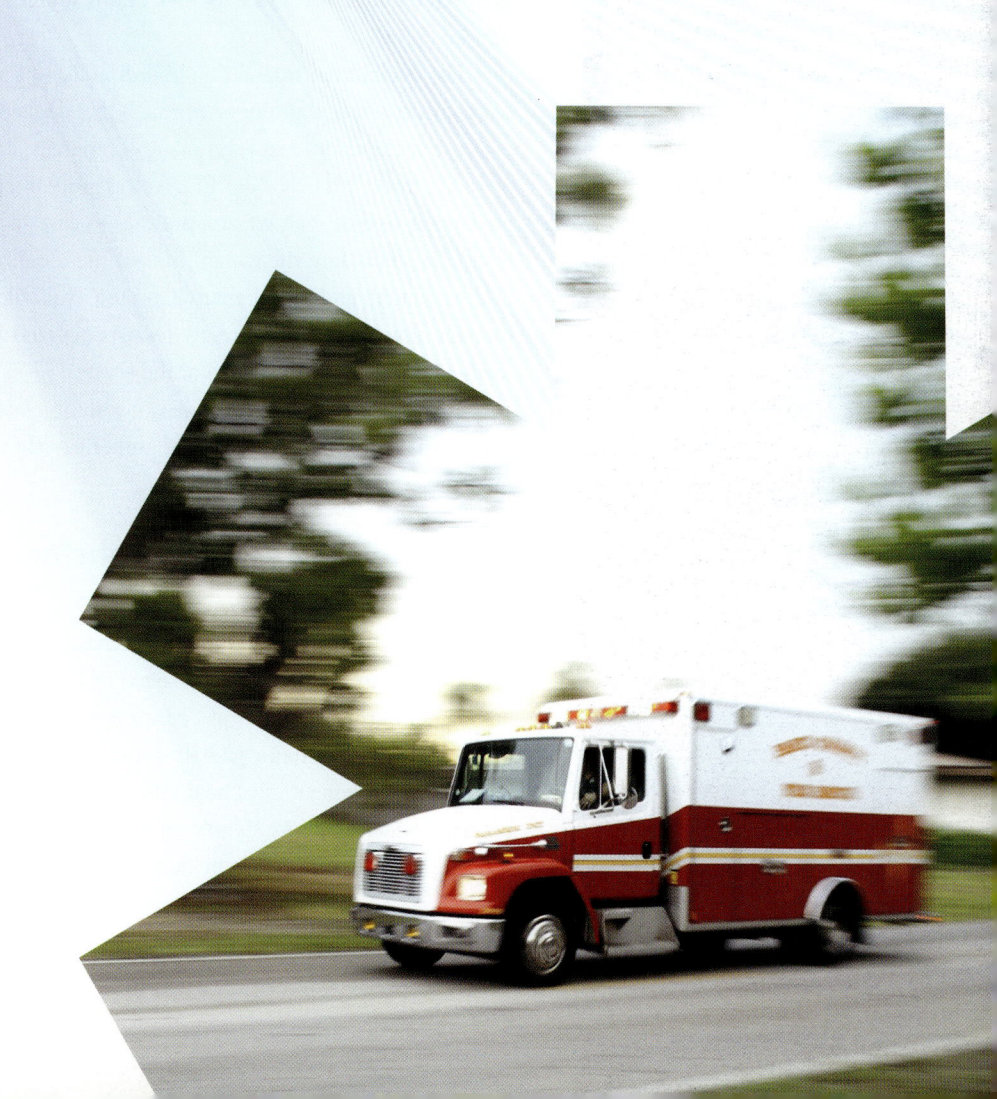

INTRODUCTION

The vast majority of injured children may be appropriately managed at local medical facilities. On occasion, it is necessary to transfer a child to a pediatric trauma center or pediatric burn center for more specialized care. The decision to transfer the child is often made after assessment and stabilization at the local emergency facility in consultation with the pediatric center. There are, however, instances in which direct transfer of the child from the scene of an injury to the pediatric trauma center or pediatric burn center is warranted. The goal of the prehospital component of the system is to minimize injury and optimize outcome by safely and rapidly transporting the injured child to the center most appropriately equipped and staffed to handle the pediatric patient's injury as defined by local, regional, state guidelines, or medical direction.

DECISION PROCESS

The decision to transfer a child directly to a specialized care facility is based on two very important principles: speed and specialization. Children with significant multisystem trauma have a better outcome when those injuries are rapidly stabilized and definitively managed. The "golden hour" of trauma care applies in children as well as adults! The child's outcome also depends on the ability of the facility to provide resources that meet the child's needs. Pediatric trauma centers and pediatric burn centers have been established to provide a high level of expertise and resources that are immediately available to any injured child.

The decision to transfer a child directly to a specialized care center is one that requires a great deal of preplanning. Approach this decision with careful deliberation. Carefully evaluate local resources, physician preferences, and an established relationship with a pediatric tertiary care center to develop guidelines. Work with your medical direction physicians to establish written policies to care for injured children. Consider area resources, including the capabilities of the local medical facilities, the location of pediatric trauma centers and burn centers, and the available methods of transport. The decision to transfer an injured child directly to a specialized facility should be made by the most medically experienced person at the scene.

Ideally, make the decision in consultation with on-line medical direction. In cases where this is not possible, written guidelines should be established by the emergency medical service medical director.

Suggested Criteria for Transfer

Table A.1 provides a partial list of mechanisms of injury that are critical for transport to a specialized care facility. The presence of these criteria, plus pediatric burns, near-drowning, and head injuries with loss of consciousness, indicate that the patient should go to a facility qualified to handle major pediatric trauma.

Clinical judgment must be used in every case. Some children who meet these criteria do not have evidence of any significant injury (overtriage). On the other hand, other children with seemingly little trauma show evidence of severe injury (undertriage).

PEARLS

The goal of prehospital care is to minimize injury and optimize outcome by safely and rapidly transporting an injured child to the center most appropriately equipped and staffed to handle the pediatric patient's injuries.

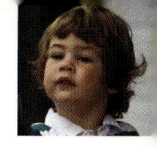

Table A.1: Suggested Criteria for Transfer to an Emergency Department Approved for Pediatrics or a Pediatric Trauma Center

Criteria
• Obstructed airway
• Need for an airway intervention
• Respiratory distress
• Shock
• Altered mental status
• Dilated pupil
• Glasgow Coma Scale <13

• Mechanisms of injury (less reliable indicators) associated with severe injuries:
  • Fall from height of 10 feet (3 meters) or more
  • Motor vehicle collision with fatalities
  • Ejection from an automobile in a MVC
  • In a MVC, significant intrusion into the passenger compartment
  • Hit by a car as a pedestrian or bicyclist
  • Fractures in more than one extremity
  • Significant injury to more than one organ system

> **PEARLS**
>
> **Pediatric transfer directly to a specialized care center requires a great deal of preplanning. Prehospital providers should be intimately involved in the process.**

Appropriate Mode of Transfer

When deciding where to transfer an injured child from the scene, you must select an appropriate method of transport. Two primary options are available: ground vehicles and helicopter. Select the mode of transport based on the distance and time to the specialty center, local resources, weather conditions, and skills of the transporting agency. As with the decision to transfer, establish direct consultation with medical direction or written protocol to provide guidance in determining the appropriate transport mode (Fig. A.1).

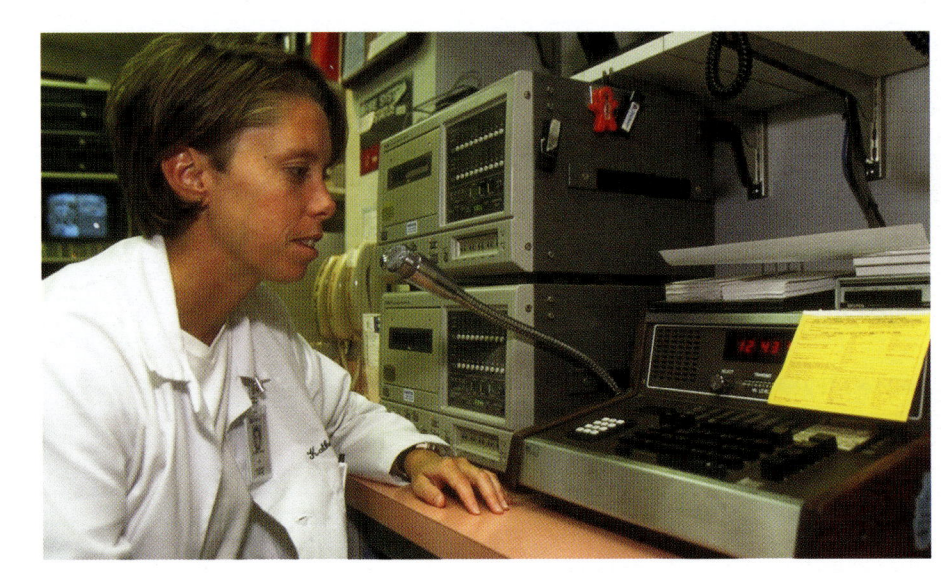

Figure A.1 *Providers should consult with medical direction to determine transfer procedures.*

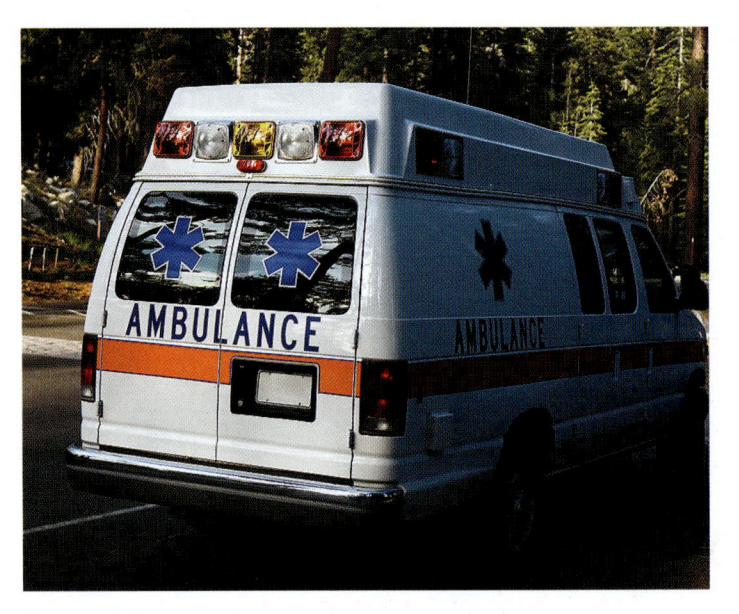

Figure A.2 *Ground transportation, such as an ambulance, is preferred when the transport distance and time are short.*

Transport by ground ambulance is preferred when the time and distance to the pediatric trauma center or pediatric burn center are short (Fig. A.2). In general, use ground ambulance for transport distances of less than 15 miles (24 km) or transport times of less than 30 minutes. Ground ambulance offers several advantages over helicopter transport. Ground transport is more cost-effective than air transport and is not generally affected by weather conditions. There is an orderly transfer of medical responsibility from the ground ambulance crew to the receiving physician when ground transport is used. There are also fewer space constraints in a ground ambulance.

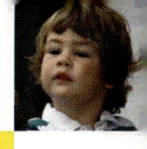

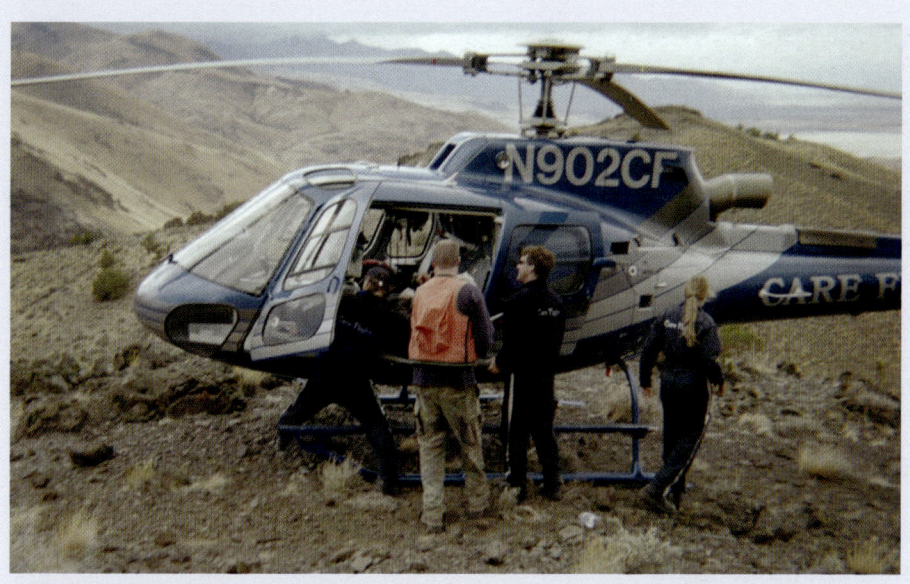

Figure A.3 *Helicopter transport should be used for transport distances of between 15 to 100 miles (24 to 161 km) or when transport time exceeds 30 minutes.*

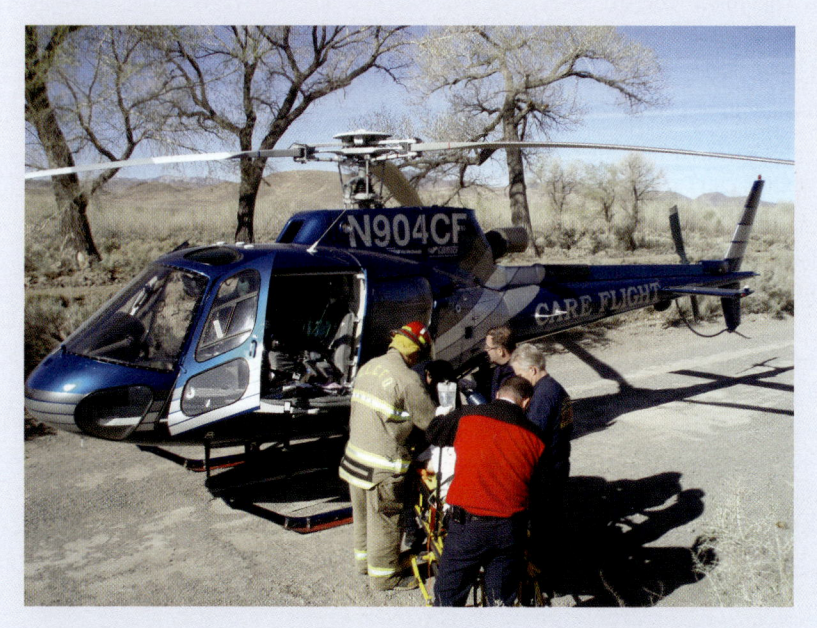

Figure A.4 *Helicopter transport may also be useful when the special skills of the crew are a consideration for the care of a pediatric patient.*

Helicopter transport is used for distances of between 15 and 100 miles (24 to 161 km) or when transport times exceed 30 minutes (Fig. A.3, A.4). Despite their limitations, helicopters are useful in situations in which speed and the special skills of the crew are a consideration for pediatric patient care. Airplane or fixed-wing transport is generally not used for direct scene transfer of children, except in the most rural environments. Airplanes are useful if the distance is in excess of 100 miles (161 km) or the weather conditions do not allow helicopter transfer. In these settings, transport the pediatric patient to the local emergency facility for initial treatment and stabilization while awaiting transport.

Use of Specialized Pediatric Care Centers

SUMMARY

1. Most children can be treated at the local emergency facility following a traumatic injury. Base any direct transfer to a pediatric trauma center on regional triage guidelines, availability of pediatric resources at the local emergency facility, or instructions from medical direction.
2. Establish guidelines for the direct transfer of significantly injured children from the scene.
3. The decision to transfer a child from the scene should be made by the person with the most medical experience on the scene in consultation with medical direction.
4. The mode of transport is determined by the time and distance to the pediatric specialty center as well as weather conditions and local resources.

Recommended Reading

American Academy of Pediatrics. "Guidelines for Air and Ground Transportation of Pediatric Patients." *Pediatrics* 78 (1986): 943–50.

American Academy of Pediatrics, Committee on Pediatric Emergency Medicine, American College of Critical Care Medicine, Society of Critical Care Medicine. "Consensus Report for Regionalization of Services for Critically Ill or Injured Children." *Pediatrics* 105 (January 2000): 152–5.

American College of Surgeons, Committee on Trauma. *Resources for Optimal Care of the Injured Patient*. Chicago: Author, 2006.

Hanson, James H. and Richard A. Orr. "The Air Medical Transfer Process of the Critically Ill or Injured Pediatric Patient." In *Principles and Direction of Air Medical Transport*, edited by Ira J. Blumen and Daniel L. Lemkin, 399–405. Salt Lake City, U.T.: Air Medical Physician Association, 2006.

Low, Ronald B. "Interfacility Transport." In *Prehospital Systems and Medical Oversight*, edited by Alexander E. Kuehl, 576–83. Dubuque, I.A.: National Association of EMS Physicians, Kendall/Hunt Publishing, 2002.

National Association of Emergency Medical Services Physicians. "Air Medical Dispatch: Guidelines for Scene Response." *Air Medical Journal* 13 (August 1994): 315–6.

B

Appendix B
Pediatric Trauma Triage and Multiple Casualty Incident Management

Roy L. Alson, PhD, MD, FACEP
Jim Augustine, MD, FACEP
David Maatman, NREMT-P/IC

Objectives

Upon completion of this chapter, you should be able to:

1. Discuss the differences between pediatric and adult major incidents.

2. Describe the process of managing pediatric casualties in a multiple casualty incident.

3. Describe the process of triage and communication for pediatric major incidents.

4. Discuss pediatric consent in major trauma incidents.

5. Discuss the psychological effects of the management of a pediatric major incident on victims, families, and prehospital providers.

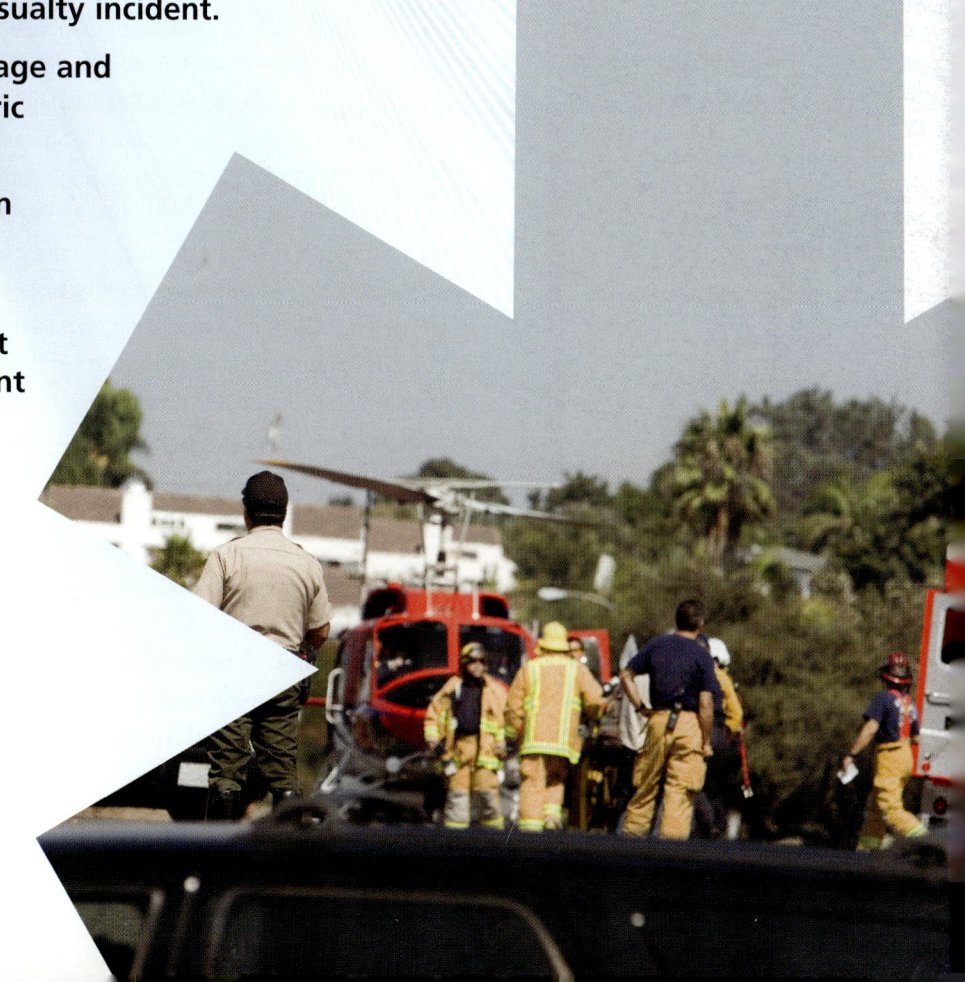

INTRODUCTION

Multiple casualty incidents often involve pediatric patients. While basic principles of a multiple casualty incident (MCI) are the same for adult and pediatric patients, there are certain aspects of the response that change with the presence of children. Pediatric patients may have different injuries and responses to injuries compared to the adult victim due to differences in anatomy and physiology. Events involving children offer distinctive management challenges. The mechanisms of pediatric injury are typically accidental, but children can be the victims of intentional violence and terrorism, as evidenced by the increasing number of school attacks and shootings.

Such events produce strong emotional responses from responsible adults and prehospital providers. A well-organized incident management system will permit an effective operation to take place, and then allow a confident evaluation and treatment of the pediatric trauma patient. The planning elements for major incidents for prehospital providers should be consistent with the National Incident Management System (NIMS), outlined in the National Response Framework.

Dealing with any major EMS incident, especially one involving multiple seriously injured children, requires a coordinated approach to facilitate both the medical and psychological evaluation of all of the involved children. The uniform approach to assessment, intervention, packaging, and transport methods, as taught in the Pediatric ITLS course, should be utilized to optimize efficiency and care.

PLANNING FOR PEDIATRIC MAJOR INCIDENTS

Any disaster event involves phases. In the pre-event phase, preplanning for an incident will ensure an effective and coordinated response to the event. Involve all levels of providers from first responders to providers in medical facilities in this planning. Identifying resources that will be available when an incident happens, developing dispatch and triage protocols, coordinating, and training all occur during this phase. Obtain necessary supplies for pediatric MCI and provide to response units. When located with other disaster supplies, ensure that these supplies are readily identifiable. The preplan process provides timely availability of all needed equipment, supplies, and personnel for the incident. In this phase, the EMS service and other community response agencies must assess the response through exercises and adjust the response plan based on the objective findings from such exercises. Risk identification (threat assessment) in the community must also include pediatric patients with special medical needs, as these types of patients are very resource-intensive. Remember that, while many multiple casualty events are relatively short term, other disasters such as storms or other events that disrupt the community might persist for days. Therefore, include provisions for additional personnel and supplies in disaster and MCI plans. Pediatric incidents will challenge communications resources more than general emergency responses. Include how to communicate with parents and families of the patients in pediatric plans. Early notification of treatment facilities is essential for a successful response. A robust communications plan is necessary. Include a Public Information Officer as an early priority in incident management strategies. You may even include one individual who has responsibility for notifying parents.

> **PEARLS**
> A well-organized incident management system will permit an effective operation and assist in a confident evaluation and treatment of the pediatric trauma patient.

> **PEARLS**
> The preplan process provides timely availability of all needed equipment, supplies, and personnel for the incident.

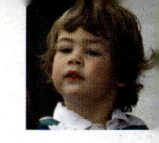

The National Response Framework specifies that an Incident Action Plan is built on four elements, with the acronym POST:

P – Priorities: regardless of the size or complexity of an event or incident, the fundamental priorities remain constant: life safety, incident stability, and conservation of property and the environment.
O – Objectives: statements of the desired outcomes or actions to achieve that are consistent with the priorities.
S – Strategies: action processes by which the objectives are met.
T – Tactics (or Tasks): specific activities that are implemented to achieve the identified strategies.

MANAGING PEDIATRIC MULTIPLE CASUALTY INCIDENTS

There are predictable incident types that will involve multiple pediatric trauma patients. Several common scenarios include: school bus collisions, chemical exposures in schools, motor vehicle collisions where a large number of children are in the same automobile, or exposure to an environmental poison. Other incidents include shooting incidents at schools and other public places in which children have been victims. The possibility of terrorism also exists.

The prehospital provider is challenged during these incidents to triage the pediatric patients with the most serious illness or injury from those who are upset, anxious, or manifesting psychological problems. Episodes of mass hysteria may occur with younger persons, with a large number of patients requesting evaluation and transportation. Resources may not be available to provide immediate transportation for all those who feel they are ill or injured. Their needs may compromise the care of those who have life-threatening injuries. In these circumstances, several incident management techniques are useful, as described in the following list.

1. Establish a member of the emergency response team who is in charge of the incident (Incident Command), and designate a Triage Group Leader. These individuals should direct all strategies and communications of the incident.
2. Physically separate potential patients, or those complaining of an illness or injury, from those who are uninjured as quickly as possible. Appropriately evaluate and triage all potential patients to prioritize further care.
3. Transport pediatric patients who are most seriously ill or injured away from the scene as rapidly as possible. Many experienced providers will prioritize pediatric patients for transportation before adult victims with a similar triage classification. If the event is large and there are many injured patients, you may need to establish a treatment area on site.
4. Appoint a prehospital provider with good communication skills to reassure the other juveniles at the scene, and try to prevent any panic reactions or undue anxiety. Ideally, sequester those that have minor injuries from the incident as soon as possible. You may find an authority recognized by the group, such as a school official, team leader, or school counselor valuable in reassuring the group and preventing undue anxiety.

> **PEARLS**
>
> Many experienced providers will prioritize pediatric patients for transportation before adult victims with a similar triage classification.

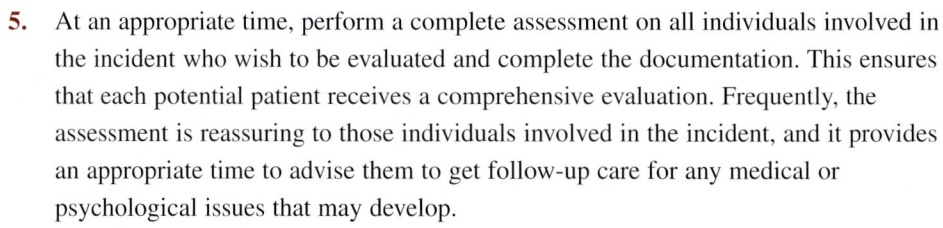

5. At an appropriate time, perform a complete assessment on all individuals involved in the incident who wish to be evaluated and complete the documentation. This ensures that each potential patient receives a comprehensive evaluation. Frequently, the assessment is reassuring to those individuals involved in the incident, and it provides an appropriate time to advise them to get follow-up care for any medical or psychological issues that may develop.

6. Appoint a prehospital leader with knowledge of the local hospitals to oversee transportation of patients and communications with the receiving hospital or hospitals. This person may be designated as the Transportation Group Leader. This individual has the important responsibility of tracking all patients removed from the scene by EMS. This information is vital when parents and other authorities seek notification of where to find the patients.

7. Designate a leader with excellent communication skills to interact with the media present at the scene, and with any officials of the school or other agency involved in the incident. This person is designated as the Public Information Officer (PIO). Establish a Joint Information Center, if needed, to integrate the release of information in a major incident.

Due to the different needs when pediatric patients are involved, manage major multiple casualty incidents according to established Incident Command System triage, treatment, and transportation management principles (Fig. B.1).

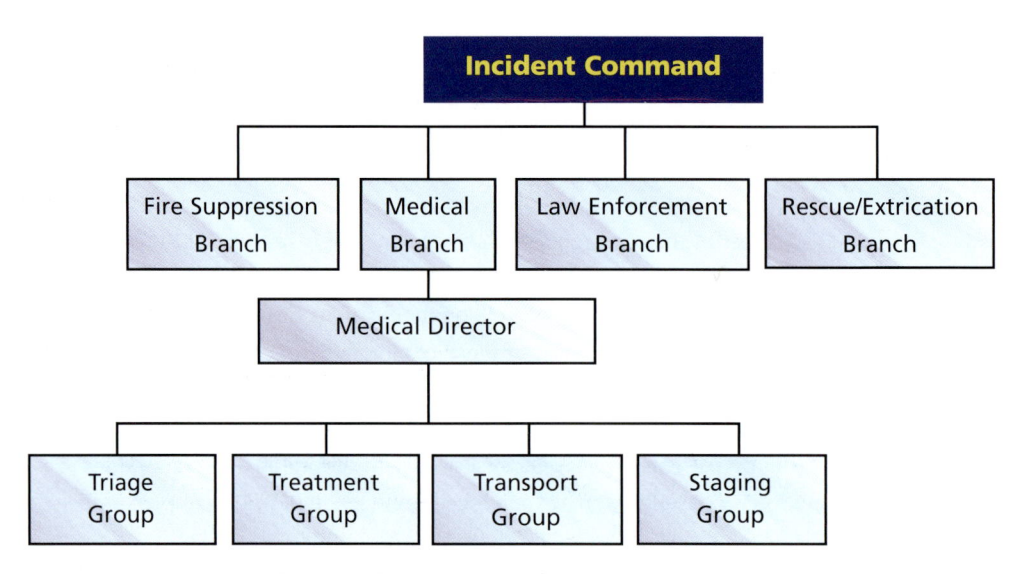

Figure B.1 *Medical Branch of the Incident Command System (ICS)*

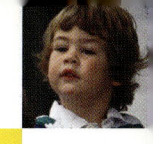

Triage Considerations

Triage is the process of sorting patients. This is something prehospital providers do on a daily basis, whether it involves deciding who is seen next in the emergency department, office, or clinic; which call the ambulance is sent to first; or which patient is treated or transported first by the prehospital team. In most cases, the priority is given to the most seriously injured or ill patient. Prehospital providers base this on their assessment of the patient, looking for immediate life threats and unstable vital signs, along with clues from the history and mechanism of injury.

There is no universally accepted triage scheme for mass casualties and disasters, nor is there any system that has been tested in real events and shown to be scientifically valid. Studies are underway that attempt to develop triage systems based upon documented patient outcomes. Thus, the current approach to triage is based upon a consensus model. It is recognized that disaster and MCI triage does differ from day-to-day operations. Disasters are defined by available resources; when demands exceed resources, rescuers begin to operate in a "disaster" mode. The premise is to do the "greatest good for the greatest number." This concept is often challenging for prehospital providers in that they are driven to provide care to those in need. When the event involves children, it is even harder because of the emotions pediatric patients evoke.

Assessment is made by "RPM" methodology using the respiratory status, perfusion status based on pulses, and the patient's mental status—the very same things that are assessed in the ITLS Primary Survey. Essentially, a patient who meets the criteria for "load and go" is a critical priority patient in a mass casualty situation (Table B.1).

> **PEARLS**
>
> Disaster assessment is made by "RPM": respiratory status, perfusion status based on pulses, and the patient's mental status—the same things that are assessed in the ITLS Primary Survey.

Table B.1: Triage Designations

Priority	Triage Class	Color Code	Intervention
1	Immediate	Red	Critical—likely to survive if simple care is given in minutes
2	Urgent	Yellow	Urgent—likely to survive if simple care is given in hours
3	Minor	Green	Critical—likely to survive even if care is delayed hours to days (walking wounded)
4	Deceased	Black	Expectant or Deceased

Some advocate inserting as the second class a catastrophic class (Priority 2, color blue), persons who will not survive without extensive and complex care. These patients would be placed in the "Expectant" category as shown in Table B.1.

Multiple tag systems have been developed to assist in this process. Many agencies use tear-off segments, bar codes, or colored cards to assist in identifying the triage class, and all have space for demographics, assessments, and interventions. Part of the problem is that each system may use different tags. Since most multiple casualty events involve multiple agencies working together, confusion can quickly happen. In order for prehospital providers to maintain familiarity with the tags, they must be simple to use, uniformly used across the operational area, and used regularly.

An important point to remember is that triage is a dynamic process. Patient condition can improve or deteriorate. Additional supplies or personnel may arrive at the event or additional patients may be located. Patients are usually triaged several times. Primary triage happens at the incident site and will determine who is transported first (or taken to the treatment area first). Secondary triage happens at the casualty collection point or treatment area and again prior to patient transport. Tertiary triage takes place at the treatment facility. The same sequence and guidelines are used at all of these levels of triage.

Triage Algorithm

The most commonly used triage algorithm in the United States is S.T.A.R.T., which was first developed by the Newport Beach Fire Department in the 1990s. In 1995, Dr. Lou Romig, a pediatric emergency physician, modified the algorithm to take into account that most pediatric cardiac arrests are respiratory in origin. In the adult triage sequence, an apneic patient in an MCI is classified as deceased (4, Black). With a pediatric patient who is apneic, ventilations are administered. If spontaneous respirations resume, the patient is considered critical (1, Red). If there is no response, the patient is considered deceased (4, Black). The Combined START – JumpSTART Algorithm is shown in Figure B.2.

The initial step in triage is to get the "Green" patients, or walking wounded, to move themselves to an area set aside by the prehospital providers as the minor area. Not all "Green" patients will follow the commands. For example, do not expect parents who are not hurt to leave an injured child. Patients with minor injuries can be taken to a site other than the emergency department when there are large numbers. Ensure that this site, an Alternate Care Facility (ACF), is staffed and equipped to assess and treat these injuries. In events that involve children, particularly those with violence, such as shootings, ensure that psychological support staff are present to help the victims and their families deal with the event. By moving the less acutely injured to the ACF, the system avoids overloading hospital emergency departments. In addition, it allows patients to meet with law enforcement, if necessary, and gives families a private and controlled environment in which they can be together. Coordination and planning for these types of pediatric events should include school officials, emergency management, fire, EMS, law enforcement, and medical and psychological support personnel.

Treatment Considerations

Overtriage is common in most multiple casualty events. Prehospital providers tend to be conservative so as not to miss any injuries. Overtriage can lead to overloading treatment areas and depletion of resources on site. It is important to treat only those injuries and conditions that require immediate treatment. In the field or in transport, do not carry out interventions that can be delayed until the patient reaches definitive care.

Treatment and transportation of pediatric trauma patients must proceed in a timely manner. Consider the climate, distance from hospital, and the patient's condition. In general, you should prioritize rapid packaging and transportation. Pediatric trauma patients will not tolerate the physical stress of a hostile environment, or the psychological rigor of hearing, seeing, and smelling the other operations occurring at the emergency scene.

Many pediatric trauma patients require spinal motion restriction (SMR). You must continually monitor young persons who are in SMR. Children in particular have a higher incidence of vomiting following any type of trauma, and, if spinal motion–restricted, may

---

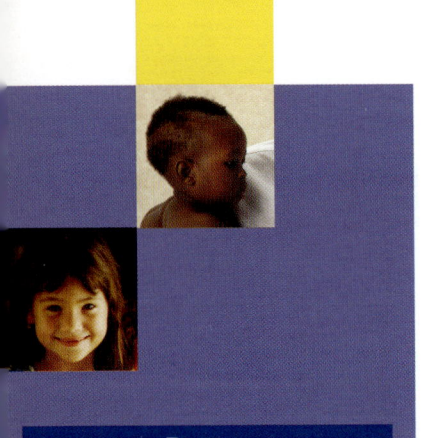

PEARLS

In the adult START triage sequence, an apneic patient in an MCI is classified as deceased (4, Black). With a pediatric patient who is apneic, ventilations are administered, and if spontaneous respirations resume, the patient is considered critical (1, Red). If there is no response, the patient is considered deceased (4, Black).

JumpSTART PEdiatric MCI Triage©

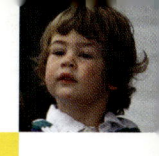

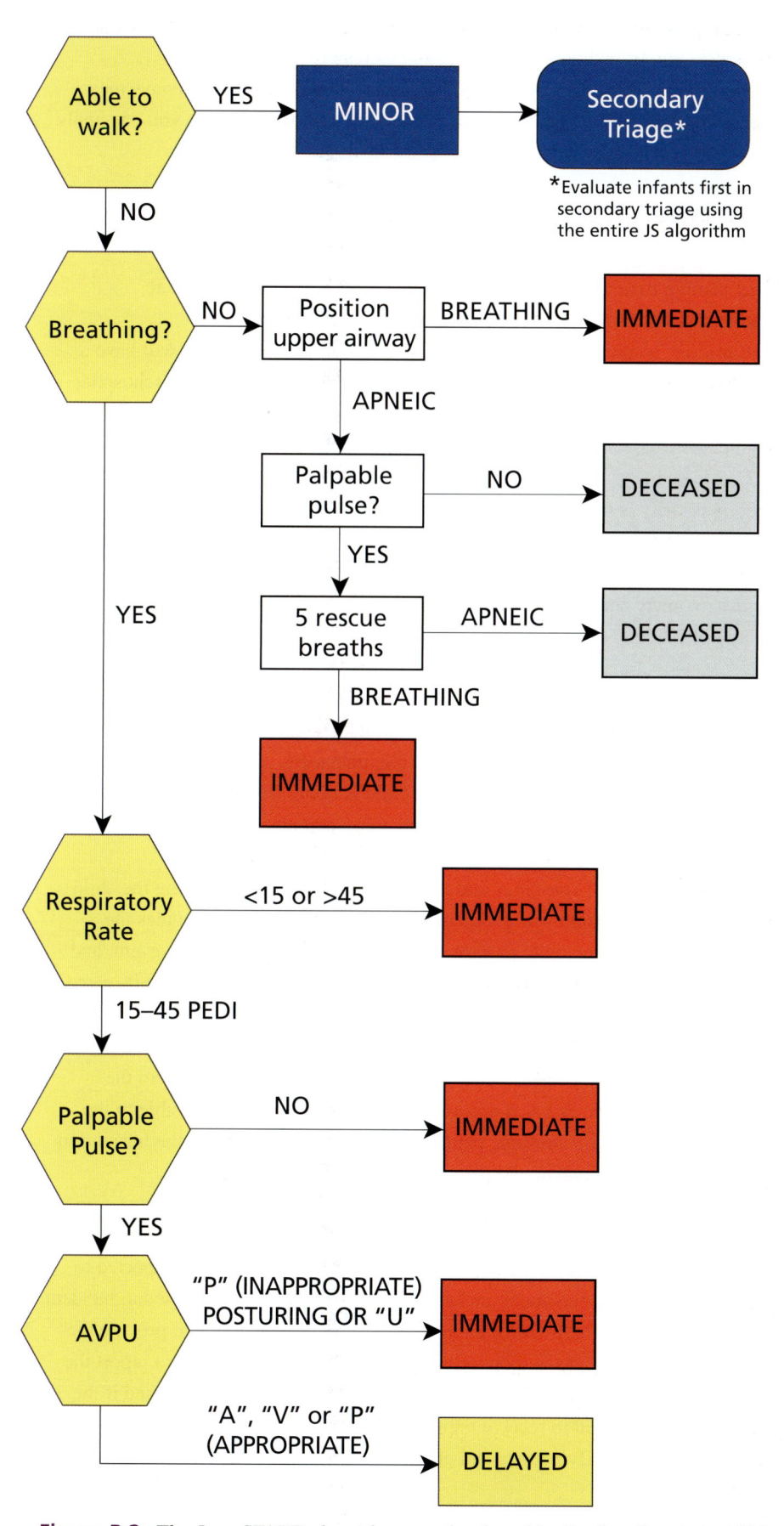

```
Able to walk? --YES--> MINOR --> Secondary Triage*
    |
   NO
    |
    v
Breathing? --NO--> Position upper airway --BREATHING--> IMMEDIATE
    |                    |
   YES                 APNEIC
    |                    |
    |                    v
    |              Palpable pulse? --NO--> DECEASED
    |                    |
    |                   YES
    |                    |
    |                    v
    |              5 rescue breaths --APNEIC--> DECEASED
    |                    |
    |                BREATHING
    |                    |
    |                    v
    |               IMMEDIATE
    v
Respiratory Rate --<15 or >45--> IMMEDIATE
    |
15–45 PEDI
    |
    v
Palpable Pulse? --NO--> IMMEDIATE
    |
   YES
    |
    v
AVPU --"P" (INAPPROPRIATE) POSTURING OR "U"--> IMMEDIATE
    |
    --"A", "V" or "P" (APPROPRIATE)--> DELAYED
```

*Evaluate infants first in secondary triage using the entire JS algorithm

Figure B.2 *The JumpSTART algorithm was developed by Dr. Lou Romig in 1995.*

Pediatric Trauma Triage and Multiple Casualty Incident Management

aspirate. Do not leave injured and spinal motion restricted children unattended. Each will require emotional support and continual airway maintenance.

On scene, it is important to stabilize the airway early (which does not always mean intubation) and control life-threatening hemorrhage. For the critical patient, you can apply all other interventions during transportation or at the hospital.

Communications Considerations

Incidents that involve traumatic injuries to children require an expanded look at communications. More resources must be dedicated to that function.

The first priority is to the pediatric patients. If conscious, these patients will have a higher level of anxiety and require repeated and consistent reassurance from prehospital providers. Provide this reassurance in the form of calm communications, a caring attitude, and, if possible and true, a message that parents are being contacted and will be with the child as soon as possible.

The second priority is the parents or guardians (legal or situational). Situational guardians include school officials, sports coaches, bus drivers, or babysitters who may have had temporary responsibilities for the involved children at the time of the incident. Communicate in a timely and professional manner with the adults who have responsibilities for the children. If parents are not present with the children at the time of the incident, the adults at the scene should make it a priority to contact them and advise what has happened, where they should go, and who else they may need to contact. In some situations, the parents may be at, or on their way to, the scene, and Incident Command must prepare to deal with those parents when they arrive. In other circumstances, Incident Command will tell the parents to report to the hospital where the child is being transported. If so, tell the emergency department personnel to prepare for incoming parents, who may have little information about what has happened and how badly injured their child is.

In older children who are conscious and medically stable, consider having the child communicate directly with parents or guardians by cellular phone. This provides the opportunity for both parent and child to have direct communication about the event, and avoids prehospital providers having to consider issues of privacy. Some EMS units carry extra cellular phones for this purpose.

The third consideration is for the emergency department personnel who will assume care and responsibility for the pediatric patients after receiving the patients from the prehospital providers. Provide as much accurate information as early as possible to the receiving facility, particularly if multiple patients are involved. This allows the hospital to mobilize the appropriate equipment and personnel.

The fourth consideration is the media. Incidents involving trauma to children, particularly with multiple pediatric patients, are intensive media events. Bus collisions, hazardous material incidents with injured children, and school incidents are expected to draw a large crowd of media personnel, including live-broadcast electronic media. Incident Command must designate a Public Information Officer, whose function is to provide the media with appropriate messages and opportunities to do their job, which is to report the news. The media is a very valuable communication method, and it should be used if the community or the parents need to receive important facts. Live media messages may be the most effective way to notify parents and others of the event, and give instructions for the appropriate response.

Pediatric Trauma Life Support

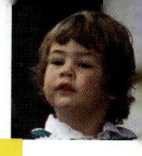

Pediatric Consent and Major Incident Management

The issue of consent for pediatric patients is a daily challenge for prehospital providers. The consent issue in a major incident is usually less complicated than in routine day-to-day operations. In major incidents, there is an anticipated higher level of concern for the pediatric patients. You may apply the legal principle of "implied consent" for evaluation and treatment. On an everyday basis, the prehospital provider is acting on behalf of society to evaluate and provide appropriate treatment for pediatric patients. Legal minors cannot otherwise provide their own legal consent, unless they are emancipated. Prehospital personnel provide three services for pediatric patients: evaluation, treatment, and transportation. When there is a call for a pediatric patient, the prehospital care system acts in a legally responsible manner when a pediatric patient assessment is performed. When that evaluation indicates that a real or potential emergency condition exists, the prehospital providers must provide that treatment. Under those circumstances, there is no need for parental consent. Transportation is provided to the appropriate receiving facility according to the needs of the patient, in line with the evaluation and treatment.

Major incidents involving children make the issue of pediatric consent even more protective of actions that protect the interests of young patients. An excellent example of this is a major commercial airline crash where there are multiple victims of varying ages. A child found in the wreckage is assumed to have significant injuries until proven otherwise. This child was temporarily separated from the parents. Prehospital providers immediately and appropriately evaluate the child. If any indication of crash-related illness or injury exists, the child is cared for and then transported without the need for first obtaining consent from any parents. Should the providers later locate the parents, providers can obtain consent for treatment retrospectively. Even if providers could not obtain this type of consent, they operated in a responsible fashion considering the potential mechanisms of injury and the primary concern for the physical well-being of the patient.

Equipment Considerations

Multiple casualty incidents often result in a shortage of packaging and treatment equipment. When this occurs, specialized pediatric equipment may not be immediately available for each child. Children cannot be expanded to fit on or into adult-sized equipment, and adult-sized equipment cannot be condensed in the field. Appropriate pediatric-sized equipment must be used for each child whenever possible. A variety of manufacturers offer equipment especially designed for children. Appropriately sized pediatric airway equipment, cervical motion restriction devices, and spinal motion restriction equipment is available. In developing MCI response plans, include appropriate pediatric equipment for the care and transportation of pediatric patients in the equipment cache. Prehospital providers should regularly train in the use of this equipment. In situations where sufficient pediatric equipment is not available, providers may employ improvised techniques, ensuring that the objectives of the interventions are met. The Skills Station chapters of this text will assist with learning to select the appropriate equipment.

> **PEARLS**
>
> In developing MCI response plans, include appropriate pediatric equipment for the care and transportation of pediatric patients in the equipment cache. Prehospital providers should regularly train in the use of this equipment.

Transportation and Destination Decision Making

Major incidents involving children with serious or critical trauma will influence triage priorities. Many prehospital providers may make treatment and transportation of children a priority over adults. It is a natural response to guide the highest level of care toward younger patients, who may be perceived as more salvageable. Incident Command and transportation officers should consider this predictable response during incident operations. If an adult and child have similar injuries (for example, a closed head injury with airway compromise), the pediatric patient will be prioritized for transport before the adult patient.

When an incident involves a family unit, pediatric priorities will influence decisions regarding institution and mode of transport. The Transportation Officer should, if possible, keep a family unit together. This facilitates information gathering and ultimately the medical care of the individual family members. Examples of incidents where this type of situation may occur include: multiple family members injured in a motor vehicle collision or carbon monoxide inhalation. Whenever possible, if it does not overwhelm the receiving hospital, take all family members to the same facility. Family members may then provide support and medical information for each other. This will be more complicated when there are separate pediatric and adult trauma facilities serving the area where the incident occurs. Make decisions based on the severity of the injuries and local protocols, or direct conversation with medical direction. If the family must be divided between institutions, obtain as much information as possible prior to transport and try to obtain the phone number of another adult relative that may be contacted to stay with the child.

If the parent refuses to be separated from the child, explain to the parent the options for care for all family patients in the incident. Compromising care for any family member has long-term implications, and missed injuries can be devastating to a child. You should not unnecessarily overload one facility in such a way that medical care for any of the family members is compromised.

PSYCHOLOGICAL EFFECTS

Major incidents involving pediatric patients can generate a higher degree of psychological stress among prehospital providers than incidents involving adults. Utilize critical incident stress debriefing teams for counseling. If this resource is not available, a counseling team from the regional pediatric trauma center may be available. Appropriate debriefing of emergency personnel is very important for pediatric cases, and to prevent long-term psychological trauma, home problems, or unnecessary job anxiety related to future pediatric patients.

PEARLS

Whenever possible, if it does not overwhelm the receiving hospital, take all family members to the same facility.

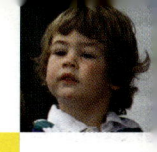

SUMMARY

To effectively manage major pediatric trauma incidents, utilize the following steps:

1. Appropriately identify an event as a multiple casualty incident that involves pediatric patients.
2. Establish Incident Command and appropriate sectors.
3. Call for needed medical and rescue resources for pediatric patients.
4. Perform adequate and appropriate triage, stressing the ABCs and level of perfusion and consciousness.
5. If possible, designate a medical person in charge of each pediatric patient.
6. Perform evaluation and treatment with appropriately trained personnel to perform patient care and airway control.
7. Do not leave injured and spinal motion restricted children unattended. They require emotional support and continual airway maintenance.
8. It is necessary to professionally communicate and interact with parents and other adults from responsible agencies. Media communications may also be a priority.
9. When multiple family members are injured in the same incident, attempt to transport those members to the same facility. Medical direction may be helpful in choosing correct destinations in multiple patient incidents.
10. Appropriately timed hospital notification enhances medical care and patient turnover to receiving hospitals.
11. Stress the repeated evaluation of perfusion and mental status (the most important physical findings) in incident documentation for pediatric trauma patients.
12. Debrief after the incident to ask questions, minimize stress, and apply the lessons to the next incident.
13. Provide counseling and psychological support for response and prehospital providers after the event.

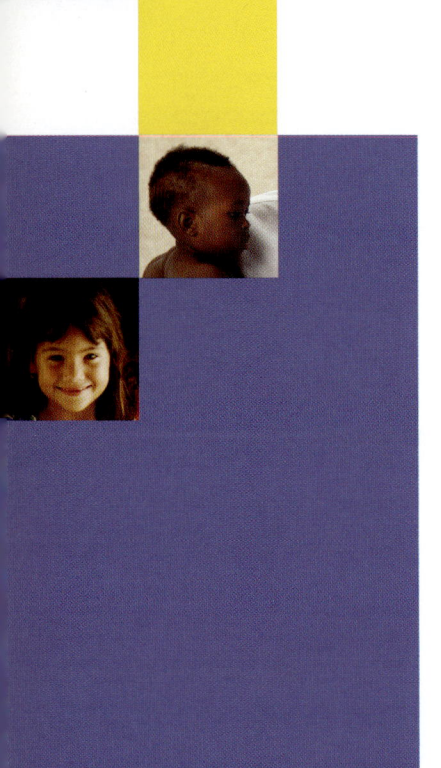

Recommended Reading

Agency for Healthcare Research and Quality. *Pediatric Terrorism and Disaster Preparedness: A Resource for Pediatricians*. AHRQ Publication No. 06(07)-0056. Rockville, M.D.: Author, 2006.

Auf der Heide, Erik. "Triage." In *Disaster Response: Principles of Preparation and Coordination*, 104–21. St. Louis: Mosby Year-Book, 1989.

Augustine, Jim. "Keep the Kids Together: Triage for Incidents Involving Children." *EMS Magazine* 35(April 2006): 30–2.

Augustine, Jim. "Patient Tracking at an MCI: Critical Needs for Tracking to Facilitate Customer Service." *EMS Magazine* 36 (July 2007): 26–9.

Campbell, John Emory, ed. "Multicasualty Incidents and Triage." In *International Trauma Life Support for Prehospital Providers*, 6th ed., 400–07. Upper Saddle River, N.J.: Pearson/Prentice Hall, 2008.

Ralston, Mark, Mary Fran Hazinski, Arno L. Zaritsky, Stephen M. Schexnayder, and Monica E. Kleinman, eds. *Pediatric Advanced Life Support Provider Manual*. Dallas: American Heart Association, 2007.

JumpSTART. Combined JumpSTART algorithm. http://www.jumpstarttriage.com/ (accessed November 1, 2007).

The National Response Framework and the National Incident Management System. http://www.fema.gov/pdf/emergency/nrf/nrf-nims.pdf (accessed November 1, 2007)

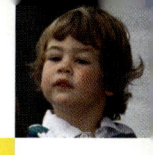

PHOTO & ILLUSTRATION CREDITS

ITLS would like to acknowledge the individuals and organizations who have allowed their images to be used in *Pediatric Trauma Life Support for Prehospital Care Providers*.

Images may not be reproduced or reprinted without the permission of International Trauma Life Support.

Chapter 1

Figure 1.6:   Courtesy of the Emergency Medical Services for Children Program
Figure 1.7:   Courtesy of John Mohler, RN
Figure 1.8a: Andrew Larson Studios
Figure 1.8b: Elizabeth Lee, Lee Medical Studios
Figure 1.13: Courtesy of the Emergency Medical Services for Children Program
Figure 1.14: Courtesy of Chris Hitney
Figure 1.15: Courtesy of David Maatman, NREMT-P/IC
Figure 1.16: Courtesy of John Mohler, RN
Figure 1.17: Larry Hamill, Hamill Photography

Chapter 2

Figure 2.1:   Larry Hamill, Hamill Photography
Figure 2.3:   Larry Hamill, Hamill Photography
Figure 2.4:   Courtesy of the Emergency Medical Services for Children Program
Figure 2.5:   Courtesy of the Emergency Medical Services for Children Program
Figure 2.6:   Courtesy of the Emergency Medical Services for Children Program
Figure 2.7:   Larry Hamill, Hamill Photography

Chapter 3

Figure 3.1:   Larry Hamill, Hamill Photography
Figure 3.2:   Larry Hamill, Hamill Photography
Figure 3.3:   Larry Hamill, Hamill Photography
Figure 3.4:   Larry Hamill, Hamill Photography
Figure 3.5:   Larry Hamill, Hamill Photography
Figure 3.6:   Larry Hamill, Hamill Photography
Figure 3.7:   Larry Hamill, Hamill Photography
Figure 3.8:   Larry Hamill, Hamill Photography
Figure 3.9:   Larry Hamill, Hamill Photography
Figure 3.10: Courtesy of the Emergency Medical Services for Children Program
Figure 3.11: Larry Hamill, Hamill Photography
Figure 3.12: Larry Hamill, Hamill Photography
Figure 3.13: Larry Hamill, Hamill Photography
Figure 3.14: Larry Hamill, Hamill Photography
Figure 3.15: Larry Hamill, Hamill Photography

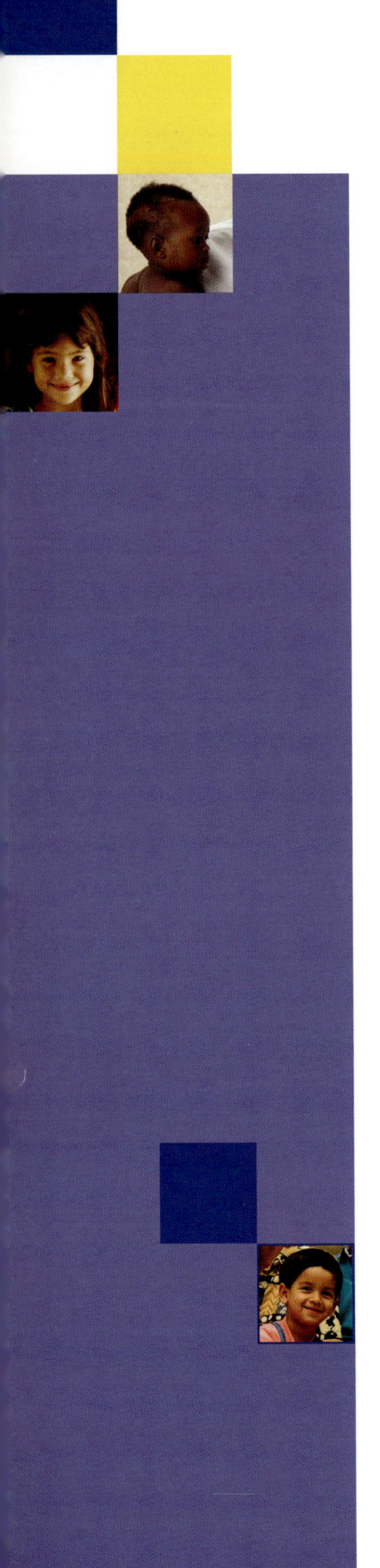

Chapter 4

Figure 4.1: Elizabeth Lee, Lee Medical Studios
Figure 4.2: Elizabeth Lee, Lee Medical Studios
Figure 4.3: Larry Hamill, Hamill Photography
Figure 4.4: Larry Hamill, Hamill Photography
Figure 4.5: Courtesy of the Emergency Medical Services for Children Program
Figure 4.6: Larry Hamill, Hamill Photography
Figure 4.7: Larry Hamill, Hamill Photography
Figure 4.8: Sue Clemons Tysiak, photographer
Figure 4.9: Larry Hamill, Hamill Photography
Figure 4.10: Ted Blackwelder Photography
Figure 4.11: Courtesy of Bob Page, AAS, NREMT-P, CCEMT-P, NCEE

Chapter 5

Figure 5.1: Elizabeth Lee, Lee Medical Studios
Figure 5.2: Elizabeth Lee, Lee Medical Studios
Figure 5.3: Courtesy of the Emergency Medical Services for Children Program
Figure 5.4: Larry Hamill, Hamill Photography
Figure 5.5: Ted Blackwelder Photography
Figure 5.6: Elizabeth Lee, Lee Medical Studios
Figure 5.7: Elizabeth Lee, Lee Medical Studios
Figure 5.8a: Elizabeth Lee, Lee Medical Studios
Figure 5.8b: Elizabeth Lee, Lee Medical Studios
Figure 5.8c: Elizabeth Lee, Lee Medical Studios
Figure 5.9: Elizabeth Lee, Lee Medical Studios
Figure 5.10a: Elizabeth Lee, Lee Medical Studios
Figure 5.10b: Elizabeth Lee, Lee Medical Studios
Figure 5.11: Courtesy of Bob Page, AAS, NREMT-P, CCEMT-P, NCEE

Chapter 6

Figure 6.1: Larry Hamill, Hamill Photography
Figure 6.2: Ted Blackwelder Photography
Figure 6.3: Courtesy of the Emergency Medical Services for Children Program
Figure 6.4: Courtesy of the Emergency Medical Services for Children Program
Figure 6.5: Courtesy of the Emergency Medical Services for Children Program
Figure 6.6: Larry Hamill, Hamill Photography
Figure 6.7: Courtesy of Bob Page, AAS, NREMT-P, CCEMT-P, NCEE
Figure 6.8: Larry Hamill, Hamill Photography
Figure 6.9: Elizabeth Lee, Lee Medical Studios
Figure 6.10: Courtesy of the Emergency Medical Services for Children Program
Figure 6.11: Elizabeth Lee, Lee Medical Studios
Figure 6.12: Elizabeth Lee, Lee Medical Studios
Figure 6.13: Reprinted with permission from Mediscan for Medical-On-Line Ltd.
Figure 6.14: Ted Blackwelder Photography

Chapter 7

Figure 7.1: Larry Hamill, Hamill Photography
Figure 7.2: Larry Hamill, Hamill Photography
Figure 7.3: Larry Hamill, Hamill Photography
Figure 7.4: Courtesy of the Emergency Medical Services for Children Program

Chapter 8

Figure 8.1: Courtesy of Mary McNicholas
Figure 8.2: Ted Blackwelder Photography
Figure 8.3: Courtesy of the Emergency Medical Services for Children Program
Figure 8.4: Ted Blackwelder Photography

Chapter 9

Figure 9.1: Elizabeth Lee, Lee Medical Studios
Figure 9.2: Courtesy of Kyee Han, MBBS, FRCS, FFAEM
Figure 9.3: Courtesy of the Emergency Medical Services for Children Program

Chapter 10

Figure 10.1: Elizabeth Lee, Lee Medical Studios
Figure 10.4: Elizabeth Lee, Lee Medical Studios
Figure 10.5: Elizabeth Lee, Lee Medical Studios
Figure 10.6: Courtesy of Bob Page, AAS, NREMT-P, CCEMT-P, NCEE
Figure 10.7: Courtesy of Kyee Han, MBBS, FRCS, FFAEM
Figure 10.8: Courtesy of Roy Alson, PhD, MD, FACEP
Figure 10.9: Andrew Larson Studios

Chapter 11

Figure 11.1: Courtesy of Ann Marie Dietrich, MD, FACEP, FAAP
Figure 11.2: Larry Hamill, Hamill Photography
Figure 11.3: Courtesy of David Maatman, NREMT-P/IC
Figure 11.4: Ted Blackwelder Photography
Figure 11.5: Ted Blackwelder Photography
Figure 11.6: Ted Blackwelder Photography
Figure 11.7: Courtesy of Kyee Han, MBBS, FRCS, FFAEM

Chapter 12

Figure 12.1: Ted Blackwelder Photography
Figure 12.2: Courtesy of the Emergency Medical Services for Children Program
Figure 12.3: Courtesy of John Mohler, RN
Figure 12.4: Ted Blackwelder Photography
Figure 12.5: Ted Blackwelder Photography
Figure 12.6: Ted Blackwelder Photography
Figure 12.7: Ted Blackwelder Photography
Figure 12.8: Courtesy of the Emergency Medical Services for Children Program
Figure 12.9: Ted Blackwelder Photography
Figure 12.10: Ted Blackwelder Photography

Figure 12.11: Ted Blackwelder Photography
Figure 12.12: Ted Blackwelder Photography

Chapter 13

Figure 13.2: Courtesy of John Mohler, RN
Figure 13.3: Reprinted with permission from Mediscan for Medical-On-Line Ltd.
Figure 13.4: Reprinted with permission from Mediscan for Medical-On-Line Ltd.
Figure 13.5: Larry Hamill, Hamill Photography
Figure 13.6: Courtesy of John Mohler, RN
Figure 13.7: Courtesy of John Mohler, RN
Figure 13.8: Courtesy of the Emergency Medical Services for Children Program

Chapter 14

Figure 14.1: Courtesy of the Emergency Medical Services for Children Program
Figure 14.2: Courtesy of the Emergency Medical Services for Children Program
Figure 14.3: Elizabeth Lee, Lee Medical Studios
Figure 14.4: Courtesy of the Emergency Medical Services for Children Program
Figure 14.5: Elizabeth Lee, Lee Medical Studios
Figure 14.6a: Andrew Larson Studios
Figure 14.6b: Andrew Larson Studios

Chapter 16

Figure 16.1: Elizabeth Lee, Lee Medical Studios
Figure 16.2: Reprinted with permission from Mediscan for Medical-On-Line Ltd.
Figure 16.3: Courtesy of Bob Page, AAS, NREMT-P, CCEMT-P, NCEE

Chapter 17

Figure 17.2: Courtesy of the Emergency Medical Services for Children Program
Figure 17.3: Larry Hamill, Hamill Photography

Chapter 18

Figure 18.9: Larry Hamill, Hamill Photography

Chapter 19

Figure 19.1: Larry Hamill, Hamill Photography
Figure 19.8: Courtesy of the Emergency Medical Services for Children Program
Figure 19.9: Courtesy of John Mohler, RN
Figure 19.10: Courtesy of the Emergency Medical Services for Children Program
Figure 19.11: Elizabeth Lee, Lee Medical Studios
Figure 19.12: Elizabeth Lee, Lee Medical Studios

Chapter 20

Figure 20.1: Courtesy of the Emergency Medical Services for Children Program
Figure 20.2: Courtesy of the Emergency Medical Services for Children Program
Figure 20.3: Courtesy of the Emergency Medical Services for Children Program
Figure 20.4: Courtesy of the Emergency Medical Services for Children Program

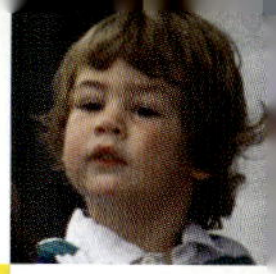

Figure 20.5: Courtesy of the Emergency Medical Services for Children Program
Figure 20.6: Elizabeth Lee, Lee Medical Studios
Figure 20.7: Reprinted with permission from Mediscan for Medical-On-Line Ltd.
Figure 20.8: Elizabeth Lee, Lee Medical Studios

Appendix A

Figure A.1: Larry Hamill, Hamill Photography
Figure A.3: Courtesy of John Mohler, RN
Figure A.4: Courtesy of John Mohler, RN

Appendix B

Figure B.2: Courtesy of Lou Romig, MD, FACEP, FAAP

All images not listed above are royalty-free stock photographs.

Unless otherwise noted, all tables, graphs, and flow charts were designed by Norcom, Inc. for International Trauma Life Support's *Pediatric Trauma Life Support for Prehospital Care Providers.*

ACKNOWLEDGMENTS

ITLS would like to thank all of the individuals who served as models for images that appear in the textbook:

T.J. Adelman
Shawn Adelman
Alex Hitney
Courtney McNicholas
Megan McNicholas
Ben Murphy
Aaron Michael Page
Ashley Ann Page

ITLS would also like to acknowledge the following individuals for their assistance in coordinating the photography and illustrations:

Scot Allen, BS. FF III/EMT-P
Janice P. Ciszek
Patricia G. Lee, MD, FACEP
Bob Page, AAS, NREMT-P, CCEMT-P, NCEE

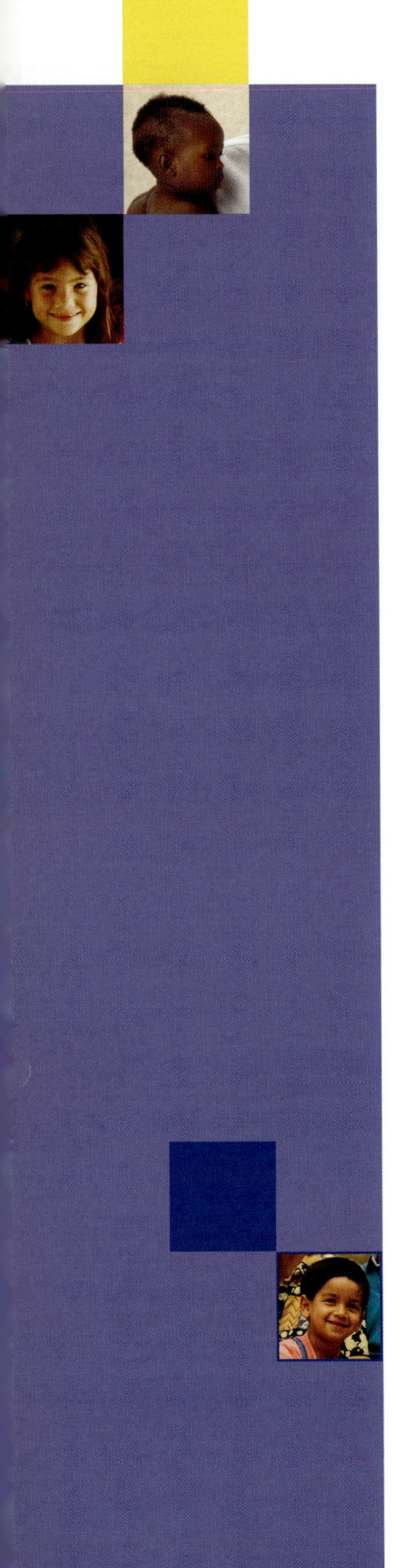

INDEX

A

Abdomen
- anatomy, 67, 113
- examination of, 34, 47, 116
- muscles, 113
- palpation, 30
- quadrants, 113, 116
- spinal trauma, 144-145

Abdominal aorta, 113

Abdominal trauma, 112-120
- anatomy, 67, 113
- assessment, 114-116
- case study, 112, 117-118
- diaphragmatic injuries, 78
- gunshot wounds, 8, 116
- pathophysiology, 113
- primary survey, 114-115
- secondary survey, 116
- signs and symptoms, 114-116

Acute epidural hematoma, 126

Acute subdural hematoma, 126

Adolescents, 3, 7, 9, 12, 13, 16

Ages
- cricothyroidotomy, 56
- endotracheal tube depth, 57-58
- fall injuries, 30-31
- mechanisms of injury, 31-34
- normal weights, 43
- vital signs, 43

Air transport, 263

Air, swallowing, 113

Airway
- abdominal trauma, 115
- anatomy, 52-54
- burns, 190, 196, 198, 200
- case presentation, 52, 62-63
- head trauma, 129
- inhalation injuries, 200
- initial assessment, 54-57
- neonatal resuscitation, 234-235, 236, 238-240
- physiology, 52-54
- primary survey, 54
- secondary survey, 62
- spinal trauma, 141-142
- submersion injuries, 191-192
- transportation decisions, 57
- trauma, 51-64

Airway management skills, 83-94
- assessment, 84, 88
- bag-valve-mask ventilation, 86-87
- BIAD, 59-60
- blind nasotracheal intubation, 90
- needle cricothyroidotomy, 90-91
- needle decompression, 92-94
- oral intubation, 88-89
- oropharyngeal airway, 85
- pediatric equipment, 58-61, 88, 90, 92
- supplemental oxygen, 56, 58, 61

Airway obstruction
- burns, 178, 180
- dry drowning, 192
- edema, 52-53
- foreign bodies, 52
- respiratory arrest, 206

Allergies, history of, 31, 45

Altered mental status (*see also* Level of consciousness)
- head trauma, 128
- hypoxia, 57, 98
- initial assessment, 28
- nontraumatic causes, 30
- ongoing assessment, 34, 48
- shock, 98
- spinal trauma, 140

Ambulances, 262

American Academy of Pediatrics, 12, 234, 248

Amputations, 160, 166-167

Anatomy
- abdomen, 67-68, 113
- airway, 52-53
- chest, 67-68
- head, 122-123, 126
- skin, 173-176

Ankle, immobilization of, 164

Anoxic brain injury, 123, 194

Aorta, 8, 67, 68, 77-78, 113

Apnea
- assessment, 28, 41, 69, 141
- causes of, 141, 205
- in children with special health care needs, 248
- in infancy, 236, 239, 243
- neonates, 236, 239, 243
- ventilation, 54, 69, 86

282 Pediatric Trauma Life Support

Arrhythmias, 194-195
Asherman Chest Seal, 70-71, 92, 94
Asphyxia, 79, 192
Aspiration, 58-59, 85-86, 90, 108, 191-192, 194, 196, 205, 237, 238, 251
Assessments (*see also* specific injuries; specific types)
- children in car seats, 143-144, 153-156
- detailed exam, 33-34
- initial, 27-30, 40-43
- ongoing exam, 34-35, 48-49
- patient assessment diagram, 26
- preparation for, 24
- primary survey, 25-33. 40-47
- secondary survey, 33-34, 46-48

Atropine, 19, 243
AVPU system, 28, 33, 41, 46, 128

B

Backboards, 19, 30, 44, 127, 142-143, 150-156, 164
Bag-valve-mask ventilation
- airway obstruction, 55-58, 178
- apneic episodes, 29, 42, 193, 240
- initial assessments, 28-29, 42
- neonatal, 235, 239, 240, 242-244
- pediatric device sizes, 19
- spinal trauma, 141-142, 144
- thoracic trauma, 74, 77
- traumatic cardiopulmonary arrest, 206, 208
- use of, 28-29, 42, 86-87

Basilar skull fracture, 34, 125
Battle's sign, 34, 46, 125, 132
Behavioral changes, 57, 127, 128, 133, 223
Benzodiazepines, 61, 131
Bicarbonate, 19, 244
Bicycles, 10-12, 14, 15, 16, 27, 112, 114, 116, 135, 140, 159
Bites, 183, 214
Blind insertion airway devices (BIAD), 42, 59-60
Blind nasotracheal intubation, 90
Blistering, 174-175
Blood loss (*see also* Hemorrhages)
- amputations, 160, 166-167
- control of, 66, 78, 81, 122, 131, 160, 167, 207
- hypovolemia, 74, 96, 99, 141, 160
- internal, 67, 74-76, 78, 81, 115
- neonatal, 122, 243
- prevention of, 96, 97, 99, 100, 122, 160
- shock, 66, 81, 96-100, 101-102, 104, 122, 131, 160, 207

Blood pressure
- by age, 25, 99
- normal levels, 25, 99
- shock, 66, 96-97

Blood sample tube, 19
Blood sugar, neonatal, 244
Blunt trauma, 8, 43, 70, 74, 78, 79, 112-114, 116, 125, 159, 165, 232, 233
Body surface area (BSA)
- Lund Browder chart, 176-177
- rule of nines, 176

Bone marrow, 100, 108
Bones (*see also* Fractures)
- intraosseous infusions, 100-101, 107-108, 144, 180, 208, 242
- pediatric anatomy, 8, 100, 158, 161-162, 243

Bradycardia, 57, 99, 127, 130, 192, 236, 239, 230
Brain
- anoxia, 194, 197
- edema, 127
- fixation points, 8
- hematomas, 126-127
- pathophysiology, 122-123
- primary brain injury, 123
- secondary brain injury, 123

Brain death, 197
Breathing
- assessments, initial, 28-29, 31-33, 42, 54-57
- assessments, ongoing, 34-35, 48-49
- burns, 178-179, 180, 182
- head trauma, 129, 131
- oxygen use, 84
- pain, 115
- pneumothorax, 29, 30, 32, 35, 43, 45, 48, 56, 70, 72
- shock, 98, 100
- spinal trauma, 141, 144
- submersion injuries, 191-192, 194, 195

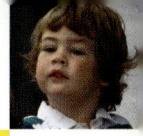

Bronchial tree, 61, 68, 78, 182
Broselow tape, 24, 25, 89
Burn centers, 181, 260, 262
Burns, 171-188
- anatomy, 173-176

Index 283

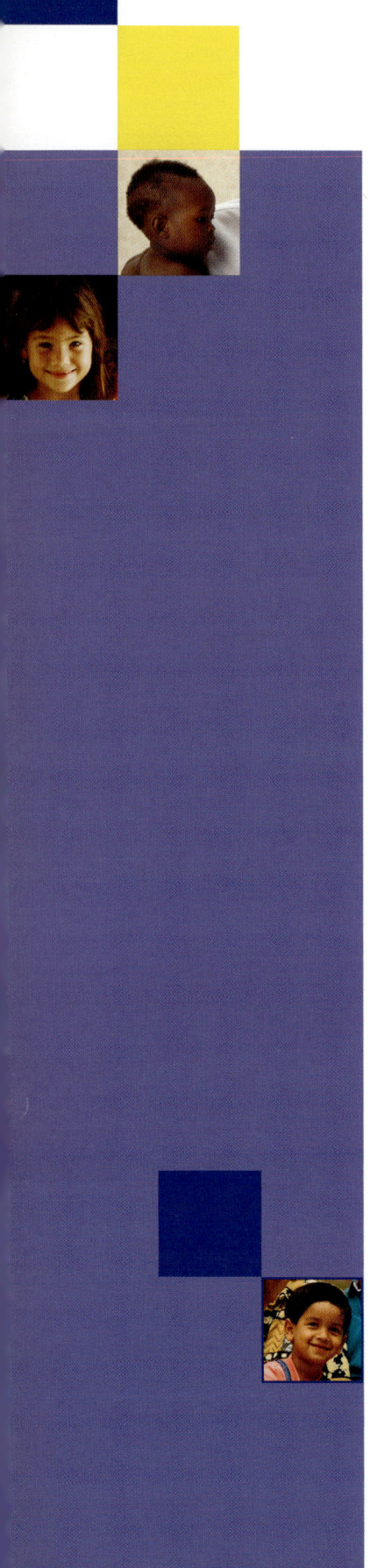

care during transport, 181
chemical, 172, 178, 181
cigarette, 214
circumferential, 176
classification, 176
depths of, 174-176
electrical, 183
extent of injuries, 176-177
fluid resuscitation, 182
inhalation injuries, 182
level of consciousness, 178
lightning injuries, 183
management, 181-183
pharmacologic therapy, 182
physiology, 173-176
prevention of, 184
primary survey, 178-181
rule of nines, 176
scene size-up, 178
secondary survey, 181
smoke detectors, 184

C

Capillary refill, 29, 99, 101, 121, 169, 194
Capnography, 32, 49, 59, 60, 61, 69, 76, 77, 86, 87, 90, 131, 208, 240
Capnometry, 33, 35, 46, 60
Car seats (see also Child passenger restraint devices)
    assessment of children in, 10, 143-144, 153-156
    extrication, 115, 143, 155-156
    immobilization in, 143, 155
    mechanisms of injury, 10, 115
Carbon dioxide, 52, 124
Carbon monoxide
    description, 179, 182
    level of consciousness, 179
    oxygen, 179, 182
Cardiac arrest (see Traumatic cardiopulmonary arrest)
Cardiac monitoring
    electrical injuries, 180
    pediatric equipment, 19, 49
    submersion injuries, 195
    thoracic trauma, 77-78
    ventriculoperitoneal shunts, 255-256
Cardiac tamponade, 68, 74-76

Cardiopulmonary resuscitation (CPR)
    burns patients, 179, 183
    neonates, 240-242
    pediatric trauma patients, 32, 45, 179, 183, 203-210
    public education, 198
    submersion injuries, 194, 197
    traumatic cardiopulmonary arrest, 203-210
Caregivers (see Parents)
Case studies
    abdominal trauma, 112
    airway, 52
    assessment of the pediatric patient, 24
    burns, 172
    child abuse, 212
    children with special health care needs (CSHCN), 248
    death of a child, 222
    extremity trauma, 158
    head trauma, 122
    injured child, 2
    newborn trauma, 232
    shock and fluid resuscitation, 96
    spinal trauma, 138
    submersion injuries, 190
    thoracic trauma, 66
    traumatic cardiopulmonary arrest, 204
Catheters, 19, 58, 72, 90-91, 92-94, 100, 107, 238, 242, 251-255
Central venous access devices, 252-253
Cerebral blood flow, 123-124
Cerebral edema, 127
Cerebral hematoma, 127
Cerebrospinal fluid (CSF), 123-124, 125, 132, 254
Cervical collars, 18-20, 30, 35, 44, 48, 142-143, 150-153, 155-156
Cervical spine
    abdominal trauma, 115
    airway management, 28, 41, 69, 129, 141, 142, 178
    burns, 178
    control of, 18, 28, 30, 41, 44, 58, 98, 128-129, 130, 140-141, 142-143, 150-156, 160, 178, 193, 195, 196, 206, 238
    fixation point, 8
    head trauma, 128-130, 140, 141
    initial assessments, 28, 41, 69, 98, 128,

160, 178, 193
  intubation and control of, 142
  location, 12, 138-139
  manual control, 28, 41, 140, 150, 154, 155-156, 178, 193, 206-207
  motion restriction, 18, 28, 30, 41, 44, 58, 69, 98, 128-129, 130, 140-141, 142-143, 150-156, 160, 178, 193, 195, 196, 206, 238
  pediatric motion restriction devices, 30, 44, 130, 142-143, 151-153, 154, 160, 195, 239, 273
  submersion injuries, 193, 195, 196
Chemical burns, 172, 178, 181
Chest compressions, neonates, 240-242
Chest injuries (*see* Thoracic trauma)
Child abuse, 211-220
  care and safety issues, 215
  case study, 217-218
  characteristic marks, 214
  definition, 212
  family members, 216-217
  fractures, 79
  head trauma, 127-128, 214
  pediatric burns, 172-173, 214
  prehospital considerations, 216
  questionable submersion events, 196
  red flags, 214
  rib fractures, 79
Child passenger restraint devices (*see also* Car seats)
  assessment of children in, 10, 143-144, 153-156
  extrication, 115, 143, 155-156
  immobilization in, 143, 155
  mechanisms of injury, 10, 115
Children with Special Health Care Needs (CSHCN), 247-258
  evaluation, 249-250
  CSHCN medical equipment, 250-256
Circulating blood volume (CBV), 96, 131
Circulation (*see also* Capillary refill; Perfusion)
  abdominal trauma, 115
  airway management, 57, 61
  assessments, initial, 25, 29, 40, 43
  assessments, ongoing, 35, 48
  burns, 172, 179, 180

  extremity trauma, 160, 161, 166
  head trauma, 129-130, 131
  neonates, 240-242
  shock, 98, 99, 100
  spinal trauma, 141, 144
  submersion injuries, 194, 195, 197
  thoracic trauma, 74, 77
  traumatic cardiopulmonary arrest, 207, 208
Circumferential burns, 176
Closed fractures, 161, 164
Closed skull fractures, 125
Cold stress, neonates, 244
Cold-water drowning, 32, 194, 197
Cold-water submersion, 194, 197
Combitube, 60
Communications
  child abuse, 215-217
  confidence, 17-18
  death of a child, 226-227
  multiple casualty incidents, 266, 267-268, 272
  treatment issues by age, 3, 7
  with children, 2-7, 112, 150
Compartment syndrome, 158, 165
Compassionate Friends, 226-227
Compression injuries, 8, 79, 116
Confident approach, 17-18
Consent, parental, 273
Consumer Product Safety Commission, 198
Cricothyroid membrane, 90-91
Cricothyroidotomy, 56, 90-91
Critical incident stress debriefing (CISD), 226, 274
Crush injuries, 78, 166
Cushing's reflex, 30
Cushing's Triad, 127, 130, 256
Cyanide poisoning, 179, 182
Cyanosis, 56, 70, 72
  neonatal, 236, 240

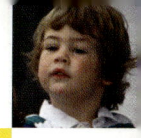

D
DCAP BTLS mnemonic, 30, 33, 43, 44, 101, 145
Death
  determination of, 225, 228
  impact of, 222-228
Decerebrate posturing, 127, 133

Index 285

Decorticate posturing, 127, 133
Decompression
　　catheter placement, 72, 74, 92-93, 242
　　pneumothorax, 29, 32-33, 35, 49, 72, 74, 79, 92-93, 207, 208, 242
Deep partial-thickness burns, 173-175
Defibrillation, 179, 208
Delivery of infant, 234-235, 236-238
Dental injuries, 46-47, 84, 214
Depressed skull fracture, 125
Dermis, 173-175
Descending aorta fixation, 8
Detailed exam, 33-34, 46-48, 77
Dextrose solutions, 19, 244
Diaphragm, 54, 67-68, 70, 78, 113, 115
Diazepam, 19, 131
Diffuse axonal injury, 127
Dislocations, 158, 161-164
Documentation
　　detailed exam, 62, 144, 161
　　mass casualty incidents, 268
　　neonatal assessment, 234, 240
　　suspicions of abuse, 197, 213, 215
　　transfer policies, 181, 260-263
Doppler ultrasonography, 233-234
Drowning, 189-202 (see also Submersion injuries)
Dry drowning, 192
Duodenum, 113
Dura mater, 126-127
Dysrhythmias, 194-195 (see also Arrhythmias)

E

Ecchymosis, 46, 116, 125, 132, 161
Edema, 52-53, 61, 88, 106, 109, 124, 127, 165, 191
Education, 12, 14, 15, 16, 184, 198 (see also Injury prevention)
Ejection injuries, 10, 261
Elbow, immobilization of, 163
Electrical injuries, 183
　　burns, 176, 178, 183
　　cardiac dysrhythmias, 179
　　cardiopulmonary arrest, 179
　　education, 184
　　fluid resuscitation, 180, 182
　　respiratory arrest, 179
Emergency departments, 18, 33, 46, 54, 61, 66, 100, 101, 106, 116, 122, 155, 180, 181, 191, 196, 207, 208, 213, 215, 216-217, 232, 242, 260-261, 270, 272 (see also Medical direction)
Emergency medical services (EMS)
　　multiple casualty incidents, 266-276
　　pediatric injuries, 7, 13
　　staging officers, 267-268
End-tidal CO_2 ($ETCO_2$), 59, 61, 77, 88-90, 127, 129, 131, 195, 208, 235, 240
Endotracheal intubation, 32, 57-59, 74, 77, 88-90, 208, 235, 238, 240, 243, 244, 252 (see also Orotracheal intubation)
　　burns, 180
　　neonates, 235, 238, 240, 243, 244
　　spinal trauma, 142
　　submersion injuries, 195
　　traumatic cardiopulmonary arrest, 208
Endotracheal tubes
　　depth by age, 58
　　pediatric, 57-59
　　sizes, 58
Epidermis, 173-175
Epidural hematomas, 126
Epiglottis, 52-53, 89
Epinephrine, 97, 208, 243, 244
Epiphyses, 158
Equipment, 18-19, 24, 27, 40, 49, 57-59, 88, 90, 92, 106, 108, 109, 152-153, 235, 242, 273 (see specific equipment)
　　CSHCN medical, 250-256
Equipment list, 19
Eschar, 175-176
Escharotomy, 175-176
Esophageal injuries, 68, 79
Estimated time of arrival (ETA), 33, 46
Events, history of, 27, 31, 45, 97, 172, 213, 215 (see also SAMPLE history)
Extracranial injuries, 125
Extremity trauma, 157-170 (see also specific injuries)
　　amputation, 166-167
　　anatomy, 158
　　assessment, 159-161
　　circumferential burns, 176
　　compartment syndrome, 165
　　dislocations, 161-164
　　examination, 161

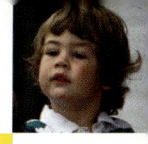

    fractures, 161-164
    open wounds, 160, 161, 162, 166-167
    pelvis stabilization, 164
    physiology, 158
    primary survey, 159-161
    secondary survey, 161
    sensory testing, 161, 162, 165
    splinting, 162-164
    sprains, 165
    strains, 165
    strength testing, 161
Extrications, 33, 101, 114, 116, 143, 153-156, 178,
Eye contact, 4, 140
Eye opening, 31, 129

F

Facial expressions, 4, 21
Falls, 112-113
    case study, 24, 35-37, 158, 248, 256
    child abuse, 213
    frequency of injuries, 14, 15, 16, 66, 77, 78, 112, 140, 150, 159, 167-169, 213
    in children with special health care needs, 248, 256
    transfer guidelines, 261
Families, 2, 5, 12, 17, 18, 21, 31, 45, 213-217, 222-228, 266, 270, 274 (*see also* Parents)
Fear, 2, 3, 5, 15, 17, 214, 216, 223, 225
Femur injuries, 164, 169
Fetal distress, 233, 234
Fetus, trauma to, 232, 233, 234
Fibula, immobilization of, 164
Finger amputations, 44, 166-167
Fire scenes, 54, 172, 178, 186
Firearms, 13, 15, 16 (*see also* Gunshot wounds)
First-degree burns, 173-175
Flail chest, 10, 68, 70, 73-74, 77, 205,
Fluid boluses
    abdominal trauma, 116
    administration of, 33, 81, 101, 106-110
    burns, 180
    equipment, 106, 108, 109
    setup, 109
    shock, 61, 77, 100-101, 131
    submersion injuries, 195
    traumatic cardiopulmonary arrest, 208

Fluid resuscitation, 95-110
    abdominal trauma, 116
    anatomy, 96-97, 106, 108
    burn management, 180, 182
    formulae, 97
    equipment, 106, 108, 109
    infusion rates, 97
    intraosseous (IO) infusion, 33, 100-101, 107-110
    intravenous (IV) access, 33, 100, 101, 106-107, 109-110
    neonatal, 243
    ongoing exam, 35, 48
    pathophysiology, 96-97
    peripheral cannulation, 106-107
    primary survey, 33
    shock, 61, 77, 100-101, 131, 144
    submersion injuries, 195, 196
    traumatic cardiopulmonary arrest, 208
Focused exam
    extremity trauma, 160
    performance of, 30, 44
Fontanel, 34, 46, 127, 132, 214, 255
Foot, immobilization of, 164
Foreign objects
    abdominal trauma, 116
    airway obstruction, 56, 84
    head trauma, 125, 130
    penetrating injuries, 8-9, 32, 35, 45, 49, 79, 116, 125, 130
    removal, 79, 116, 125, 130
Fractures
    anatomy, 158
    case study, 158, 167-169
    child abuse, 214
    electrical injuries, 183
    extremity trauma, 110, 159, 161-162
    falls, 12, 30
    greenstick, 161-162
    intraosseous (IO) infusion, 101, 107, 243
    lower extremities, 164
    pelvis, 164, 233
    rib, 56, 68, 73, 79, 113, 116
    signs and symptoms, 34, 162
    skull, 34, 123, 125, 126, 132
    spinal trauma, 133-134
    torus, 161-162
    transfer guidelines, 181, 261

Index 287

treatment, 162-164
Waddell's triad, 10-11
Freshwater aspiration, 191, 194,
Full-thickness burns, 173-175

G

Gag reflex, 84, 85, 129
General impressions
    importance of, 27, 31, 45, 98, 140
    initial assessments, 27, 40, 98, 140
    shock, 98
    submersion injuries, 193
Glasgow Coma Score (GCS)
    assessment, 30-31, 44
    components of, 30-31,
    head trauma, 129, 133
    initial assessment, 30-31, 44
    Pediatric, 30-31, 44, 129
    spinal trauma, 141
    transfer guidelines, 261
Glucose analyzer, 19, 108, 132, 244
Golden Hour, 32, 260
Greenstick fracture, 158, 161-162 (*see also* Fractures)
Grief reactions, 222-225
Ground rules for teaching and evaluation, 49-50
Ground transport, 261-262
Growth plates, 108, 158
Grunting, 28, 42, 56, 69, 115, 178
Guarding, abdominal, 34, 47, 115
Gunshot wounds, 8, 13, 21 (*see also* Firearms)

H

Hand, immobilization of, 164
Head trauma, 121-136
    anatomy, 122-123
    assessment, 128-131
    bicycle injuries, 11-12
    brain injuries, 123-124
    case study, 122, 134-135
    child abuse, 214
    examination of, 30, 34, 43, 46-47, 132
    fluid replacement, 131
    immobilization devices, 130, 142, 153-154, 255, 256
    initial assessment, 128-130
    intracranial pressure (ICP), 123-134
    level of consciousness, 128
    neurological exam, 133
    occult, 128, 144
    pathophysiology, 122-123
    pharmacologic therapy, 133
    primary brain injury, 123
    primary survey, 128-131
    secondary brain injury, 123
    secondary survey, 132
    pupils, 30, 33, 34, 46-47, 48, 127, 129, 133, 144, 196, 197, 256, 261
    scalp lacerations, 99, 100, 122, 125
    securing of, 130, 142, 151, 153-154
    skull fracture, 125
    submersion injuries, 193, 194, 196, 197
    types of, 123-127
Heart
    cardiac arrest, 52, 179, 192, 194, 205, 207, 270
    cardiac tamponade, 74-76
    electrical injuries, 183
    fetal, 233-234
    location of, 67
    myocardial contusions, 78
    neonatal chest compressions, 242
    submersion injuries, 195
    thoracic trauma, 65-82
    traumatic asphyxia, 79
    traumatic cardiopulmonary arrest, 203-210
Heart rates (*see also* Arrhythmias; Circulation; Dysrhthmias; Pulses)
    assessment, 33, 35, 57, 66
    by age, 25
    neonates, 25, 240
    spinal trauma, 141
    tachycardia, 115
Height, measurement, 24-25, 177, 249
Helicopter transfers, 17, 101, 261, 263
Helmets, 12, 14
Hematomas
    epidural, 126
    subdural, 126-127
Hemorrhages, 79, 85, 113, 115, 126, 127, 130, 207, 239, 240, 243, 272 (*see also* Blood loss)
Hemorrhagic shock, 99, 205, 207
Hemothorax, 35, 48, 56, 67, 68, 74-75, 77, 242
Herniation, brain, 124, 127, 129, 144, 256
High-voltage injuries, 179, 180, 183,
Hip, immobilization of, 164

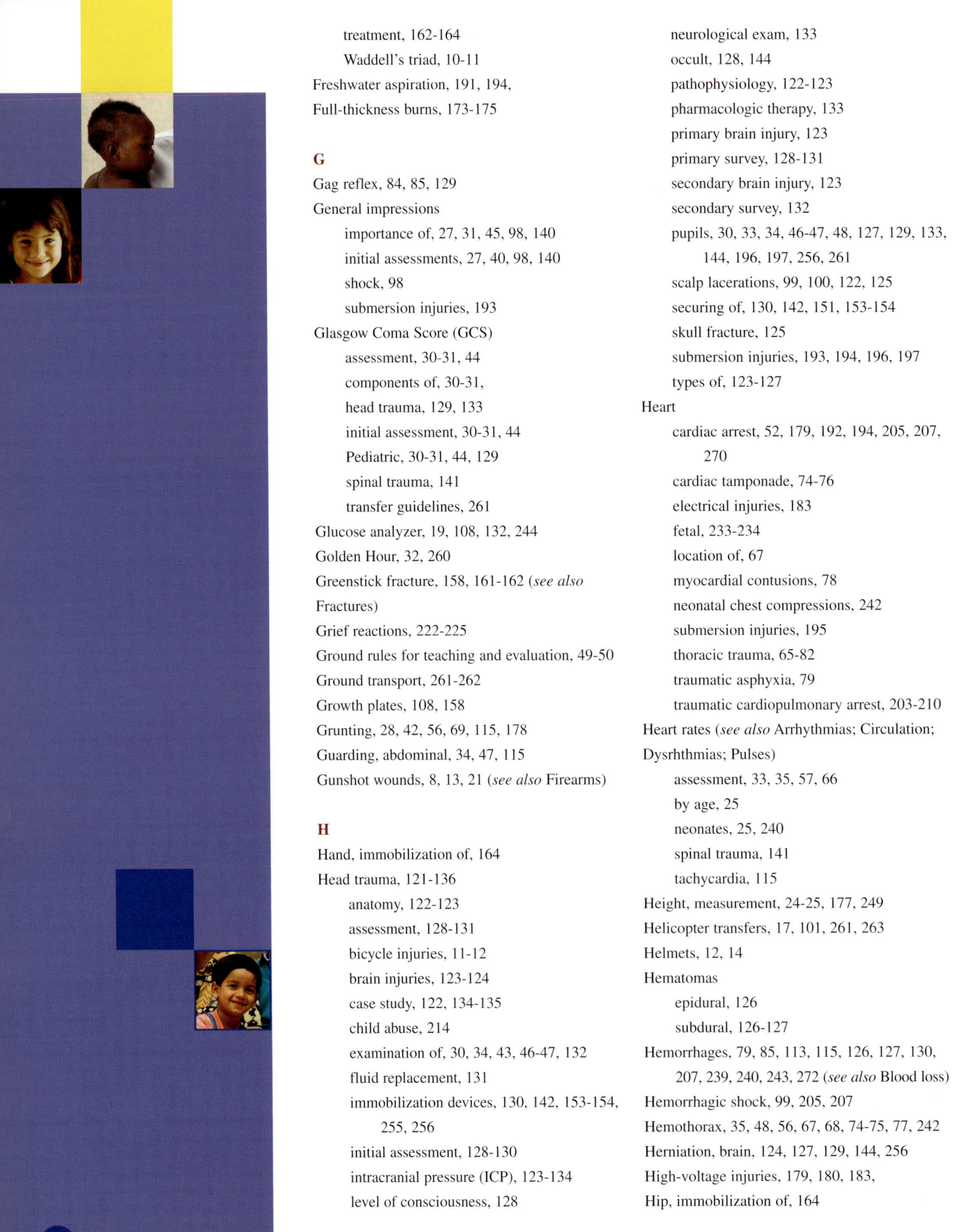

History,
    allergies, 31, 45
    events, 27, 31, 45, 97, 172, 213, 215
    illness, 31, 45
    SAMPLE, 31, 33, 45, 46, 130
Humerus, immobilization of, 164
Hyperventilation, herniation and, 124
Hypotension
    cardiac tamponade, 74
    hypovolemia, 30, 115
    initial assessments, 30
    shock, 30, 99, 115, 130
    tension pneumothorax, 70
Hypothermia
    airway management, 54
    burns patients, 178, 180
    cardiac arrhythmias, 195
    management of, 101, 196
    neonates, 244
    submersion injuries, 194, 195, 196, 197
Hypovolemia
    in children, 96
    massive hemothorax, 74
    shock, 101, 141
    submersion injuries, 191
    vascular access, 101
Hypoxia
    behavioral changes, 30, 57
    bradycardia, 57
    brain injuries, 123, 124, 129, 130, 131,
    mental status, 30, 57, 98
    recognition of, 32
    submersion injuries, 191, 194, 195
    traumatic cardiopulmonary, 205, 206, 207

I

Illnesses, history of, 31, 45 (*see also* History; SAMPLE history)
Immersion injuries, 196, 214
Immersion syndrome, 190, 192
Immobilization (*see also* Backboards; Cervical spine; Spinal motion restriction; specific body parts)
    car seat, 143, 153-156
    extremity trauma, 162-164
    head, 153-154
IV access sites, 107
    pediatric devices, 142-143, 150, 154

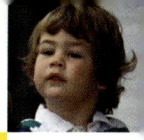

spinal, 142-143, 149-156
Immunization status, 31, 45 (*see also* Allergies, history of; History, SAMPLE; SAMPLE history)
Impaled object stabilization, 32, 35, 45, 49, 79, 116, 125, 130
Impalement injuries, 79, 116 (*see also* Penetrating injuries)
Incident command system (ICS), 267-268, 272, 274
Infants (*see also* Neonates; Newborns)
    apnea, 236, 239, 243
    breathing, 234-237, 238-240
    communication with, 3-4
    injury prevention, 14
    mechanisms of injury, 14
    ventilation rates, 239-240
    vital signs, 25
Inferior vena cava, 67, 113, 252
Inhalation injuries, 35, 48, 176, 179, 181, 182,
Initial assessment, 18, 25, 26, 27-30, 33, 34, 40-43, 46
    abdominal trauma, 114-115
    airway management, 54-57
    burns, 178-179
    car seats, 143
    extremity trauma, 160
    head trauma, 128-130
    neonates, 136
    shock, 98-99
    spinal trauma, 140-141
    submersion injuries, 193-194
    thoracic trauma, 69-75
    traumatic cardiopulmonary arrest, 206-207
Injury prevention, 14-16, 197-198
    adolescents, 16
    burns, 184, 197-198
    caregivers' role in, 14-16
    drowning, 197-198
    helmets, 12
    infants, 14
    injuries by age group, 14-16
    preschool children, 15
    school age children, 15-16
    submersion injuries, 197-198
    toddlers, 14
International Trauma Life Support (ITLS)
    confident approach, 17

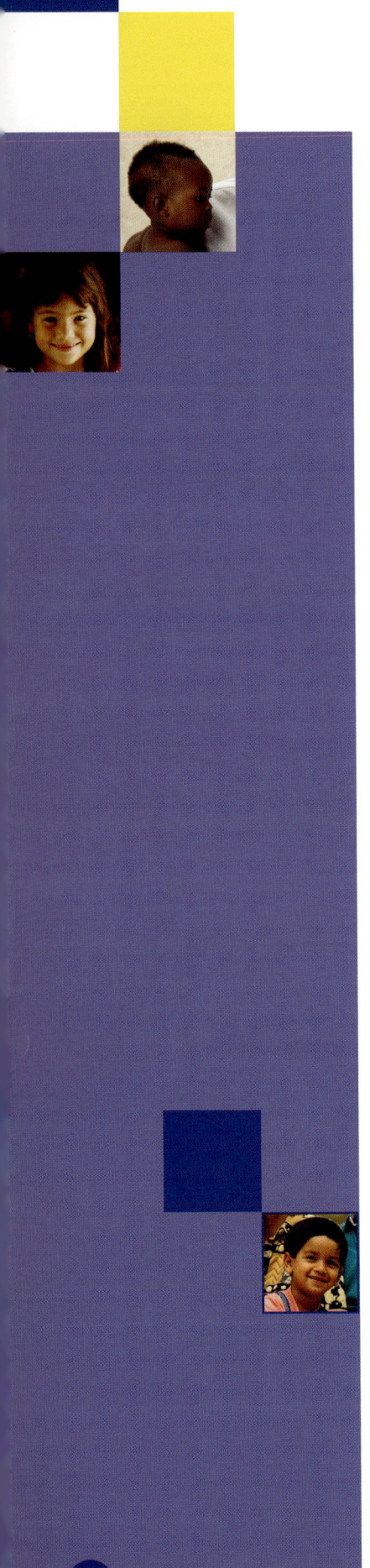

    ongoing exam, 34-35, 48-49
    patient assessment, 24-35, 40-49
    primary survey, 25-33, 40-46
    secondary survey, 33-34, 46-48
Interventions, critical (*see also* specific interventions)
    abdominal trauma, 115-116
    airway management, 57-61
    assessments, 31-33, 45
    burn patients, 179-181
    during transport, 32-33, 45
    extremity trauma, 160-161
    head trauma, 130-131
    on-scene, 32, 45
    shock 100-101
    spinal trauma, 142-144
    submersion injuries, 194-196
    thoracic trauma, 77
    traumatic cardiopulmonary arrest, 208
Intra-abdominal bleeding, 8, 67, 78, 79, 112, 115, 207
Intracranial injuries, 125-127
Intracranial pressure (ICP)
    assessment, 30, 44, 123-125, 129, 130
    fontanel bulge, 132
    initial assessment, 129
    intercranial volume, 123-125
    rapid trauma assessment, 30, 44
    seizures, 131
    shunts, 255-256
Intraosseous (IO) infusion
    choice of, 100-101
    fluid resuscitation, 33, 100-101, 107-110
    in newborns, 242-243
    insertion of lines, 100-101, 107-109
    location, 101
    method, 100-101, 107-110
    pediatric needle sizes, 19, 108, 242
Intravascular fluid replacement, 100-101
Intravenous (IV) access (*see also* Fluid boluses; Fluid resuscitation)
    fluid resuscitation, 100-101, 208
    immobilization of sites, 107
    insertion of lines, 106-107
    neonates, 243
    pediatric equipment, 19, 106
Intravenous solutions, 19, 33, 101, 116, 131, 180, 182, 243 (*see also* specific solutions)

Intravenous catheters, 19, 72
Intubation, 32, 57-59, 74, 77, 88-90, 208, 235, 238, 240, 243, 244, 252 (*see also* Endotracheal intubation; Orotracheal intubation)
    blind nasotracheal, 90
Irrigation of burns, 178, 187
Irritability, 31, 127, 129, 255
Isotonic fluid, 104, 243
ITLS
    confident approach, 17
    ongoing exam, 34-35, 48-49
    patient assessment, 24-35, 40-49
    primary survey, 25-33, 40-46
    secondary survey, 33-34, 46-48

J
Jaw thrust maneuver, modified, 28, 41, 55, 84, 129, 193
Joint injuries, 161, 162, 164, 165, 175, 181
Jugular venous distention, 28, 35, 42, 48
JumpSTART, 270-271

K
Kidneys
    electrical injuries, 183
    fixation points, 8
    location of, 113
    traumatic injuries, 113
King LT-D airway, 59-60
Knee, immobilization of, 164

L
Labor, trauma and, 232-234
Lacerations, 33, 35, 48, 97,
    head, 11, 30, 123, 132
    liver, 113
    neonates, 241
    open fractures, 161
    scalp, 99, 122, 123
Larygneal mask airway (LMA), 59-60
Laryngoscopes, pediatric 19, 88-89, 180
Larynx, 52-53
Law enforcement, 215, 216, 217, 268, 270
Legal issues, 273
    child abuse, 215, 216
Length-based tape, 24-25, 89
Lethargy, 126, 127, 255 (*see also* Level of

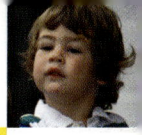

consciousness)
Level of consciousness (LOC)
    abdominal trauma, 114, 115
    airway management, 56, 84
    assessments, 25, 28, 33, 40-41, 46
    AVPU, 28, 33, 41, 46, 128
    burns, 178, 179
    extremity trauma, 160
    head trauma, 1286, 127, 128, 130
    initial assessments, 28, 40-41,
    neonates, 136
    shock, 98,
    spinal trauma, 140, 143
    submersion injuries, 193, 196
    thoracic trauma, 69
    traumatic cardiopulmonary arrest, 206
Lidocaine, 19
Ligamentous injuries, 165
Lightning injuries, 176, 179, 180, 181, 183
Linear skull fracture, 125
Liver, 8, 97, 113, 115, 116
Load-and-go, 31-32, 45, 57, 77, 98, 130, 169, 208, 224, 269
Log rolling, 30, 44, 49, 150, 154, 195,
Low-voltage electrical burns, 183
Lower trachea fixation, 8
Lubricating jelly, 19
Lumbar spine fixation, 19
Lund Browder chart, 176-177
Lungs (see also Aspiration; Breathing; Respiration)
    dry drowning, 192
    initial assessment, 29, 42
    location of, 67
    neonates, 236, 242,
    preterm infants, 236
    rapid trauma survey, 207
    secondary survey, 181
    submersion injuries, 191-192, 193-194,
    traumatic injuries, 70, 181
    wet drowning, 191

M

Masks, pediatric, 19, 29, 41, 55, 84, 86-97
Meal, last, 31, 45 (see also History; SAMPLE history)
Mechanisms of injury, 7-16 (see also specific injuries)
    amputations, 166
    assessment, 27, 30, 31, 35, 40, 45, 67
    blunt trauma, 8
    burns, 172, 174
    by age, 13-16
    child abuse, 97, 128, 172, 196, 212-214
    compression, 8, 79
    cycling, 10-12
    ejection, 10
    falls, 12-13
    firearms, 13
    fractures, 159, 161-164
    gunshot wounds, 13
    immersion, 192
    impalement, 79
    motor vehicle collisions, 9-10
    pedestrian injuries, 10
    penetrating trauma, 8
    scene size-up, 27, 40, 54
    thoracic trauma, 67
    transfer guidelines, 260-261
Meconium staining, 237-238
Medical direction (see also Emergency departments)
    communications with, 18, 33, 46, 253, 260-262, 274
    fluid resuscitation, 101, 180
    head trauma, 124, 133
    intravenous access, 106
    pharmacologic therapy, 61
    transfer guidelines, 208, 260-262, 274
Medical incident command system, 268
Medications
    anti-convulsant, 131
    history of, 31, 45 (see also History; SAMPLE history)
    intubation, 61
    neonates, 234-235, 242-244
    pediatric equipment, 19
Mental status (see Altered mental status)
Metabolic acidosis, 194
Midazolam, 61
Middle meningeal artery, 126, 132
Modified jaw thrust, 28, 41, 55, 84, 129, 193
Monitoring equipment, pediatric, 19
Motor examination, 133
Motor vehicle collisions (MVCs)
    abdominal trauma, 10-11, 114

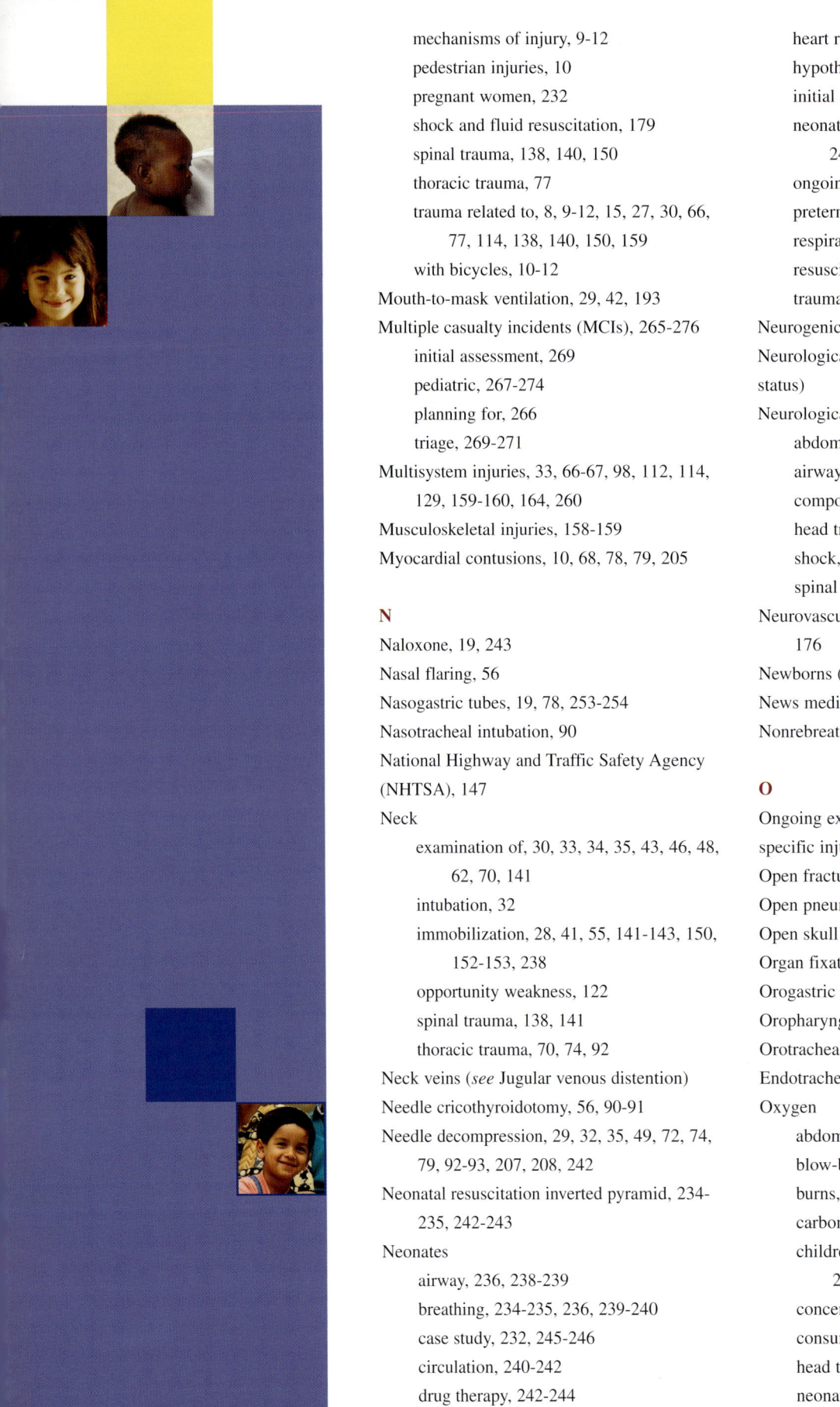

mechanisms of injury, 9-12
pedestrian injuries, 10
pregnant women, 232
shock and fluid resuscitation, 179
spinal trauma, 138, 140, 150
thoracic trauma, 77
trauma related to, 8, 9-12, 15, 27, 30, 66, 77, 114, 138, 140, 150, 159
with bicycles, 10-12
Mouth-to-mask ventilation, 29, 42, 193
Multiple casualty incidents (MCIs), 265-276
initial assessment, 269
pediatric, 267-274
planning for, 266
triage, 269-271
Multisystem injuries, 33, 66-67, 98, 112, 114, 129, 159-160, 164, 260
Musculoskeletal injuries, 158-159
Myocardial contusions, 10, 68, 78, 79, 205

N

Naloxone, 19, 243
Nasal flaring, 56
Nasogastric tubes, 19, 78, 253-254
Nasotracheal intubation, 90
National Highway and Traffic Safety Agency (NHTSA), 147
Neck
examination of, 30, 33, 34, 35, 43, 46, 48, 62, 70, 141
intubation, 32
immobilization, 28, 41, 55, 141-143, 150, 152-153, 238
opportunity weakness, 122
spinal trauma, 138, 141
thoracic trauma, 70, 74, 92
Neck veins (*see* Jugular venous distention)
Needle cricothyroidotomy, 56, 90-91
Needle decompression, 29, 32, 35, 49, 72, 74, 79, 92-93, 207, 208, 242
Neonatal resuscitation inverted pyramid, 234-235, 242-243
Neonates
airway, 236, 238-239
breathing, 234-235, 236, 239-240
case study, 232, 245-246
circulation, 240-242
drug therapy, 242-244

heart rates, 25
hypothermia prevention, 237
initial stabilization and assessment, 236-237
neonatal resuscitation pyramid, 234-235, 242-243
ongoing assessment, 244-245
preterm infants, 236, 237
respiratory rates, 25
resuscitation, 234-235, 238-244
trauma in, 231-246
Neurogenic shock, 141, 179
Neurological deterioration (*see* Altered mental status)
Neurological examinations, 30-31, 33, 34, 46, 57
abdominal trauma, 115, 144-145
airway management, 57
components of, 30-31
head trauma, 130, 141
shock, 98
spinal trauma, 141
Neurovascular function, 34, 48, 161, 162, 164, 176
Newborns (*see* Neonates)
News media, 227, 268, 272
Nonrebreather mask, 84, 179, 194

O

Ongoing exam, 25, 34-35, 48, 49, 209 (*see also* specific injuries)
Open fractures, 161, 164
Open pneumothorax, 68, 70, 74, 77
Open skull fractures, 125
Organ fixation points, 8
Orogastric tube, 61, 254
Oropharyngeal airways, 55-56, 85-86, 90
Orotracheal intubation, 32 (*see also* Endotracheal intubation; Intubation)
Oxygen
abdominal trauma, 115
blow-by method, 239, 244
burns, 179, 180, 182
carbon monoxide, 182
children with special health care needs, 248, 249, 250, 251, 255-256
concentration, 28-29, 32, 45, 55-56
consumption by pediatric patients, 54
head trauma, 123, 124, 127, 129-130, 131
neonates, 235, 236, 239-240, 242, 244

rescuer responsibility, 41
shock, 100, 205
spinal trauma, 141, 142
submersion injuries, 191, 194-197
thoracic trauma, 69, 70, 74, 77, 78, 79
use of, 28-29, 32, 35, 41, 45, 48, 55-56, 58, 61, 69, 84-85, 89, 98, 207

P

Padding, backboard, 28, 41, 142, 143, 150, 153, 154
Pain
    abdominal assessment, 113
    abdominal trauma, 114-116
    breathing, 69, 78, 115, 160
    burns, 174-175, 182
    chest pain, 69, 78, 224
    compartment syndrome, 165
    extremity trauma, 160, 162, 163-164, 165
    fear of, 3
    level of consciousness, 28, 41, 128
    pharmacologic therapy, 19, 163, 182
    response to, 28, 31, 41, 128, 129
Pancreas, 113
Paralysis, 193
Parents
    behavioral changes, 215, 222-228
    child abuse, 213, 215
    communication with, 2-7, 17, 266, 268, 270, 272
    consent, 273
    death of a child, 222-228, 244
    decision-making, 2-7, 17
    drowning prevention, 198
    during assessments, 27, 28, 31, 40, 43, 45, 133, 151, 250
    prevention of injuries, 12, 14, 15, 16, 184, 198
    transport of children, 17, 270, 274
Partial-thickness burns, 173-175
Pedestrians, 10-11, 14, 15, 27, 30, 112, 114, 140, 197, 261
Pediatric care centers, specialized, 32, 100, 102, 259-264
Pelvis
    assessment, 35, 45
    fractures, 169, 233
    immobilization of, 164

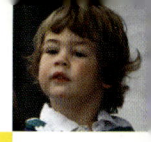

stability, 35, 43
transfer guidelines, 169
Penetrating injuries
    abdominal, 112, 116-117
    head trauma, 125, 130
    mechanism of, 8-9, 13
    neonatal, 232, 242
    thoracic, 66, 70, 74, 78, 79
Perfusion (see also Circulation)
    initial assessments, 30, 33, 84
    head trauma, 101, 123-124, 131
    intracranial, 123
    neonates, 242, 244
    shock, 81, 99, 141, 160
    thoracic trauma, 74
    triage, 269
Pericardial tamponade, 99, 205, 207, 253
Peripheral cannulation, 106-107, 109-110, 180
Peripheral perfusion, 27, 57, 75, 99
Personal floatation devices (PFD), 190
Personal protective equipment (PPE), 27, 40, 49
Pharmacologic interventions
    anti-convulsant, 131
    burns, 182
    head trauma, 133
    neonates, 234-235, 242-244
    pain, 19, 163, 182
Placenta previa, 243
Placenta, abruption of, 233, 243
Pleura, 67
Pleural spaces, 67, 70-71, 74, 78, 92-93
Pneumatic antishock garments (PASG), 77
Pneumothorax (*see also* Tension pneumothorax)
    decompression, 30, 32-33, 35, 45, 49, 72, 92-94, 206-208
    definition of, 56, 67, 74-75
    neonates, 239, 242
    open, 68, 70-71, 77
    simple, 79
    special health care needs equipment, 250-256
    tension, 29, 30, 32-33, 35, 45, 49, 68, 70-72, 74-75, 77, 78, 92-94, 99, 205-208
Points of fixation, organ, 8
Polluted water aspiration, 191
Pools, 190, 193, 198
Positive-pressure ventilation, 74, 113, 240, 242

Index 293

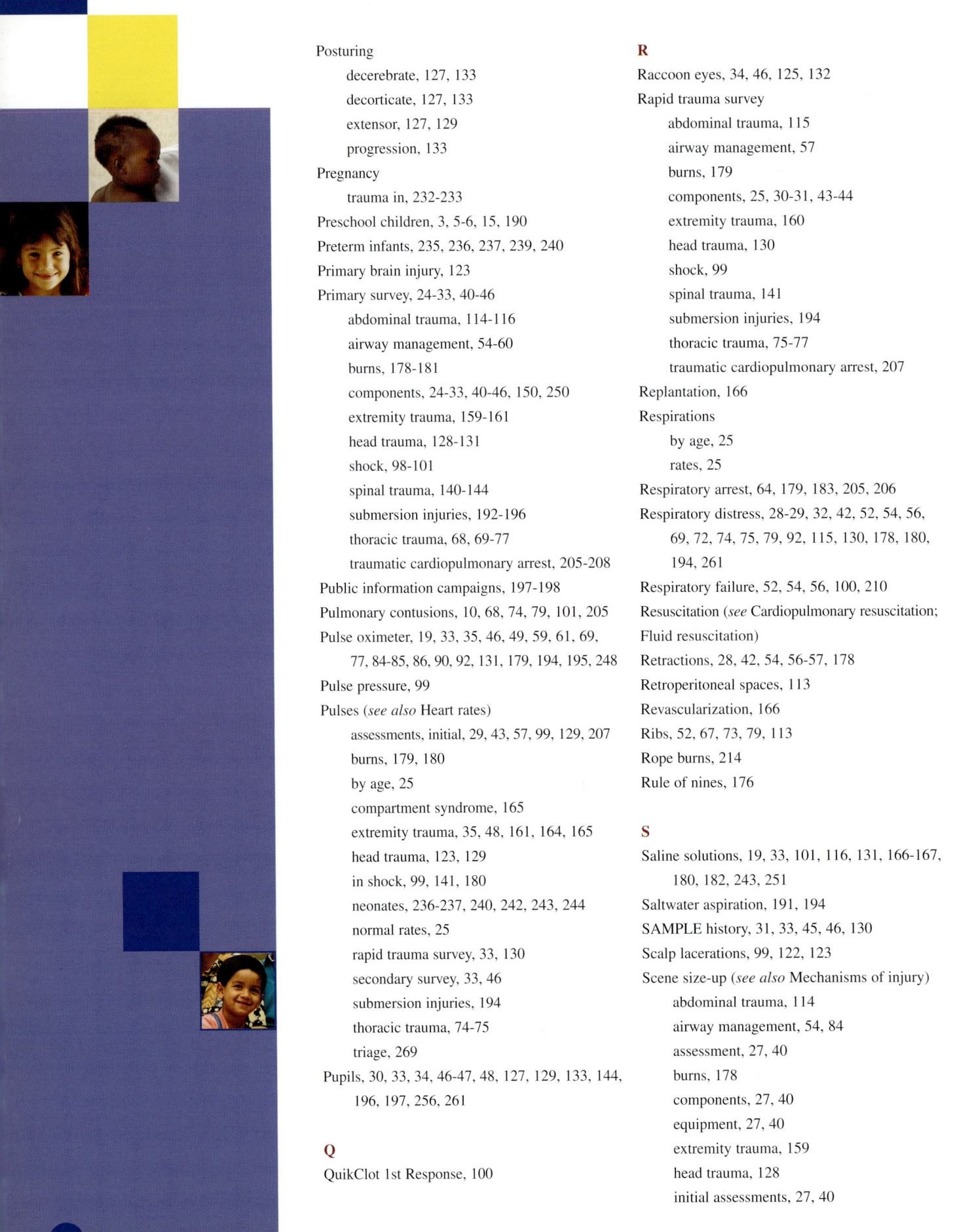

Posturing
    decerebrate, 127, 133
    decorticate, 127, 133
    extensor, 127, 129
    progression, 133
Pregnancy
    trauma in, 232-233
Preschool children, 3, 5-6, 15, 190
Preterm infants, 235, 236, 237, 239, 240
Primary brain injury, 123
Primary survey, 24-33, 40-46
    abdominal trauma, 114-116
    airway management, 54-60
    burns, 178-181
    components, 24-33, 40-46, 150, 250
    extremity trauma, 159-161
    head trauma, 128-131
    shock, 98-101
    spinal trauma, 140-144
    submersion injuries, 192-196
    thoracic trauma, 68, 69-77
    traumatic cardiopulmonary arrest, 205-208
Public information campaigns, 197-198
Pulmonary contusions, 10, 68, 74, 79, 101, 205
Pulse oximeter, 19, 33, 35, 46, 49, 59, 61, 69, 77, 84-85, 86, 90, 92, 131, 179, 194, 195, 248
Pulse pressure, 99
Pulses (*see also* Heart rates)
    assessments, initial, 29, 43, 57, 99, 129, 207
    burns, 179, 180
    by age, 25
    compartment syndrome, 165
    extremity trauma, 35, 48, 161, 164, 165
    head trauma, 123, 129
    in shock, 99, 141, 180
    neonates, 236-237, 240, 242, 243, 244
    normal rates, 25
    rapid trauma survey, 33, 130
    secondary survey, 33, 46
    submersion injuries, 194
    thoracic trauma, 74-75
    triage, 269
Pupils, 30, 33, 34, 46-47, 48, 127, 129, 133, 144, 196, 197, 256, 261

Q

QuikClot 1st Response, 100

R

Raccoon eyes, 34, 46, 125, 132
Rapid trauma survey
    abdominal trauma, 115
    airway management, 57
    burns, 179
    components, 25, 30-31, 43-44
    extremity trauma, 160
    head trauma, 130
    shock, 99
    spinal trauma, 141
    submersion injuries, 194
    thoracic trauma, 75-77
    traumatic cardiopulmonary arrest, 207
Replantation, 166
Respirations
    by age, 25
    rates, 25
Respiratory arrest, 64, 179, 183, 205, 206
Respiratory distress, 28-29, 32, 42, 52, 54, 56, 69, 72, 74, 75, 79, 92, 115, 130, 178, 180, 194, 261
Respiratory failure, 52, 54, 56, 100, 210
Resuscitation (*see* Cardiopulmonary resuscitation; Fluid resuscitation)
Retractions, 28, 42, 54, 56-57, 178
Retroperitoneal spaces, 113
Revascularization, 166
Ribs, 52, 67, 73, 79, 113
Rope burns, 214
Rule of nines, 176

S

Saline solutions, 19, 33, 101, 116, 131, 166-167, 180, 182, 243, 251
Saltwater aspiration, 191, 194
SAMPLE history, 31, 33, 45, 46, 130
Scalp lacerations, 99, 122, 123
Scene size-up (*see also* Mechanisms of injury)
    abdominal trauma, 114
    airway management, 54, 84
    assessment, 27, 40
    burns, 178
    components, 27, 40
    equipment, 27, 40
    extremity trauma, 159
    head trauma, 128
    initial assessments, 27, 40

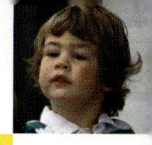

mechanisms of injury, 27, 40, 150
scene safety, 27, 40
shock, 98
spinal trauma, 140, 150
standard precautions, 27, 40
submersion injuries, 192-193
thoracic trauma, 69
traumatic cardiopulmonary arrest, 206
School-age children, 3, 6, 15-16
Seatbelts, 10, 14, 34, 47, 116, 139, 144
Second-degree burns, 173-175
Secondary brain injury, 123
Secondary survey, 25, 30, 32, 33-34, 45, 46-48
    abdominal trauma, 116-117
    airway management, 62
    burns, 181
    components, 33-34
    extremity trauma, 161
    head trauma, 144-145
    shock, 102
    spinal trauma, 140, 150
    submersion injuries, 196
    thoracic trauma, 68, 77-79
    traumatic cardiopulmonary arrest, 209
Sedation, 61, 88, 180
Seizures
    head trauma, 127, 128, 130, 131, 133, 144
    medications, 131, 133
    neonates, 243
    shunt dysfunction, 255
    submersion injuries, 191, 194, 196
Sellick maneuver, 58-59, 86, 89
Sensory examination, 133
Shaken baby syndrome, 127
Shock
    abdominal trauma, 112, 113, 115-116
    airway management, 61
    assessments, 29-30, 31-32, 33, 45
    burns, 179, 180, 182
    case study, 96, 102-103
    causes of, 66, 96-97
    extremity trauma, 160, 161
    fluid resuscitation, 61, 100-101, 105-110, 131, 180, 182, 254
    grief response, 223
    head trauma, 122, 123, 129-130, 131
    initial assessments, 98-99
    management, 95-104, 105-110

    neurogenic, 141, 179
    pathophysiology, 96-97
    pediatric, 95-104
    primary survey, 98-101
    pulse oximetry, 59
    secondary survey, 102
    spinal trauma, 141, 144
    submersion injuries, 194, 195
    tachycardia, 81, 160
    thoracic trauma, 66, 74, 75, 77, 81
    transfer guidelines, 142, 160, 179, 261
    traumatic cardiopulmonary arrest, 205, 207
    vital signs, 66, 81, 160, 180
Shoulder, immobilization of, 163
Shunts, 106, 248, 254-256
Simple pneumothorax, 72, 79
Skin
    anatomy, 173-176
    burns, 171-188
    burns, classification, 174-177
    color, 173-175
    irrigation, 178
Skull fractures, 34, 125
Skull, anatomy of, 122-123
Slings and swathes, 163-164
Smoke detectors, 184
Smoke inhalation, 179, 182
Sodium bicarbonate, 19, 244
Sodium thiosulfate, 182
Special health care needs (SHCN), 247-258
    equipment assessment, 250-256
Specialized pediatric care centers, 32, 100, 102, 259-264
Spinal trauma, 137-148
    anatomy, 138-139
    case study, 138, 145-146
    cervical collars, 150-152
    extrication, 142, 149-156
    immobilizers, 142-143, 150, 154
    level, 138-139
    motion restriction, 142-143, 149-156
    pathophysiology, 138-139
    primary survey, 140-144
    scene size-up, 140
    secondary survey, 144-145
    thoracic fractures, 139
    transfer guidelines, 142

Spinal motion restriction (SMR), 142-143, 149-156
    cervical collar application, 150-152
    equipment, 19-20, 152-154
Spleen, 97, 113, 115, 116
Splinting, 163-164
Sprains, 165
Standard precautions, 27, 40
START triage system, 270
Sternum, 67, 241-242
Strains, 165
Straps, selection of, 19, 151, 152-154, 156
Stridor, 28, 56, 58, 178, 180
Stumps, amputations, 160, 166
Stylets, pediatric, 19, 91, 108
Subdural hematomas, 126-127
Subglottic area, 52-53
Submersion injuries, 189-202
    anatomy, 191-192
    case study, 190, 199-200
    categories of, 191-192
    immersion syndrome, 192
    initial assessment, 193-194
    pathophysiology, 191-192
    prevention of, 197-198
    primary survey, 192-196
    prognosis, 198
    secondary survey, 196
Sucking chest wound, 32, 35, 45, 48, 70, 205
Sucking responses, 5
Suction
    airway assessment, 28-29, 41-42, 57, 84, 85, 88, 89, 99
    burns, 178
    catheter size by age, 58
    head trauma, 129, 131
    machines, 19
    neonates, 234, 236-238, 239, 245
    submersion injuries, 193, 195
    tracheostomies, 251-252
    traumatic cardiopulmonary arrest, 206, 208
Superficial partial-thickness burns, 173-175
Supplemental oxygen, 28, 84, 98, 100, 160, 255-256 (*see also* Oxygen)
Surfaces, falls onto, 12, 114
Swimming (*see* Submersion injuries)
Symptoms, history of, 31, 45 (*see also* History; SAMPLE history)
Syringes, 19, 90, 92, 107-110, 254

Systolic blood pressure (*see* Blood pressure)

T

Tachycardia, 29, 78, 81, 97, 99, 101, 115, 160, 194,
Tachypnea, 28, 56, 69, 98, 104, 180, 236-237
Teaching and evaluation, 49-50
Team leaders, 18, 32, 45, 49
Tenderness, abdominal, 34, 35, 43, 47, 48
Tenderness, instability, crepitus (TIC), 30, 43, 74, 161
Tendons, 165
Tension pneumothorax (*see also* Pneumothorax)
    anatomy, 70-72
    decompression of, 29, 30, 32-33, 35, 43, 45, 49, 71-72, 92-94
    initial assessments, 29, 206-207
    management, 29, 30, 32-33, 70-72, 92-94, 205-208
    needle decompression, 29, 30, 32-33, 35, 43, 45, 49, 71-72, 92-94
    rescuer responsibility, 32
    rapid trauma survey, 99, 207
    secondary survey, 78, 79
    signs and symptoms, 68, 70-72, 74-75
    transfer guidelines, 77, 208
Tertiary care centers, 260
Thermoregulation, 180, 196 (*see also* Hypothermia)
Third-degree burns, 173-176
Thoracic cavity, 67-68
Thoracic trauma, 65-82
    anatomy, 66-68
    cardiac tamponade, 74-75
    case study, 66, 80-81
    chest decompression, 29, 30, 32-33, 35, 43, 45, 49, 71-72, 92-94
    diaphragmatic injuries, 78
    esophageal injuries, 79
    flail chest, 73-74
    impaled objects, 79
    initial assessment,
    massive hemothorax, 74-75
    myocardial contusions, 78
    motor vehicle collisions, 8, 9-11, 66
    open pneumothorax, 68, 70-71, 77
    pathophysiology, 66-67
    primary survey, 68, 69-77